Toxicology

Guest Editor

JAMES A. KRUSE, MD, FCCM

CRITICAL CARE CLINICS

www.criticalcare.theclinics.com

Consulting Editor

RICHARD W. CARLSON, MD, PhD

October 2012 • Volume 28 • Number 4

SAUNDERS an imprint of ELSEVIER, Inc.

W.B. SAUNDERS COMPANY
A Division of Elsevier Inc.

Elsevier Inc. ● 1600 John F. Kennedy Blvd., ● Suite 1800 ● Philadelphia, Pennsylvania 19103-2899

http://www.theclinics.com

CRITICAL CARE CLINICS Volume 28, Number 4
October 2012 ISSN 0749-0704, ISBN-13: 978-1-4557-3846-5

Editor: Patrick Manley
Developmental Editor: Donald Mumford

Critical Care Clinics (ISSN: 0749-0704) is published quarterly by Elsevier Inc., 360 Park Avenue South, New York, NY 10010-1710. Months of issue are January, April, July, and October. Business and Editorial Offices: 1600 John F. Kennedy Blvd., Suite 1800, Philadelphia, PA 19103-2899. Customer Service Office: 6277 Sea Harbor Drive, Orlando, FL 32887-4800. Periodicals postage paid at New York, NY and additional mailing offices. Subscription prices are $193.00 per year for US individuals, $463.00 per year for US institution, $94.00 per year for US students and residents, $238.00 per year for Canadian individuals, $574.00 per year for Canadian institutions, $278.00 per year for international individuals, $574.00 per year for international institutions and $137.00 per year for Canadian and foreign students/residents. To receive student/resident rate, orders must be accompanied by name of affiliated institution, date of term, and the signature of program/residency coordinator on institution letterhead. Orders will be billed at individual rate until proof of status is received. Foreign air speed delivery is included in all *Clinics* subscription prices. All prices are subject to change without notice. POSTMASTER: Send address changes to *Critical Care Clinics*, Elsevier Periodicals Customer Service, 11830 Westline Industrial Drive, St. Louis, MO 63146. **Customer Service: 1-800-654-2452 (US). From outside of the US, call 1-314-447-8871. Fax: 1-314-447-8029. E-mail: journalscustomerservice-usa@elsevier.com (for print support) or journalsonlinesupport-usa@elsevier.com (for online support).**

Reprints. For copies of 100 or more of articles in this publication, please contact the Commercial Reprints Department, Elsevier Inc., 360 Park Avenue South, New York, NY 10010-1710. Tel.: 212-633-3813; Fax: 212-462-1935; E-mail: reprints@elsevier.com.

Critical Care Clinics is also published in Spanish by Editorial Inter-Medica, Junin 917, 1er A, 1113, Buenos Aires, Argentina.

Critical Care Clinics is covered in *MEDLINE/PubMed (Index Medicus)*, *EMBASE/Excerpta Medica, Current Concepts/ Clinical Medicine, ISI/BIOMED*, and *Chemical Abstracts*.

Printed and bound by CPI Group (UK) Ltd, Croydon, CR0 4YY

Transferred to digital print 2012

Contributors

CONSULTING EDITOR

RICHARD W. CARLSON, MD, PhD
Professor, Department of Medicine, Maricopa Medical Center; College of Medicine, University of Arizona, Phoenix, Arizona; Mayo Clinic College of Medicine, Scottsdale, Arizona

GUEST EDITOR

JAMES A. KRUSE, MD, FCCM
Clinical Professor, College of Physicians and Surgeons, Columbia University, New York, New York; Chief, Critical Care Services, Bassett Medical Center, Cooperstown, New York

AUTHORS

SOFIAN AL-KHATIB, MD
Department of Medicine, Maricopa Medical Center, Phoenix, Arizona

SRIKALA AYYAGARI, MD
Department of Hospital Medicine, University of California San Diego School of Medicine, San Diego, California

HEATHER A. BOREK, MD
Medical Toxicology Fellow, Division of Medical Toxicology, Department of Emergency Medicine, University of Virginia School of Medicine, University of Virginia Health System, Charlottesville, Virginia

RICHARD W. CARLSON, MD, PhD
Professor, Department of Medicine, Maricopa Medical Center; College of Medicine, University of Arizona, Phoenix, Arizona; Mayo Clinic College of Medicine, Scottsdale, Arizona

MARTINA M. CARTWRIGHT, PhD, RD
Adjunct Professor, Department of Nutritional Sciences, University of Arizona, Tucson, Arizona

ALEXANDER R. GARRARD, PharmD
Clinical Assistant Professor, Clinical Toxicologist, Department of Emergency Medicine, Upstate New York Poison Center, SUNY Upstate Medical University, Syracuse, New York

JORGE A. GUZMAN, MD
Head, Section of Critical Care, Director, Medical Intensive Care Unit, Respiratory Institute, Cleveland Clinic, Cleveland, Ohio

WADDAH HAJJA, MD
Department of Medicine, Maricopa Medical Center, Phoenix, Arizona

MARYAM HAZEGHAZAM, MD, PhD
Department of Psychiatry and Medicine, Maricopa Medical Center, Phoenix, Arizona

MATTHEW W. HEDGE, MD
Assistant Professor, Department of Emergency Medicine, Detroit Receiving Hospital,
Children's Hospital of Michigan Regional Poison Control Center, Wayne State University,
Detroit, Michigan

MICHAEL J. HODGMAN, MD
Clinical Assistant Professor, Medical Toxicology Consultant, Department of Emergency
Medicine, Upstate New York Poison Center, SUNY Upstate Medical University, Syracuse,
New York; Emergency and Trauma Services, Bassett Medical Center, Cooperstown,
New York

CHRISTOPHER P. HOLSTEGE, MD, FAACT, FACMT
Chief of the Division of Medical Toxicology, Associate Professor of the Departments of
Emergency Medicine & Pediatrics, Medical Director of the Blue Ridge Poison Center,
University of Virginia Health System, University of Virginia School of Medicine,
Charlottesville, Virginia

FRANK K. JACKSON
Department of Medicine, Maricopa Medical Center, Phoenix, Arizona; Midwestern
University, Glendale, Arizona

SALMAAN KANJI, PharmD
Associate Scientist, Department of Pharmacy, The Ottawa Health Research Institute;
Clinical Pharmacy Specialist, The Ottawa Hospital, Ottawa, Ontario, Canada

JAMES A. KRUSE, MD, FCCM
Clinical Professor, College of Physicians and Surgeons, Columbia University, New York,
New York; Chief, Critical Care Services, Bassett Medical Center, Cooperstown, New York

NIVEDITA N. KUMAR, MD
Department of Medicine, Legacy Salmon Creek Medical Center, Vancouver, Washington

REBECCA NA LI, MD
Department of Internal Medicine, Sutter Pacific Medical Foundation, San Rafael, California

ROBERT D. MACLEAN, PharmD
Clinical Pharmacist, Department of Pharmacy, The Ottawa Hospital, Ottawa, Ontario, Canada

NITIN PURI, MD
Department of Internal Medicine, Inova Fairfax Hospital, Virginia Commonwealth
University, Falls Church, Virginia

DAN QUAN, DO
Emergency Physician, Medical Toxicologist, Department of Emergency Medicine,
Maricopa Medical Center; Clinical Assistant Professor, Emergency Medicine, College
of Medicine, University of Arizona, Phoenix, Arizona

SHIVARAMAIAH SHASHIKUMAR, MD
Department of Medicine, St John's Mercy Medical Center; Mercy Critical Care Training Program, Fellow, Critical Care Medicine, Saint Louis University, St Louis, Missouri

DHARMASHREE SREEDHAR, MD
Department of Internal Medicine, Maricopa Medical Center, Phoenix, Arizona

EDNA WONG-MCKINSTRY, MD
Departments of Medicine and Internal Medicine, College of Medicine, University of Arizona, Tucson, Arizona

JANICE L. ZIMMERMAN, MD
Professor of Clinical Medicine, Department of Medicine, Weill Cornell Medical College, New York, New York; Medical Director, Medical Intensive Care Unit, Director, Critical Care Division, Department of Medicine, The Methodist Hospital, Houston, Texas

Contents

The critical care physician is often called to care for poisoned patients. This article reviews the general approach to the poisoned patient, specifically focusing on the utility of the toxidrome. A toxidrome is a constellation of findings, either from the physical examination or from ancillary testing, which may result from any poison. There are numerous toxidromes defined in the medical literature. This article focuses on the more common toxidromes described in clinical toxicology. Although these toxidromes can aid the clinician in narrowing the differential diagnosis, care must be exercised to realize the exceptions and limitations associated with each.

Acetaminophen poisoning remains one of the more common drugs taken in overdose with potentially fatal consequences. Early recognition and prompt treatment with *N*-acetylcysteine can prevent hepatic injury. With acute overdose, the Rumack-Matthew nomogram is a useful tool to assess risk and guide management. Equally common to acute overdose is the repeated use of excessive amounts of acetaminophen. Simultaneous ingestion of several different acetaminophen-containing products may result in excessive dosage. These patients also benefit from *N*-acetylcysteine. Standard courses of *N*-acetylcysteine may need to be extended in patients with persistently elevated plasma concentrations of acetaminophen or with signs of hepatic injury.

Cocaine, a natural alkaloid derived from the coca plant, is one of the most commonly abused illicit drugs. Cocaine is commonly abused by inhalation, nasal insufflation, and intravenous injection, resulting in many adverse effects that ensue from local anesthetic, vasoconstrictive, sympathomimetic, psychoactive, and prothrombotic mechanisms. Cocaine can affect all body systems and the clinical presentation may primarily result from organ toxicity. Among the most severe complications are seizures, hemorrhagic and ischemic strokes, myocardial infarction, aortic dissection, rhabdomyolysis, mesenteric ischemia, acute renal injury and multiple organ failure.

Digitalis toxicity produces a toxidrome characterized by gastrointestinal, neurologic, electrolyte, and nonspecific cardiac manifestations. Chronic toxicity remains much more difficult to recognize compared with an acute presentation because of the nonspecific manifestations; therefore, serum glycoside levels are essential for diagnosis in this population. The mainstay of management continues to be rapid toxidrome identification followed by digoxin-specific antibody fragment therapy with supportive care. Several controversies still remain, including therapy for patients dependent on hemodialysis, appropriateness of calcium therapy for hyperkalemia, ideal agents for arrhythmia therapy, and the potential utility of plasmapheresis for removal of bound digoxin-antibody fragment complexes.

Jorge A. Guzman

Carbon monoxide (CO) poisoning is the leading cause of death as a result of unintentional poisoning in the United States. CO toxicity is the result of a combination of tissue hypoxia-ischemia secondary to carboxyhemoglobin formation and direct CO-mediated damage at a cellular level. Presenting symptoms are mostly nonspecific and depend on the duration of exposure and levels of CO. Diagnosis is made by prompt measurement of carboxyhemoglobin levels. Treatment consists of the patient's removal from the source of exposure and the immediate administration of 100% supplemental oxygen in addition to aggressive supportive measures. The use of hyperbaric oxygen is controversial.

Richard W. Carlson, Nivedita N. Kumar, Edna Wong-Mckinstry, Srikala Ayyagari, Nitin Puri, Frank K. Jackson, and Shivaramaiah Shashikumar

In susceptible patients, alcohol withdrawal syndrome (AWS) is often precipitated by other medical or surgical disorders, and AWS can adversely affect the course of these underlying conditions. Although the mortality rate of AWS has decreased over the past few decades, significant risk for morbidity and death remain if management is complicated by a variety of conditions. This review of AWS focuses on the scope of the clinical problem, historical features, pathophysiology, clinical presentation, and approaches to therapy, with particular emphasis on severe AWS that requires management in the intensive care unit.

Matthew W. Hedge

The topic of central nervous system intoxicants encompasses a multitude of agents. This article focuses on three classes of therapeutic drugs, with specific examples in which overdoses require admission to the intensive care unit. Included are some of the newer antidepressants, the atypical neuroleptic agents, and selected anticonvulsant drugs. The importance of understanding pertinent physiology and applicable supportive care is emphasized.

Martina M. Cartwright, Waddah Hajja, Sofian Al-Khatib, Maryam Hazeghazam, Dharmashree Sreedhar, Rebecca Na Li, Edna Wong-McKinstry, and Richard W. Carlson

Ketoacidotic syndromes are frequently encountered in acute care medicine. This article focuses on ketosis and ketoacidotic syndromes associated with intoxications, alcohol abuse, starvation, and certain dietary supplements as well as inborn errors of metabolism. Although all of these various processes are characterized by the accumulation of ketone bodies and metabolic acidosis, there are differences in the mechanisms, clinical presentations, and principles of therapy for these heterogeneous disorders. Pathophysiologic mechanisms that account for these disorders are presented, as well as guidance regarding identification and management.

Critters and creatures can strike fear into anyone who thinks about dangerous animals. This article focuses on the management of the most common North American scorpion, arachnid, hymenoptera, and snake envenomations that cause clinically significant problems. Water creatures and less common animal envenomations are not covered in this article. Critical care management of envenomed patients can be challenging for unfamiliar clinicians. Although the animals are located in specific geographic areas, patients envenomed on passenger airliners and those who travel to endemic areas may present to health care facilities distant from the exposure.

Accidental or intentional ingestion of substances containing methanol and ethylene glycol can result in death, and some survivors are left with blindness, renal dysfunction, and chronic brain injury. However, even in large ingestions, a favorable outcome is possible if the patient arrives at the hospital early enough and the poisoning is identified and appropriately treated in a timely manner. This review covers the common circumstances of exposure, the involved toxic mechanisms, and the clinical manifestations, laboratory findings, and treatment of methanol and ethylene glycol intoxication.

Toxicology

CRITICAL CARE CLINICS

Preface

Toxicology

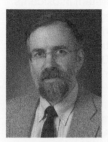

James A. Kruse, MD
Guest Editor

Patients with serious toxic ingestions, drug overdoses, envenomations, and other forms of poisoning are frequently admitted to intensive care units (ICUs), either because they are critically ill at the time of hospital admission or because they have the potential for rapid deterioration in their condition. As such, known or suspected intoxications constitute a common reason for admission to medical and mixed medical–surgical ICUs, and occasionally as initially unsuspected or otherwise comorbid factors in critically ill or injured patients admitted to ICUs caring exclusively for patients with surgical problems.

This issue of *Critical Care Clinics* includes 10 reviews pertaining to toxicologic topics relevant to the ICU setting. The first title, by Drs Holstege and Borek, reviews the general approach to the poisoned patient, specifically focusing on the recognition of particular constellations of clinical findings and simple screening laboratory tests, which have been named toxic syndromes or "toxidromes." As the authors point out, early recognition of occult intoxication can be key to a favorable outcome. The second article, by Drs Hodgman and Garrard, reviews one of the most common and potentially very serious drug overdoses, namely, acetaminophen poisoning. Ingestion of an otherwise lethal dose of acetaminophen is potentially survivable with no sequelae if the patient presents to the hospital soon after the ingestion, but only if the diagnosis is recognized and appropriate antidotal treatment is properly administered in a timely manner. The next topic, by Dr Zimmerman, covers one of the most commonly abused illicit drugs, cocaine, which can be associated with diverse life-threatening complications.

Drs Kanji and MacLean next review the topic of cardiac glycoside intoxication. This form of poisoning can occur from intentional or accidental overdose, including occasional iatrogenic overdoses and less commonly in association with ingestion of various species of plants. While less common than acetaminophen or cocaine intoxication, cardiac glycoside poisoning can be life-threatening and there is specific effective antidotal therapy. Dr Guzman covers the pathophysiology, clinical recognition, and treatment of carbon monoxide poisoning, the leading cause of death due to unintentional poisoning in the United States. Dr Carlson and colleagues provide an extensive review

Crit Care Clin 28 (2012) xi–xii
http://dx.doi.org/10.1016/j.ccc.2012.08.001
0749-0704/12/$ – see front matter © 2012 Elsevier Inc. All rights reserved.

of alcohol withdrawal. The resulting syndrome, in contrast to the other topics herein, generally occurs after a period of abstinence rather than at the time of intoxication. However, the topic is of immense relevance because of its prevalence and potential seriousness, both within and outside the ICU.

Dr Hedge's article covers a number of specific central nervous system intoxicants. The huge number of toxic agents that could be included in this category necessitated limiting the included substances to some of the newer antidepressants, which are now commonly involved in intentional drug overdoses seen in the ICU setting, as well as the atypical neuroleptic agents and selected anticonvulsant drugs. Dr Cartwright and colleagues provide a unique review of both toxigenic and metabolic causes of ketosis and ketoacidotic syndromes, including recommendations for their identification and management. Envenomations requiring ICU admission are uncommon in the United States, but do occur and can threaten life and limb. Dr Quan reviews the most serious envenomations by arthropods and snakes indigenous to North America. The final topic details the clinical recognition and management of methanol and ethylene glycol poisoning.

James A. Kruse, MD
Clinical Professor
College of Physicians and Surgeons
Columbia University
New York, NY 10027, USA

Chief, Critical Care Services
Bassett Medical Center
One Atwell Road
Cooperstown, NY 13326, USA

E-mail address:
james.kruse@bassett.org

Toxidromes

Christopher P. Holstege, MD[a,b,]*, Heather A. Borek, MD[a]

KEYWORDS

- Toxidrome • Syndrome • Poisoning • Toxicology

KEY POINTS

- A toxidrome is a constellation of findings, either from the physical examination or from ancillary testing, which may result from any given poison. It serves to clue the clinician into the correct diagnosis.
- Common toxidromes include: anticholinergic toxidrome, cholinergic toxidrome, opioid toxidrome, sympathomimetic toxidrome.
- Even though these toxidromes can aid the clinician in narrowing the differential diagnosis, care must be exercised to realize the exceptions and limitations associated with each.

Poisonings are commonly encountered in critical care medicine.[1] Patients can be exposed to potential toxins either accidentally (eg, drug interactions or occupational exposures) or intentionally (eg, substance abuse or suicide attempt). The outcome following a poisoning depends on numerous factors, such as the dose taken, the characteristics of the substance, the time to presentation to the health system, and the preexisting health status of the patient. If a poisoning is recognized early and appropriate supportive care is initiated quickly, most outcomes will be favorable.

This article introduces the basic concepts for the initial approach to the poisoned patient and the initial steps in stabilization. Next, it introduces some key concepts in diagnosing the poisoning with focus on the various classic toxidromes, including those based on physical examination, laboratory analysis, and the ECG.

INITIAL CLINICAL EVALUATION

All patients presenting with toxicity or potential toxicity should be managed supportively regardless of the perceived toxidrome encountered.[2,3] The patient's airway

[a] Division of Medical Toxicology, Department of Emergency Medicine, Blue Ridge Poison Center, University of Virginia Health System, University of Virginia School of Medicine, PO Box 800774, Charlottesville, VA 22908-0774, USA; [b] Division of Medical Toxicology, Department of Pediatrics, Blue Ridge Poison Center, University of Virginia Health System, University of Virginia School of Medicine, PO Box 800774, Charlottesville, VA 22908-0774, USA
* Corresponding author. Division of Medical Toxicology, Department of Emergency Medicine, Blue Ridge Poison Center, University of Virginia Health System, University of Virginia School of Medicine, PO Box 800774, Charlottesville, VA 22908-0774.
E-mail address: ch2xf@virginia.edu

Crit Care Clin 28 (2012) 479–498
http://dx.doi.org/10.1016/j.ccc.2012.07.008
0749-0704/12/$ – see front matter © 2012 Elsevier Inc. All rights reserved.

should be patent and adequate ventilation assured. If necessary, endotracheal intubation should be performed with assisted ventilation initiated. Too often, physicians are lulled into a false sense of security when a poisoned patient's oxygen saturations are adequate on high-flow oxygen. If the patient has either inadequate ventilation (eg, from profound sedation) or a poor gag reflex, the patient may be at risk for subsequent carbon dioxide narcosis with worsening acidosis or aspiration.

The initial treatment of hypotension consists simply of adequate administration of intravenous (IV) fluids. Close monitoring of the patient's pulmonary status should be performed to assure that pulmonary edema does not develop as fluids are infused. The health care providers should place all potentially unstable overdose patients on continuous cardiac monitoring and pulse oximetry, and perform frequent neurologic reassessments. In all patients with altered mental status, the patient's blood glucose level should be checked. Poisoned patients should receive a large-bore peripheral IV line and all symptomatic patients should have a second line placed in either the peripheral or central venous system. Placement of a urinary catheter should be considered early in the care of hemodynamically unstable poisoned patients to monitor urinary output as an indicator of adequate perfusion.

Identification of the constellation of signs, symptoms, laboratory findings, and ECG changes that define a specific toxicologic syndrome, or toxidrome, may narrow a differential diagnosis to a specific class of poisons and guide subsequent management.[4,5] Select toxidromes that may be diagnosed via the physical examination may be found in **Table 1**. Many toxidromes have several overlapping features. For example, anticholinergic findings are highly similar to sympathomimetic findings, with an exception being the effects on sweat glands: anticholinergic agents produce warm, flushed dry skin, whereas sympathomimetic agents produce diaphoresis. Toxidrome findings may also be affected by individual variability, comorbid conditions, and coingestants. For example, tachycardia associated with sympathomimetic or anticholinergic toxidromes may be absent in a patient who is concurrently taking beta-adrenergic receptor antagonist medications. Additionally, although toxidromes may be applied to classes of drugs, some individual agents within these classes may have one or more toxidrome findings absent.[6] For instance, meperidine is an opioid analgesic but does not induce miosis, which helps define the classic opioid toxidrome. When accurately identified, the toxidrome may provide invaluable information for diagnosis and subsequent treatment, although the many limitations impeding acute toxidrome diagnosis must be carefully considered.[7]

Table 1	
Selected physical examination toxidromes	
Toxidrome	**Signs and Symptoms**
Anticholinergic	Mydriasis, tachycardia, anhidrosis, dry mucous membranes, hypoactive bowel sounds, altered mental status, delirium, hallucinations, urinary retention
Cholinergic	Diarrhea, diaphoresis, involuntary urination, miosis, bradycardia, bronchospasm, bronchorrhea, emesis, lacrimation, salivation
Opioid	Sedation, miosis, decreased bowel sounds, decreased respirations, bradycardia
Sympathomimetic	Agitation, mydriasis, tachycardia, hypertension, hyperthermia, diaphoresis

PHYSICAL EXAMINATION TOXIDROMES
Anticholinergic Toxidrome

Anticholinergic agents act by inhibiting muscarinic receptors.[8] Muscarinic receptors primarily are associated with the parasympathetic nervous system, which innervates numerous organ systems, including the eye, heart, respiratory system, skin, gastrointestinal tract, and bladder. Sweat glands, innervated by the sympathetic nervous system, also are modulated by muscarinic receptors.

Following exposure to a muscarinic antagonist, findings consistent with anticholinergic syndrome develop on physical examination. Characteristic manifestations of the anticholinergic syndrome have long been taught using the old medical adage "dry as a bone, blind as a bat, red as a beet, hot as a hare, and mad as a hatter," which correspond with anhidrosis, mydriasis, flushing, hyperthermia, and delirium, respectively.

Depending on the dose and time postexposure, several of central nervous system (CNS) effects may manifest.[9] Restlessness, apprehension, abnormal speech, confusion, agitation, tremor, picking movements, ataxia, stupor, and coma have all been described following exposure to various anticholinergic agents. When manifesting delirium, the individual often stares into space, mutters, and fluctuates between occasional lucid intervals with appropriate responses and periods of vivid hallucinations. Phantom behaviors, such as plucking or picking in the air or at garments, are characteristic. Hallucinations are prominent and may be benign, entertaining, or terrifying to the patient experiencing them. Exposed patients may have conversations with hallucinated figures or they may misidentify persons they typically know well. Simple tasks typically performed well by the exposed person may become difficult. Motor coordination, perception, cognition, and new memory formation are altered.

Mydriasis causes photophobia. Impairment of near vision occurs because of loss of accommodation and reduced depth of field secondary to ciliary muscle paralysis and pupillary enlargement. Tachycardia may occur. Exacerbated heart rate responses to exertion are also expected. Systolic and diastolic blood pressure may show moderate elevation. A decrease in precapillary tone may cause skin flushing. Intestinal motility slows and secretions from the stomach, pancreas, and gallbladder decrease resulting in decreased bowel sounds. Nausea and vomiting may occur. All glandular cells become inhibited, and dry mucus membranes of the mouth and throat are noted. Inhibition of sweating results in dry skin, which is best examined in the axilla or groin due to the high concentration of muscarinic sweat glands in these areas. Urination may be difficult and urinary retention may occur. Urinary retention may contribute to an anticholinergic patient's agitation and early urinary catheter placement is recommended. The exposed patient's temperature may become elevated from the inability to sweat and dissipate heat. In warm climates this may result in marked hyperthermia.

Cholinergic Toxidrome

A true cholinergic toxidrome is the opposite of the anticholinergic toxidrome depicted previously. Cholinergic agents activate muscarinic acetylcholine receptors. However, the clinical syndrome encountered by many cholinergic agents may vary considerably because many muscarinic agonists are also agonists of other receptors. For example, organophosphates, considered classic cholinergic agents, do not only cause muscarinic activation, but also activate the sympathetic system.[10]

Acetylcholine is a neurotransmitter found throughout the nervous system, including the CNS, the autonomic ganglia (sympathetic and parasympathetic), the postganglionic parasympathetic nervous system, and at the skeletal muscle motor end plate.[11] Acetylcholine binds to and activates muscarinic and nicotinic receptors. The enzyme, acetylcholinesterase (AChE), regulates acetylcholine activity within the synaptic cleft. Acetylcholine binds to the active site of AChE where the enzyme rapidly hydrolyzes acetylcholine to choline and acetic acid. These hydrolyzed products rapidly dissociate from AChE so that the enzyme is free to act on another molecule. Organophosphates and carbamate insecticides act as AChE inhibitors by binding at the enzyme's active site. The inhibited enzyme is unable to inactivate acetylcholine. As a result, excessive acetylcholine stimulation occurs. Subsequently, not only are the muscarinic receptors activated but also are the nicotinic receptors leading to both activation of the sympathomimetic system and stimulation of the neuromuscular junction. Nicotine poisoning is clinically similar to an organophosphate or carbamate poisoning. Nicotine directly stimulates the nicotinic receptors and, therefore, stimulates the sympathetic and parasympathetic ganglia.

A pure cholinergic toxidrome affects nearly every organ system.[12] The respiratory system effects of cholinergic agents tend to be dramatic and are considered to be the major factor leading to the death of the victim.[13] Profuse watery nasal discharge, nasal hyperemia, marked salivation, and bronchorrhea have all been described. Prolonged expiratory phase, cough, and wheezing may manifest as a consequence of lower respiratory tract bronchorrhea and bronchoconstriction. Bradydysrhythmias and hypotension may be seen. Lacrimation, blurred vision, and miosis can occur. The sweat glands are innervated by sympathetic muscarinic receptors and profuse diaphoresis can occur. Cholinergic innervation causes an increase in gastric and intestinal motility and a relaxation of reflex anal sphincter tone. As a result, profuse watery salivation and gastrointestinal hyperactivity with resultant nausea, vomiting, abdominal cramps, tenesmus, and uncontrolled defecation are characteristic features of a cholinergic toxidrome. Cholinergic stimulation of the detrusor muscle causes contraction of the urinary bladder and relaxation of the trigone and sphincter muscles resulting in involuntary urination. Mnemonics that have been used to describe the cholinergic toxidrome include DUMBBELS (defecation, urination, miosis, bronchorrhea, bronchoconstriction, emesis, lacrimation, and salivation) or SLUDGE (salivation, lacrimation, urination, defecation, gastrointestinal dysfunction, and emesis).

Seizures are frequently seen in severe cholinergic poisoning, due to the CNS effects of excess acetylcholine.[14] Stimulation of the nicotinic receptors at the motor end plate can initially result in fasiculations but can rapidly progress to a flaccid paralysis (similar to the depolarizing paralytic agent succinylcholine). The propensity to cause seizures as well as paralysis puts cholinergic patients at risk for nonconvulsive status epilepticus.

Atropine is the initial drug of choice in symptomatic cholinergic patients.[15] Atropine acts as a muscarinic receptor antagonist and blocks neuroeffector sites on smooth muscle, cardiac muscle, secretory gland cells, peripheral ganglia, and in the CNS. Atropine is, therefore, useful in alleviating bronchoconstriction and bronchorrhea, tenesmus, abdominal cramps, nausea and vomiting, bradydysrythmias, and seizure activity. Atropine can be administered by either the IV, intramuscular, or endotracheal route. The dose varies with the type of exposure, but generally is higher than doses used in Advanced Cardiac Life Support protocols for symptomatic bradycardia. For the mildly and moderately symptomatic adult, 2 mg is administered every 5 minutes to desired clinical effect. In the severely poisoned patient, dosages will need to be increased and given more rapidly. Tachycardia is not a contraindication to atropine administration in these patients and may be due to sympathetic system stimulation. Drying of the respiratory secretions and resolution of bronchoconstriction are the therapeutic end points used to determine the appropriate dose of atropine. This will be clinically apparent because the patient will have ease of respiration, improved ventilator mechanics, and decreased airway pressures if receiving positive pressure ventilation. Atropine has no effect on the nicotinic receptors and, therefore, has no effect on the autonomic ganglia and neuromuscular junction. Therefore, muscle weakness, fasciculations, tremors, and paralysis associated with organophosphate, carbamate, and nicotine poisoning are not indications for further atropine dosing. It does have a partial effect on the CNS and is helpful in resolving or preventing seizures.

Pralidoxime chloride is used to treat organophosphate poisoned patients only and does not have a role for carbamate or nicotine poisoning. It reactivates AChE by exerting a nucleophilic attack on the phosphorus resulting in an oxime–phosphate bond that splits from the AChE, leaving the regenerated enzyme. This reactivation is clinically most apparent at skeletal neuromuscular junctions, with less activity at muscarinic sites. Pralidoxime must, therefore, be administered concurrently with adequate atropine doses. The recommended dose of pralidoxime is 1 to 2 g, for adults, by the IV route. Slow administration over 15 to 30 minutes has been advocated to minimize side effects. These side effects include hypertension, headache, blurred vision, epigastric discomfort, nausea, and vomiting. Rapid administration can result in laryngospasm, muscle rigidity, and transient impairment of respiration. Pralidoxime is rapidly excreted by the kidney with a half-life of approximately 90 minutes. Therefore, a continuous infusion is often recommended after the loading dose to maintain therapeutic levels.[16] Currently, the World Health Organization recommends a bolus of greater than 30 mg/kg followed by an infusion of greater than 8 mg/kg per hour. Due to the high risk of seizures in symptomatic cholinergic-poisoned patients, empiric treatment with benzodiazepines is also recommended.

Opioid Toxidrome

Opioid syndrome is commonly encountered in medicine. Opiates are the naturally derived narcotics, such as morphine and codeine, found in opium. Opium is isolated from the poppy plant, *Papaver somniferum*. Opioids are a broader class that include opiates and include all substances that bind to opioid receptors. Opioids include the semisynthetic and synthetic compounds such as hydrocodone, hydromorphone, oxycodone, methadone, and fentanyl. These drugs all have potent analgesic and sedative properties but different pharmacokinetic properties.

Opioids exert their clinical effects by binding to three major classes of opioid receptors: mu (μ), kappa (κ), and delta (δ); or OP_3, OP_2, and OP_1, respectively. Various opioids have different affinity profiles with respect to opioid receptors, which explains the differences in the clinical effects. For example, mu receptors are primarily responsible for the sensation of euphoria, and specific opioids are preferred for abuse due to their potent mu-receptor agonism.

Opioid poisoning can have widespread clinical manifestations depending on the agent used, dose, method of delivery, and the presence of coingestants. The classic toxidrome consists of miosis plus respiratory and CNS depression. Although pinpoint pupils are often associated with opioid poisoning, one should not rely on them exclusively in making the diagnosis. Gastrointestinal motility is decreased, resulting in decreased or absent bowel sounds on physical examination. CNS and respiratory depression can lead to several potentially serious secondary effects, including anoxic brain injury, aspiration pneumonia, and rhabdomyolysis.

Several opioids cause additional nonclassic signs and symptoms that may confound the clinical diagnosis. For example, tramadol, propoxyphene, and meperidine may cause seizures.[17,18] Propoxyphene causes cardiac conduction abnormalities (eg, prolongation of the QRS interval) and dysrhythmias.[19] Methadone is known to cause QT interval prolongation. Movement disorders may also be seen with drugs such as fentanyl, including life-threatening chest wall rigidity. Certain opioids, such as meperidine, fentanyl, and tramadol, have serotonergic properties and may lead to a serotonin syndrome when combined with other serotonin agonists.[20] Adulterants or contaminants may confound the clinical presentation of a patient presenting with opioid toxicity. For example, clenbuterol-contaminated heroin produced an outbreak of an atypical clinical illness consisting of tachycardia, palpitations, hypokalemia, and hyperglycemia.[21] The opioid toxidrome may be mimicked by nonopioid agents such as clonidine, oxymetazoline, and antipsychotic drugs.

Opioid poisoning may be reversed with several opioid antagonists (eg, naloxone or naltrexone). Naloxone is commonly used in comatose patients as a therapeutic and diagnostic agent. The standard dosage regimen is to administer from 0.4 to 2 mg slowly, preferably intravenously. The IV dose should be readministered at 5 minute intervals until the desired endpoint is achieved: restoration of respiratory function, ability to protect the airway, and an improved level of consciousness. If the IV route of administration is not viable, alternative routes include intramuscular, intraosseous, intranasal, or inhalational (ie, via nebulization). A patient may not respond to naloxone administration for a variety of reasons: insufficient dose of naloxone, the absence of an opioid exposure, a mixed overdose with other CNS and respiratory depressants, or for medical or traumatic reasons.

Naloxone can precipitate profound withdrawal symptoms in opioid-dependant patients. Symptoms include agitation, vomiting, diarrhea, piloerection, diaphoresis, and yawning. Caution should be exercised in administration of naloxone and only the amount necessary to restore adequate respiration and airway protection should be used. Naloxone's clinical efficacy can last for as little as 45 minutes. Therefore, patients are at risk for recurrence of sedation, particularly for patients exposed to methadone or sustained-release opioid products. Patients should be observed for resedation for at least 4 hours after reversal with naloxone. Naloxone is renally eliminated and the elimination kinetics are not easily predicted in patients with renal failure; therefore, patients with renal impairment should be observed for resedation for a longer period of time. If a patient does resedate it is reasonable to administer naloxone as an infusion. An infusion of two-thirds the effective initial bolus per hour is usually effective with patients monitored closely for the potential development of withdrawal symptoms or worsening sedation as the drug is either metabolized or absorbed, respectively.

Sympathomimetic Toxidrome

Norepinephrine is the neurotransmitter for postganglionic sympathetic (adrenergic) fibers that innervate skin, eyes, heart, lungs, gastrointestinal tract, exocrine glands, and some neuronal tracts in the CNS. Physiologic responses to activation of the adrenergic system are complex and depend on the type of receptor (α1, α2, β1, β2), some of which are excitatory and others that have opposing inhibitory responses. Stimulation of the sympathetic nervous system produces CNS excitation (agitation, anxiety, tremors, delusions, and paranoia), tachycardia, seizures, hypertension, mydriasis, hyperpyrexia, and diaphoresis. In severe cases, cardiac arrhythmias and coma may occur.

Hyperthermic Toxidromes

Toxin-induced hyperthermia syndromes include sympathomimetic hyperthermia, uncoupling syndrome, serotonin syndrome, neuroleptic malignant syndrome, malignant hyperthermia, and anticholinergic poisoning.[22] Sympathomimetics, such as amphetamines and cocaine, may produce hyperthermia due to excess serotonin and dopamine resulting in thermal deregulation.[23] Treatment is primarily supportive and may include active cooling and administration of benzodiazepine agents. Uncoupling syndrome occurs when the process of oxidative phosphorylation is disrupted, leading to heat generation and a reduced ability to aerobically generate adenosine-5'-triphosphate. Severe salicylate poisoning is a characteristic intoxication that has been associated with uncoupling.[24] Serotonin syndrome occurs when there is a relative excess of serotonin at both peripheral and central serotonergic receptors.[25] Patients may present with hyperthermia, alterations in mental status, and neuromuscular abnormalities (rigidity, hyperreflexia, and clonus) although there may be individual variability in these findings. It is associated with drug interactions, such as the combination of monoamine oxidase inhibitors and meperidine, but may also occur with single-agent therapeutic dosing or overdose of serotonergic agents. The serotonin antagonist cyproheptadine has been advocated to treat serotonin syndrome in conjunction with benzodiazepines and other supportive treatments, such as active cooling. However, cyproheptadine may only be administered orally and its true efficacy is not well known, which limits its overall utility. Neuroleptic malignant syndrome is a condition caused by relative deficiency of dopamine within the CNS.[26] It has been associated with dopamine receptor antagonists and the sudden withdrawal of dopamine agonists such as levodopa-carbidopa products. Clinically it may be difficult to distinguish from serotonin syndrome and other hyperthermic emergencies. Clinically, patients develop hyperthermia, rigidity, autonomic instability, and mental status changes. Elevations in creatine kinase activity and white blood cell count can be seen. Bromocriptine, amantadine, and dantrolene have been used for treatment in some reports, but true efficacy has not been fully delineated. Malignant hyperthermia occurs when genetically susceptible individuals are exposed to depolarizing neuromuscular blocking agents or volatile general anesthetics.[27] Treatment consists of removing the inciting agent, supportive care, and dantrolene administration. Finally, anticholinergic poisoning may result in hyperthermia through impairment of normal cooling mechanisms such as sweating. Supportive care, including active cooling and benzodiazepines, is the primary treatment of this condition. Overall, differentiating between the various hyperthermic toxidromes may be challenging and additional causes of hyperthermia, such as heat stroke and/or exhaustion and infection, should also be explored. In most toxin-induced hyperthermic syndromes, treatment includes benzodiazepine administration, active cooling, and general supportive care.

LABORATORY TOXIDROMES

When used appropriately, diagnostic tests may be of help in the management of the intoxicated patient. When a specific toxin, or even a class of toxins, is suspected, requesting qualitative or quantitative levels may be appropriate. In the suicidal patient, whose history is generally unreliable, or in the unresponsive patient, where no history is available, the clinician may gain further clues about to the cause of a poisoning by responsible diagnostic testing.

Toxins Inducing an Osmole Gap

The serum osmole gap is a common laboratory test that may be useful when evaluating poisoned patients. This test is most often discussed in the context of evaluating the patient suspected of toxic alcohol (eg, ethylene glycol, methanol, or isopropanol) intoxication. Though this test may have utility in such situations, it has many pitfalls and limitations that limit its effectiveness.

Osmotic concentrations may be expressed in terms of either osmolality (milliosmoles per kilogram of solvent [mOsm/kg]) or osmolarity (milliosmoles per liter of solution [mOsm/L]).[28] Osmolality can be measured (Osm_m) by use of an osmometer, a tool that most often uses the technique of freezing point depression.[29] Serum osmolarity (Osm_C) may be estimated clinically by any of several equations,[30] involving the patient's serum glucose, sodium, and urea nitrogen, which normally account for almost all of the measured osmolality.[31] One of the most commonly used of these calculations is expressed as:

$$Osm_C = 2(sodium) + (urea\ nitrogen)/2.8 + (glucose)/18$$

The numerical factor in the sodium term (which is expressed in millimoles per liter) accounts for corresponding anions that contribute to osmolarity; whereas, the numerical factors in the other two terms convert their concentrations units from milligrams per deciliter to millimoles per liter.[32] Finding the osmolar contribution of any other osmotically active substances that is reported in milligrams per deciliter (eg, urea nitrogen and glucose) is accomplished by dividing by one-tenth of the substance's molecular weight in daltons.[32] For urea nitrogen this conversion factor is 2.8 and for glucose it is 18. Similarly, additional terms, along with corresponding conversion factors, may be added to this equation to account for ethanol and the various toxic alcohols (assuming they have been measured and their results are expressed in milligrams per deciliter) as:

$$Osm_C = 2(sodium) + (urea\ nitrogen)/2.8 + (glucose)/18 + (ethanol)/4.6$$
$$+ (methanol)/3.2 + (ethylene\ glycol)/6.2 + (isopropanol)/6.0$$

The difference between the measured (Osm_M) and calculated (Osm_C) osmotic concentrations is the osmole gap[32]:

$$Osmole\ gap = Osm_M - Osm_C$$

One problem with this equation is that the units are different because the measured form is in units of osmolality (milliosmoles per kilogram) and the calculated form is in units of osmolarity (milliosmoles per liter). This unit difference is generally not considered significant for clinical purposes and the gap may be expressed in either units.[30]

If a significant elevation of the osmole gap is discovered, the difference in the two values may represent presence of foreign substances in the blood.[30] A list of possible causes of an elevated osmole gap is listed in **Box 1**. Unfortunately, what constitutes a normal osmole gap is widely debated. Conventionally, a normal gap has been defined as less than or equal to10 mOsm/kg. The original source of this value is an article from Smithline and Gardner,[33] which declared this number as pure convention. Further clinical study has not shown this assumption to be correct. Glasser and colleagues[34] studied 56 healthy adults and reported that the normal osmole gap ranges from −9 to +5 mOsm/kg. A study examining a pediatric emergency department population (n = 192) found a range from −13.5 to 8.9.[35] Another study, by Aabakken and colleagues,[36] looked at the osmole gaps of 177 patients admitted to their emergency department and reported their range (mean ± 2SD) to be from −10 to 20 mOsm/kg. A vital point brought forth by the authors of this study, however, is that the day-to-day coefficient of variation for their laboratory in regard to sodium was 1%. They concluded that this level of imprecision translates to an analytical standard deviation of 9.1 mOsm/kg in regard to the osmole gap. This analytical imprecision alone may account for the variation found in osmole gaps of many patients. This concern that even small errors in sodium, urea nitrogen, glucose, and osmolality assays can result in large variations of the osmole gap has been voiced by other

Box 1
Causes of an elevated osmole gap
Toxic alcohols
Ethanol
Isopropanol
Methanol
Ethylene glycol
Drugs and excipients
Mannitol
Propylene glycol
Glycerol
Osmotic contrast dyes
Other chemicals
Ethyl ether
Acetone
Trichloroethane
Disease or illness
Chronic renal failure
Lactic acidosis
Diabetic ketoacidosis
Alcoholic ketoacidosis
Starvation ketoacidosis
Circulatory shock
Hyperlipidemia
Hyperproteinemia

researchers.[37] Overall, the clinician should recognize that there is likely a wide range of variability in a patient's baseline osmole gap.

There are several concerns in regard to using the osmole gap as a screening tool in the evaluation of the potentially toxic-alcohol poisoned patient. The lack of a well-established normal range is particularly problematic. For example, a patient may present with an osmole gap of 9 mOsm/kg—a value considered normal by the traditionally accepted upper normal limit of 10 mOsm/kg. If, however, this patient had an osmole gap of −5 mOsm/kg just before ingestion of a toxic alcohol, the patient's osmole gap must have increased by 14 mOsm/kg to reach the new gap of 9 mOsm/kg. If this increase was due to ethylene glycol, it would correspond to a toxic level of 86.8 mg/dL.[38] In addition, if a patient's ingestion of a toxic alcohol occurred at a time distant from the actual blood sampling, the osmotically active parent compound will have been metabolized to the acidifying metabolites. These metabolites do not influence the osmole gap because they are anions that displace bicarbonate and are accounted for by the doubled-sodium term in the equation; hence no osmole gap elevation will be detected.[30,39] Therefore, it is possible that a patient may present at a point after ingestion with only a moderate rise in their osmole gap and anion gap. Steinhart[40] reported a patient with ethylene glycol toxicity who presented with an osmole gap of 7.2 mOsm/L due to a delay in presentation. Darchy and colleagues[37] presented two other cases of significant ethylene glycol toxicity with osmole gaps of 4 and 7 mOsm/L, respectively. The lack of an abnormal osmole gap in these cases was speculated to be due to either metabolism of the parent alcohol or a low baseline osmole gap that masked the toxin's presence.

The osmole gap should be used with caution as an adjunct to clinical decision making and not as a primary determinant to rule out toxic alcohol ingestion. If the osmole gap obtained is particularly large, it suggests an agent from **Box 1** may be present. A "normal" osmole gap should be interpreted with caution; a negative study may, in fact, not rule out the presence of such an ingestion—the test result must be interpreted within the context of the clinical presentation. If such a poisoning is suspected, appropriate therapy should be initiated presumptively (ie, ethanol infusion, 4-methylpyrazole, hemodialysis) while confirmation from serum levels of the suspected toxin are pending.

Toxins Inducing an Anion Gap Metabolic Acidosis

Obtaining a basic metabolic panel in all poisoned patients is generally recommended. When low serum bicarbonate is discovered on a metabolic panel, the clinician should determine if an elevated anion gap exists. The equation most commonly used for the serum anion gap calculation is[41]:

$$\text{Anion gap} = Na^+ - (Cl^- + HCO3^-)$$

The primary cation (sodium) and primary anions (chloride and bicarbonate) are represented in the equation.[42] Other serum cations are not commonly included in this calculation, because either their concentrations are relatively low (eg, potassium), or they may not have been assayed (eg, magnesium), or assigning a number to represent their respective contribution is difficult (eg, cationic serum proteins).[43] Similarly, there are a multitude of other serum anions (eg, sulfate, phosphate, or organic anions) that are also difficult to measure or to quantify in terms of charge-concentration units (milliequivalents per liter).[42,43] The anion gap represents these "unmeasured" ions. The normal range for the anion gap has conventionally been accepted to be 8 to 16 mEq/L,[43] but more recent changes in the technique for measuring chloride have resulted in a lowered range, closer to 6 to 14 mEq/L.[42] Practically speaking, an increase in the anion gap beyond an accepted normal range, accompanied by metabolic acidosis, represents an increase in unmeasured endogenous (eg, lactate) or exogenous (eg, salicylate) anions.[41] A list of the more common causes of this phenomenon is organized in the classic MUDPILES mnemonic (methanol, uremia, diabetic ketoacidosis [may also include alcoholic or starvation ketoacidosis], paraldehyde, isoniazid and iron, lactic acidosis, ethylene glycol, and salicylates). The P has been removed from the classic acronym because the drug paraldehyde is no longer available (**Box 2**).

It is imperative that clinicians who care for poisoned patients initially presenting with an increased anion gap metabolic acidosis investigate the cause of that acidosis. Many symptomatic poisoned patients may have an initial mild metabolic acidosis on presentation due to elevation of serum lactate. This can occur for a variety of reasons, including acidosis related to tissue hypoperfusion or a recent seizure. However, with adequate supportive care including hydration and oxygenation, the anion gap acidosis should improve. If, despite adequate supportive care, an anion gap metabolic acidosis worsens in a poisoned patient, the clinician should consider

Box 2
Potential toxic causes of increased anion gap metabolic acidosis
Methanol
Uremia
Diabetic ketoacidosis
Iron, inhalants (ie, carbon monoxide, cyanide, toluene), isoniazid, ibuprofen
Lactic acidosis
Ethylene glycol, ethanol (alcoholic) ketoacidosis
Salicylates, starvation ketoacidosis, sympathomimetics

either toxins that form acidic metabolites (eg, ethylene glycol, methanol, or ibuprofen) or toxins which cause lactic acidosis by interfering with aerobic energy production (eg, cyanide or iron).[44]

ELECTROCARDIOGRAPHIC TOXIDROMES

Interpretation of the ECG in the poisoned patient can challenge even the most experienced clinician. There are numerous drugs that can cause ECG changes. The incidence of ECG changes in the poisoned patient is unclear and the significance of various changes may be difficult to define.[45] Despite the fact that drugs have widely varying indications for therapeutic use, many unrelated drugs share common ECG effects if taken in overdose. Potential toxins can be placed into broad classes based on their cardiac effects. Two such classes, also known as ECG toxidromes, include agents that block the cardiac potassium efflux channels (resulting in QT interval prolongation) and agents that block cardiac fast sodium channels (resulting in QRS interval prolongation). The recognition of specific ECG changes associated with other clinical data (toxidromes) potentially can be life saving.

QT Prolongation

Studies suggest that approximately 3% of all noncardiac prescriptions are associated with the potential for QT prolongation. Myocardial repolarization is driven predominantly by outward movement of potassium ions. Blockade of the outward potassium currents by drugs prolongs the action potential.[46] This subsequently results in QT interval prolongation and the potential emergence of T or U wave abnormalities on the ECG.[47] The prolongation of repolarization causes the myocardial cell to have less charge difference across its membrane, which may result in the activation of the inward depolarization current (early after-depolarization) and promote triggered activity. These changes may lead to reentry and subsequent ventricular tachycardia, most often as the torsades de pointes variant of polymorphic ventricular tachycardia.[48] The QT interval is simply measured from the beginning of the QRS complex to the end of the T wave. Within any ECG tracing, there is lead-to-lead variation of the QT interval. In general, the longest measurable QT interval on an ECG is regarded as determining the overall QT interval for a given tracing.[49] The QT interval is influenced by the patient's heart rate. Several formulas have been developed to correct the QT interval for the effect of heart rate (QTc) using the RR interval (RR), with Bazett's formula ($QTc = QT/\sqrt{RR}$) being the most commonly used. QT prolongation is considered to occur when the QTc interval is greater than 440 milliseconds in men and 460 milliseconds in women, with arrhythmias most commonly associated with values greater than 500 milliseconds. The potential for an arrhythmia for a given QT interval will vary from drug to drug and patient to patient.[50] Bradycardia in the setting of drug-induced QT prolongation is more likely to degrade into torsades de pointes than in a patient with the same numerical QT with a tachycardic rate. Drugs associated with QT prolongation are listed in **Box 3**.[51] Other causes involved in possible prolongation of the QT interval include congenital long QT syndrome, mitral valve prolapse, hypokalemia, hypocalcemia, hypomagnesemia, hypothermia, myocardial ischemia, neurologic catastrophes, and hypothyroidism.[52]

QRS Prolongation

The ability of drugs to induce cardiac Na^+ channel blockade and thereby prolong the QRS complex has been well described in numerous literature reports.[53] This Na^+ channel blockade activity has been described as a membrane stabilizing effect, a local anesthetic effect, or a quinidine-like effect. Cardiac voltage-gated sodium channels reside in the cell membrane and open in conjunction with cell depolarization. Sodium channel blockers bind to the transmembrane Na^+ channels and decrease the number available for depolarization. This creates a delay of Na^+ entry into the cardiac myocyte during phase 0 of depolarization. As a result, the upslope of depolarization is slowed and the QRS complex widens.[54] In some cases, the QRS complex may take the pattern of recognized bundle branch blocks.[55,56] In the most severe cases, the QRS prolongation becomes so profound that it is difficult to distinguish between ventricular and supraventricular rhythms.[57,58] Continued prolongation of the QRS may result in a sine wave pattern and eventual asystole. It has been theorized that the Na^+ channel blockers can cause slowed intraventricular conduction, unidirectional block, the development of a reentrant circuit, and resulting ventricular tachycardia.[59] This can then degenerate into ventricular fibrillation. Differentiating a prolongation of the QRS complex due to Na^+ channel blockade in the poisoned patient versus other nontoxic causes can be difficult. Rightward axis deviation of the terminal 40 milliseconds of the QRS axis has been associated with tricyclic antidepressant poisoning.[60,61] However, the occurrence of this finding in other Na^+ channel blocking agents is unknown. Myocardial Na^+ channel blocking drugs comprise a diverse group of pharmaceutical agents (**Box 4**). Patients poisoned with these agents will have a variety of clinical presentations. For example, sodium channel blocking medications such as diphenhydramine, propoxyphene, and cocaine may also produce anticholinergic, opioid, and sympathomimetic syndromes, respectively.[19,62,63] In addition, specific drugs may affect not only the myocardial Na^+ channels but also calcium influx and potassium efflux channels.[64,65] This may result in ECG changes and rhythm disturbances not related entirely to the drug's Na^+ channel blocking activity. All the agents listed in **Box 4**, however, are similar in that they may induce myocardial Na^+ channel blockade and may respond to therapy with hypertonic saline or sodium bicarbonate.[19,58,63] It is, therefore, reasonable to treat poisoned patients that have a prolonged QRS interval, particularly those with hemodynamic instability, empirically with 1 to 2 mEq/kg of sodium bicarbonate. A shortening of the QRS can confirm the presence of a sodium channel blocking agent. Also, it can improve inotropy and help prevent arrhythmias.[53]

There are other drug-induced ECG changes that may be seen, depending on the agent ingested. For example, lithium may result in nonspecific T-wave inversions or flattening, and beta-blockers may cause bradycardia and heart blocks. Physicians managing patients who have taken overdoses of medications should be aware of the various ECG changes that potentially can occur in the overdose setting.

Box 3
Potassium efflux channel blocking drugs

Antihistamines
   Astemizole
   Clarithromycin
   Diphenhydramine
   Loratidine
   Terfenadine
Antipsychotics
   Chlorpromazine
   Droperidol
   Haloperidol
   Mesoridazine
   Pimozide
   Quetiapine
   Risperidone
   Thioridazine
   Ziprasidone
Arsenic trioxide
Bepridil
Chloroquine
Citalopram
Clarithromycin
Class IA antiarrhythmics
   Disopyramide
   Quinidine
   Procainamide
Class IC antiarrhythmics
   Encainide
   Flecainide
   Moricizine
   Propafenone
Class III antiarrhythmics
   Amiodarone
   Dofetilide
   Ibutilide
   Sotalol
Cyclic antidepressants
   Amitriptyline
   Amoxapine

Desipramine

Doxepin

Imipramine

Nortriptyline

Maprotiline

Erythromycin

Fluoroquinolones

Ciprofloxacin

Gatifloxacin

Levofloxacin

Moxifloxacin

Sparfloxacin

Halofantrine

Hydroxychloroquine

Levomethadyl

Methadone

Pentamidine

Quinine

Tacrolimus

Venlafaxine

WORD OF CAUTION: URINE DRUG SCREENING

Many clinicians regularly obtain urine drug screening on patients with an altered sensorium or on those suspected of a drug overdose. Such routine urine drug testing, however, is of questionable benefit. Kellermann and colleagues[66] found little impact of urine drug screening on patient management. Similarly, Mahoney and colleagues[67] concluded that toxic screening added little to treatment or disposition of overdose patients. In a study of over 200 overdose patients, Brett[68] showed that, although unsuspected drugs were routinely detected, the results rarely led to changes in management and likely never affected outcome. In a similar large study of trauma patients, Bast and colleagues[69] noted that a positive drug screen had minimal impact on patient treatment.

Some investigators do argue in favor of routine testing. Fabbri and colleagues[70] countered that comprehensive screening may aid decisions on patient disposition, resulting in fewer admissions to the hospital and less demand on critical care units. However, the screen used in their retrospective study tested for over 900 drugs and is not available to most clinicians. Milzman and colleagues[71] argued in favor of screening trauma victims, stating that the prognosis of intoxicated patients is unduly poor secondary to low Glasgow coma scale scores, although patient treatment and disposition did not seem to be affected.[71]

The effect of such routine screening in management changes is low because most of the therapy is supportive and directed at the clinical scenario (ie, mental status, cardiovascular function, and respiratory condition). Interpretation of the results can be difficult even when the objective for ordering a comprehensive urine screen is

---

Box 4
Sodium channel blocking drugs

Amantadine

Carbamazepine

Chloroquine

Class IA antiarrhythmics

   Disopyramide

   Quinidine

   Procainamide

Class IC antiarrhythmics

   Encainide

   Flecainide

   Propafenone

Citalopram

Cocaine

Cyclic antidepressants

Diltiazem

Diphenhydramine

Hydroxychloroquine

Loxapine

Orphenadrine

Phenothiazine

   Mesoridazine

   Thioridazine

Propranolol

Propoxyphene

Quinine

Verapamil

---

adequately defined. Most assays rely on antibody identification of drug metabolites, with some drugs remaining positive days after use and thus potentially not related to the patient's current clinical picture. The positive identification of drug metabolites is likewise influenced by chronicity of ingestion, fat solubility, and coingestions. In one such example, Perrone and colleagues[72] showed a cocaine retention time of 72 hours following its use. Conversely, many drugs of abuse are not detected on most urine drug screens, including gamma-hydroxybutyrate (GHB), fentanyl, and ketamine. The recent increase in Internet-acquirable drugs, such as synthetic cannabinoids (eg, "spice" and "K2") and synthetic amphetamines, such as mephedrone and methylene-dioxypyrovalerone ("bath salts"), are not detected on typical health system drug screens.

Interpretation is further confounded by false positive and false negative results. George and Braithwaite[73] evaluated five popular rapid urine screening kits and found all lacked significant sensitivity and specificity. The monoclonal antibodies used in these immunoassays may detect epitopes from multiple drug classes. For example, a relatively new antidepressant, venlafaxine, produced false-positive results via cross-reactivity with the anti-phencyclidine ("PCP") antibodies used in the urine RapidTest d.a.u. assay (Siemens Health care Diagnostics, Tarrytown, NY, USA).[74] False-positive benzodiazepine results were found in patients receiving the nonsteroidal antiinflammatory drug oxaprozin who were screened using the EMIT (DuPont Medical Products, Wilmington, DE, USA) and TDx (Abbott Laboratories, North Chicago, IL, USA) urine immunoassays.[75] Conversely, antibodies used in the immunoassays may not detect all drugs classified within a specific drug class. For example, the EMIT II Plus Opiate (Dade Behring, Deerfield, IL, USA) urine immunoassay will not detect physiologic doses of methadone. This assay detects codeine and its metabolites, morphine and morphine-3-glucuronide. It can also detect hydrocodone, which is structurally related to morphine; but also meperidine (in high doses), even though it is structurally unrelated to morphine. Additionally, cross-reactivity of certain prescription and certain over-the-counter medications used in therapeutic amounts for true illness may elicit positive screens. Diphenhydramine has been documented to interfere with the EMIT II urine immunoassay for propoxyphene.[76] Additionally, codeine will give positive opioid screen, which may be incorrectly attributed to morphine or heroin use.

The utility of ordering urine drug screens is fraught with significant testing limitations, including false-positive and false-negative results. Many authors have shown that the test results rarely affect management decisions. Routine drug screening of those with altered mental status, abnormal vital signs, or suspected ingestion rarely guides patient treatment or disposition.

SUMMARY

Critical care physicians often care for poisoned patients. Many of these patients will do well with simple observation and never develop significant toxicity. However, for patients who present with serious toxic effects or after potentially fatal ingestions, prompt action must be taken. As many poisons have no true antidote and the poison involved may initially be unknown, the first step is competent supportive care. Attention to supportive care, vital signs, and prevention of complications are the most important steps. Taking care of these issues will often be all that is necessary to assure recovery.

Identifying the poison, either through history, identifying a toxidrome, or laboratory analysis may help direct care or patient disposition and should be attempted. There are several antidotes available that can be life saving and prompt identification of patients who may benefit from these should be attempted.

REFERENCES

1. Holstege CP, Dobmeier SG, Bechtel LK. Critical care toxicology. Emerg Med Clin North Am 2008;26(3):715–39.
2. Lawrence DT, Bechtel L, Walsh JP, et al. The evaluation and management of acute poisoning emergencies. Minerva Med 2007;98(5):543–68.
3. Zimmerman JL. Poisonings and overdoses in the intensive care unit: general and specific management issues. Crit Care Med 2003;31(12):2794–801.
4. Nice A, Leikin JB, Maturen A, et al. Toxidrome recognition to improve efficiency of emergency urine drug screens. Ann Emerg Med 1988;17(7):676–80.
5. Lin TJ, Nelson LS, Tsai JL, et al. Common toxidromes of plant poisonings in Taiwan. Clin Toxicol 2009;47(2):161–8.

6. Boyle JS, Bechtel LK, Holstege CP. Management of the critically poisoned patient. Scand J Trauma Resusc Emerg Med 2009;17(1):29.
7. Erickson TB, Thompson TM, Lu JJ. The approach to the patient with an unknown overdose. Emerg Med Clin North Am 2007;25(2):249–81.
8. Estelle F, Simons R. H1-receptor antagonists: safety issues. Ann Allergy Asthma Immunol 1999;83(5):481–8.
9. Scott J, Pache D, Keane G, et al. Prolonged anticholinergic delirium following antihistamine overdose. Australas Psychiatry 2007;15(3):242–4.
10. Kwong TC. Organophosphate pesticides: biochemistry and clinical toxicology. Ther Drug Monit 2002;24(1):144–9.
11. Rusyniak DE, Nanagas KA. Organophosphate poisoning. Semin Neurol 2004; 24(2):197–204.
12. Hoffmann U, Papendorf T. Organophosphate poisonings with parathion and dimethoate. Intensive Care Med 2006;32(3):464–8.
13. Eddleston M, Mohamed F, Davies JO, et al. Respiratory failure in acute organophosphorus pesticide self-poisoning. QJM 2006;99(8):513–22.
14. Hsieh BH, Deng JF, Ger J, et al. Acetylcholinesterase inhibition and the extrapyramidal syndrome: a review of the neurotoxicity of organophosphate. Neurotoxicology 2001;22(4):423–7.
15. Aygun D. Diagnosis in an acute organophosphate poisoning: report of three interesting cases and review of the literature. Eur J Emerg Med 2004;11(1):55–8.
16. Medicis JJ, Stork CM, Howland MA, et al. Pharmacokinetics following a loading plus a continuous infusion of pralidoxime compared with the traditional short infusion regimen in human volunteers. J Toxicol Clin Toxicol 1996;34(3):289–95.
17. Beaule PE, Smith MI, Nguyen VN. Meperidine-induced seizure after revision hip arthroplasty. J Arthroplasty 2004;19(4):516–9.
18. Spiller HA, Villalobos D, Krenzelok EP, et al. Prospective multicenter study of sulfonylurea ingestion in children. J Pediatr 1997;131(1 Pt 1):141–6.
19. Stork CM, Redd JT, Fine K, et al. Propoxyphene-induced wide QRS complex dysrhythmia responsive to sodium bicarbonate—a case report. J Toxicol Clin Toxicol 1995;33(2):179–83.
20. Gillman PK. Monoamine oxidase inhibitors, opioid analgesics and serotonin toxicity. Br J Anaesth 2005;95(4):434–41.
21. Centers for Disease Control and Prevention (CDC). Atypical reactions associated with heroin use–five states, January–April 2005. MMWR Morb Mortal Wkly Rep 2005;54(32):793–6.
22. Rusyniak DE, Sprague JE. Hyperthermic syndromes induced by toxins. Clin Lab Med 2006;26(1):165–84.
23. Jaehne EJ, Salem A, Irvine RJ. Pharmacological and behavioral determinants of cocaine, methamphetamine, 3,4-methylenedioxymethamphetamine, and para-methoxyamphetamine-induced hyperthermia. Psychopharmacology (Berl) 2007; 194(1):41–52.
24. Katz KD, Curry SC, Brooks DE, et al. The effect of cyclosporine A on survival time in salicylate-poisoned rats. J Emerg Med 2004;26(2):151–5.
25. Isbister GK, Buckley NA, Whyte IM. Serotonin toxicity: a practical approach to diagnosis and treatment. Med J Aust 2007;187(6):361–5.
26. Seitz DP, Gill SS. Neuroleptic malignant syndrome complicating antipsychotic treatment of delirium or agitation in medical and surgical patients: case reports and a review of the literature. Psychosomatics 2009;50(1):8–15.
27. Stowell KM. Malignant hyperthermia: a pharmacogenetic disorder. Pharmacogenomics 2008;9(11):1657–72.

28. Kruse JA, Cadnapaphornchai P. The serum osmole gap. J Crit Care 1994;9(3): 185–97.
29. Erstad BL. Osmolality and osmolarity: narrowing the terminology gap. Pharmacotherapy 2003;23(9):1085–6.
30. Glaser DS. Utility of the serum osmol gap in the diagnosis of methanol or ethylene glycol ingestion. Ann Emerg Med 1996;27(3):343–6.
31. Worthley LI, Guerin M, Pain RW. For calculating osmolality, the simplest formula is the best. Anaesth Intensive Care 1987;15(2):199–202.
32. Suchard JR. Osmolal gap. In: Dart RC, Caravati EM, White IM, et al, editors. Medical toxicology. 3rd edition. Philadelphia: Lippincott Williams & Wilkins; 2004. p. 106–9.
33. Smithline N, Gardner KD Jr. Gaps—anionic and osmolal. JAMA 1976;236(14): 1594–7.
34. Glasser L, Sternglanz PD, Combie J, et al. Serum osmolality and its applicability to drug overdose. Am J Clin Pathol 1973;60(5):695–9.
35. McQuillen KK, Anderson AC. Osmol gaps in the pediatric population. Acad Emerg Med 1999;6(1):27–30.
36. Aabakken L, Johansen KS, Rydningen EB, et al. Osmolal and anion gaps in patients admitted to an emergency medical department. Hum Exp Toxicol 1994;13(2):131–4.
37. Darchy B, Abruzzese L, Pitiot O, et al. Delayed admission for ethylene glycol poisoning: lack of elevated serum osmol gap. Intensive Care Med 1999;25(8): 859–61.
38. Hoffman RS, Smilkstein MJ, Howland MA, et al. Osmol gaps revisited: normal values and limitations. J Toxicol Clin Toxicol 1993;31(1):81–93.
39. Eder AF, McGrath CM, Dowdy YG, et al. Ethylene glycol poisoning: toxicokinetic and analytical factors affecting laboratory diagnosis. Clin Chem 1998;44(1): 168–77.
40. Steinhart B. Case report: severe ethylene glycol intoxication with normal osmolal gap—"a chilling thought." J Emerg Med 1990;8(5):583–5.
41. Chabali R. Diagnostic use of anion and osmolal gaps in pediatric emergency medicine. Pediatr Emerg Care 1997;13(3):204–10.
42. Ishihara K, Szerlip HM. Anion gap acidosis. Semin Nephrol 1998;18(1):83–97.
43. Gabow PA. Disorders associated with an altered anion gap. Kidney Int 1985; 27(2):472–83.
44. Judge BS. Metabolic acidosis: differentiating the causes in the poisoned patient. Med Clin North Am 2005;89(6):1107–24.
45. Wells K, Williamson M, Holstege CP, et al. The association of cardiovascular toxins and electrocardiographic abnormality in poisoned patients. Am J Emerg Med 2008;26(8):957–9.
46. Anderson ME, Al-Khatib SM, Roden DM, et al. Cardiac repolarization: current knowledge, critical gaps, and new approaches to drug development and patient management. Am Heart J 2002;144(5):769–81.
47. Sides GD. QT interval prolongation as a biomarker for torsades de pointes and sudden death in drug development. Dis Markers 2002;18(2):57–62.
48. Nelson LS. Toxicologic myocardial sensitization. J Toxicol Clin Toxicol 2002;40(7): 867–79.
49. Chan TC, Brady WJ, Harrigan RA, editors. ECG in emergency medicine and acute care. Phildelphia: Elsevier-Mosby; 2005.
50. Yap YG, Camm AJ. Drug induced QT prolongation and torsades de pointes. Heart 2003;89(11):1363–72.

51. De Ponti F, Poluzzi E, Cavalli A, et al. Safety of non-antiarrhythmic drugs that prolong the QT interval or induce torsade de pointes: an overview. Drug Saf 2002;25(4):263–86.
52. Priori SG, Cantu F, Schwartz PJ. The long QT syndrome: new diagnostic and therapeutic approach in the era of molecular biology. Schweiz Med Wochenschr 1996;126(41):1727–31.
53. Kolecki PF, Curry SC. Poisoning by sodium channel blocking agents. Crit Care Clin 1997;13(4):829–48.
54. Harrigan RA, Brady WJ. ECG abnormalities in tricyclic antidepressant ingestion. Am J Emerg Med 1999;17(4):387–93.
55. Heaney RM. Left bundle branch block associated with propoxyphene hydrochloride poisoning. Ann Emerg Med 1983;12(12):780–2.
56. Fernandez-Quero L, Riesgo MJ, Agusti S, et al. Left anterior hemiblock, complete right bundle branch block and sinus tachycardia in maprotiline poisoning. Intensive Care Med 1985;11(4):220–2.
57. Brady WJ, Skiles J. Wide QRS complex tachycardia: ECG differential diagnosis. Am J Emerg Med 1999;17(4):376–81.
58. Clark RF, Vance MV. Massive diphenhydramine poisoning resulting in a wide-complex tachycardia: successful treatment with sodium bicarbonate. Ann Emerg Med 1992;21(3):318–21.
59. Joshi AK, Sljapic T, Borghei H, et al. Case of polymorphic ventricular tachycardia in diphenhydramine poisoning. J Cardiovasc Electrophysiol 2004;15(5):591–3.
60. Wolfe TR, Caravati EM, Rollins DE. Terminal 40-ms frontal plane QRS axis as a marker for tricyclic antidepressant overdose. Ann Emerg Med 1989;18(4):348–51.
61. Berkovitch M, Matsui D, Fogelman R, et al. Assessment of the terminal 40-millisecond QRS vector in children with a history of tricyclic antidepressant ingestion. Pediatr Emerg Care 1995;11(2):75–7.
62. Zareba W, Moss AJ, Rosero SZ, et al. Electrocardiographic findings in patients with diphenhydramine overdose. Am J Cardiol 1997;80(9):1168–73.
63. Kerns W II, Garvey L, Owens J. Cocaine-induced wide complex dysrhythmia. J Emerg Med 1997;15(3):321–9.
64. Bania TC, Blaufeux B, Hughes S, et al. Calcium and digoxin vs calcium alone for severe verapamil toxicity. Acad Emerg Med 2000;7(10):1089–96.
65. Dorsey ST, Biblo LA. Prolonged QT interval and torsades de pointes caused by the combination of fluconazole and amitriptyline. Am J Emerg Med 2000;18(2):227–9.
66. Kellermann AL, Fihn SD, LoGerfo JP, et al. Impact of drug screening in suspected overdose. Ann Emerg Med 1987;16(11):1206–16.
67. Mahoney JD, Gross PL, Stern TA, et al. Quantitative serum toxic screening in the management of suspected drug overdose. Am J Emerg Med 1990;8(1):16–22.
68. Brett A. Toxicologic analysis in patients with drug overdose. Arch Intern Med 1988;148(9):2077.
69. Bast RP, Helmer SD, Henson SR, et al. Limited utility of routine drug screening in trauma patients. South Med J 2000;93(4):397–9.
70. Fabbri A, Marchesini G, Morselli-Labate AM, et al. Comprehensive drug screening in decision making of patients attending the emergency department for suspected drug overdose. Emerg Med J 2003;20(1):25–8.
71. Milzman DP, Boulanger BR, Rodriguez A, et al. Pre-existing disease in trauma patients: a predictor of fate independent of age and injury severity score. J Trauma 1992;32(2):236–43.

72. Perrone J, De Roos F, Jayaraman S, et al. Drug screening versus history in detection of substance use in ED psychiatric patients. Am J Emerg Med 2001;19(1): 49–51.
73. George S, Braithwaite RA. A preliminary evaluation of five rapid detection kits for on site drugs of abuse screening. Addiction 1995;90(2):227–32.
74. Sena SF, Kazimi S, Wu AH. False-positive phencyclidine immunoassay results caused by venlafaxine and O-desmethylvenlafaxine. Clin Chem 2002;48(4): 676–7.
75. Camara PD, Audette L, Velletri K, et al. False-positive immunoassay results for urine benzodiazepine in patients receiving oxaprozin (Daypro). Clin Chem 1995;41(1):115–6.
76. Schneider S, Wennig R. Interference of diphenhydramine with the EMIT II immunoassay for propoxyphene. J Anal Toxicol 1999;23(7):637–8.

A Review of Acetaminophen Poisoning

Michael J. Hodgman, MD[a,b,*], Alexander R. Garrard, PharmD[a]

KEYWORDS

- Acetaminophen poisoning • Acetaminophen overdose • N-acetylcysteine
- Hepatotoxicity • Fulminant hepatic failure • Liver transplant • Paracetamol

KEY POINTS

- Acetaminophen is the leading cause of acute liver failure in the United States. Liver toxicity may result from an acute overdose as well as from chronic excessive ingestion.
- N-acetyl cysteine (NAC) is an effective antidote for acetaminophen overdose. Early treatment with NAC prevents the formation of a toxic metabolite that leads to hepatic injury. NAC is also an effective therapy to aid in the recovery of the hepatic injury as a consequence of acetaminophen.
- Obtaining an accurate time of ingestion is essential to interpreting an acetaminophen level in an acute exposure on the Rumack-Matthews Nomogram line. The nomogram line cannot be used to assess the risk of hepatotoxicity in a chronic acetaminophen exposure.
- The King's College Hospital criteria is the most often used to determine which patients are to die from fulminant hepatic failure. Other criteria have been proposed including phosphate, lactate, and a MELD score.

Acetaminophen (APAP) is a safe and effective analgesic and antipyretic.[1] It is widely available as a single-component medication and also as a component of a plethora of combination over-the-counter and prescription medications. More than 28 billion doses of APAP-containing products were dispensed in 2005.[2] With more than 89 million prescriptions, hydrocodone/APAP was the most commonly dispensed medication in 2003.[3] Despite its safety when used properly, APAP is one of the more common overdoses reported to poison centers. Serious toxicity results in hepatic injury, which may progress to fulminant hepatic failure (FHF) and death.[4] In 2009, the American Association of Poison Control Centers' National Poison Data System reported 401 deaths caused by APAP or an APAP combination product.[5] APAP is the most common cause of acute liver failure (ALF) in the United States, accounting for nearly half of the cases of

The authors have no financial disclosures or conflicts of interest to disclose.
[a] Department of Emergency Medicine, Upstate New York Poison Center, SUNY Upstate Medical University, Suite 202, 250 Harrison Street, Syracuse, NY 13202, USA; [b] Emergency and Trauma Services, Bassett Medical Center, Cooperstown, NY 13326, USA
* Corresponding author.
E-mail address: hodgmanm@upstate.edu

Crit Care Clin 28 (2012) 499–516
http://dx.doi.org/10.1016/j.ccc.2012.07.006
0749-0704/12/$ – see front matter © 2012 Elsevier Inc. All rights reserved.
criticalcare.theclinics.com

ALF in the US Acute Liver Failure Study Group.[6,7] Additionally, a significant number of cases of ALF of unknown cause may be unrecognized APAP toxicity, suggested by the presence of APAP protein adducts.[8] In children, APAP is much less frequently the cause of acute liver failure.[9]

APAP toxicity may be the consequence of either an acute overdose or from repeated excessive dosing (repeated supratherapeutic ingestion [RSTI]).[10] Unintentional toxicity may also occur from the concurrent use of several different medications that each contains APAP. The Acute Liver Failure Study Group found nearly equal proportions of patients with APAP hepatotoxicity caused by intentional versus unintentional overdose. Unintentional overdoses were often caused by RSTI and tended to present later with signs of hepatic injury apparent on presentation.[11] Concerns that combination APAP-opioid products are a risk factor for APAP hepatotoxicity from RSTI led the Food and Drug Administration to recently request that manufacturers of prescription drugs limit the APAP content of each unit dose to 325 mg. They have until early 2014 to comply with this requirement.[12] Earlier this year, in an effort to avoid dosing errors in children receiving liquid formulations of APAP, manufacturers agreed to a uniform strength of 160 mg/5 mL.[13] Another potential challenge for clinicians is the recent introduction of an intravenous (IV) APAP product, Ofirmev, in the United States and the risk of iatrogenic toxicity.[14]

PHARMACOLOGY AND TOXICITY

APAP is rapidly absorbed from the gastrointestinal (GI) tract with peak concentrations achieved within 90 minutes of a therapeutic dose. The presence of food in the stomach may delay the peak but not the extent of absorption.[15] Distribution is rapid with a volume of distribution (V_d) of about 0.9 L/kg and minimal protein binding at therapeutic concentrations.[16] The half-life of APAP is 2.0 to 2.5 hours. With hepatic injury, the half-life is prolonged to more than 4 hours.[4,16]

APAP undergoes extensive hepatic metabolism. Approximately 85% of a therapeutic dose undergoes phase II conjugation to sulfated and glucuronidated metabolites that are renally eliminated. Of these two pathways, glucuronidation is predominant in adults, whereas sulfation predominates in children up to about 12 years of age.[17] Up to 10% of APAP undergoes phase I oxidation to a reactive intermediate, N-acetyl-para-benzoquinone imine (NAPQI), which is normally conjugated with glutathione to nontoxic cysteine and mercapturate metabolites.[18] Cytochrome 2E1 is the primary cytochrome p450 (CYP) enzyme responsible for this oxidation. At supratherapeutic doses of APAP (>4 g), sulfation becomes saturated with proportional increases in both glucuronidation and, more significantly, oxidation to NAPQI.[16,18] Smaller proportions of APAP are eliminated unchanged in the urine and by ring oxidation to a catechol derivative (**Fig. 1**).[18]

At toxic doses of APAP, the continued production of NAPQI eventually results in the depletion of glutathione. Once glutathione stores have been depleted by about 70%, NAPQI binds to cellular proteins and leads to cell injury.[19] Glutathione depletion is only one of a cascade of intracellular events that includes mitochondrial oxidative stress, generation of reactive oxygen and nitrogen species, activation of stress proteins and gene transcription mediators, and mobilization of the liver's innate immune system. The balance between these numerous pathways ultimately determines whether there is recovery or cell death.[20,21] Mitochondrial failure seems to be the terminal event heralding cell death.[21] Although apoptotic pathways are activated, cell death is typically necrotic because mitochondrial failure precludes ordered cell death. The role of these various pathways in hepatocellular injury remains an area of active research. Zone 3

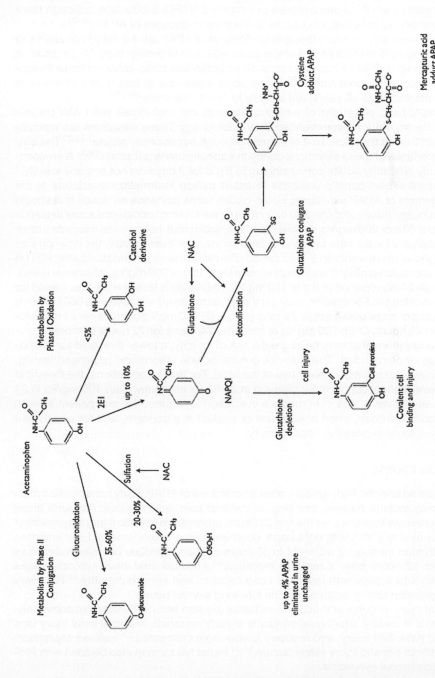

Fig. 1. Metabolism of APAP. NAC N-acetylcysteine.

hepatocytes, rich in CYP 2E1, are most susceptible to injury and this leads to the characteristic centrilobular pattern of hepatic necrosis seen with APAP. Patients on CYP2E1-inducing agents, such as ethanol, isoniazid, or St. John's wort, may be at an increased risk of toxicity because of increased NAPQI production, although there is no compelling data that this occurs at therapeutic dosages of APAP.[22–24]

Recommended maximum therapeutic dosages of APAP are 4 g daily in an adult and 50 to 75 mg/kg/d in children.[15] A single acute ingestion of greater than 7.5 g in an adult or 150 mg/kg in children has been considered potentially toxic, although these thresholds are probably conservative.[25] Single acute ingestions of less than 200 mg/kg in young children (age <6 years) are unlikely to result in toxicity.[26–28]

Asymptomatic elevations of aminotransferases are sometimes seen with chronic use at the maximum recommended daily dose of 4 g. These elevations are typically less than 3 times the upper limit of normal, although occasionally greater.[29,30] The clinical importance of these elevations during therapeutic use is uncertain.[29,31] A prospective study in healthy adults consuming up to 8 g/d for 3 days did not find any toxicity.[1]

A recent expert panel's guideline to assist poison information specialists in the management of APAP exposures also provides some guidance on doses that should be of concern. Adults and children older than 6 years with an accidental acute ingestion of at least 10 g or 200 mg/kg, whichever is less, within an 8-hour period warrants further evaluation at a health care facility. For children younger than 6 years, the criterion was 200 mg/kg or more within an 8-hour period. The referral recommendations after RSTI in adults and children older than 6 years were at least 10 g or 200 mg/kg, whichever is less, in a single 24-hour period or 6 g or 150 mg/kg, whichever is less, per 24-hour period for 48 hours or longer. For children younger than 6 years, the criteria following RSTI were (1) 200 mg/kg or more over a single 24-hour period, (2) 150 mg/kg or more per 24 hours for the past 48 hours, or (3) 100 mg/kg or more per 24 hours for 72 hours or more.[32]

For populations that may be at greater risk of toxicity, a lower threshold for evaluation was recommended. These at-risk groups include pregnancy, prolonged fasting, chronic alcoholism, and chronic use of isoniazid. For these populations, the threshold for referral is ingestion of more than 4 g in 24 hours or greater than 100 mg/kg in 24 hours, whichever is less.[32] Immediate evaluation is required for any patient with an intentional overdose, when child abuse or neglect is a concern, and for any patient with symptoms suggesting hepatic injury.

CLINICAL COURSE

There are no specific findings early after an overdose of APAP. Early nonspecific symptoms may include nausea, vomiting, abdominal pain, and malaise. Although these symptoms may improve over the first 24 hours, progressive hepatic injury may manifest as early as day 2 to 3 with right upper quadrant pain and tenderness. Liver enzymes typically start increasing within 24 to 36 hours after an overdose but may increase as early as 12 hours after a massive ingestion.[33] Maximal liver injury typically peaks between 3 to 5 days with jaundice, coagulopathy, and encephalopathy.[34] Recovery or progression to FHF occurs over the following several days.

Renal injury, oliguria, and acute renal failure are also seen, although less commonly. The onset is usually after hepatic injury is already apparent. Maximal renal injury lags beyond peak liver injury, and recovery is also more protracted.[25] Isolated nephrotoxicity without hepatic injury rarely occurs.[35,36] Renal failure may also be seen with FHF and hepatorenal syndrome.

The mental status is typically clear after an APAP overdose unless altered by a co-ingested centrally active drug. On rare occasions, however, massive APAP overdoses may result in coma.[37,38] Metabolic acidosis is another uncommon finding early in the course of APAP poisoning. This early metabolic acidosis may be a lactic acidosis or very rarely caused by a product of the gamma-glutamyl cycle, 5-oxoproline.[38,39] Lactic acidosis also occurs late secondary to hepatic failure with an inability to clear lactate.

ASSESSMENT

With acute ingestions of APAP, the Rumack-Mathews nomogram is a valuable tool to assess the risk of hepatotoxicity (**Fig. 2**). This nomogram was originally constructed in the 1970s as a tool to discriminate those patients likely to suffer hepatotoxicity, defined as an aminotransferase more than 1000 IU/L, from those who would not. A line between 200 μg/mL at 4 hours after ingestion and 25 μg/mL at 16 hours, known as the *200 line*, defined this group at risk.[4,23,40] Fifty-eight percent of patients with an APAP level above this line developed hepatotoxicity and 5% died.[40,41] A parallel line at 150 μg/mL at 4 hours, also known as the *treatment line* or *150 line*, was used in the US National Multicenter Open Study of Oral *N*-Acetylcysteine (NAC) for the Treatment of APAP Overdose and is the treatment line most commonly used in the United States.[23,42]

The nomogram is only useful for acute ingestions when the time of ingestion is known. If there is any uncertainty regarding ingestion time, the worst-case scenario ingestion time should be used. Levels performed before 4 hours will indicate whether APAP has been ingested but cannot be plotted on the nomogram to assess the risk of toxicity. Likewise, the nomogram was constructed with patient data only to about 16 hours and has been validated for use only to 24 hours after acute overdose.[40,42] The nomogram is not valid for patients who present beyond 24 hours after an acute overdose, patients with an unknown time of ingestion, patients with a history of a staggered overdose, and patients with a history of repeated supratherapeutic ingestion. In one small series, 44% of patients presenting with an APAP overdose could not be assessed using the Rumack-Matthew nomogram.[10]

After an acute overdose, a 4-hour APAP level, or as soon thereafter as feasible, should be obtained and plotted on the Rumack-Matthew nomogram to assess risk. Other tests to consider include serum aminotransferase levels, electrolyte and renal function assays, and blood prothrombin time. These tests are especially useful for patients who present more than 8–10 hours after an acute overdose as well as in

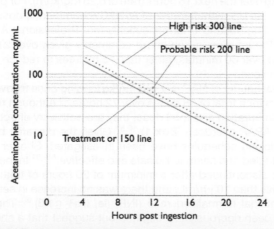

Fig. 2. Rumack-Matthew Nomogram. (*Data from* Rumack BH. Acetaminophen hepatotoxicity: the first 35 years. J Toxicol Clin Toxicol 2002;40(1):3–20.)

any patient with a history of RSTI or staggered overdose. One in 70 patients presenting with drug overdose will have an unanticipated detectable APAP level and, of these, 1 in 500 will have a potentially hepatotoxic level.[43] The incidence of an unexpected elevated APAP level is even higher in patients who are unable to provide a history.[44] Given the consequences of missed APAP poisoning, routine screening in patients who present with known or possible drug overdose seems reasonable.

MANAGEMENT

NAC is an effective antidote for APAP poisoning. When administered early after an acute APAP overdose, NAC provides cysteine for the replenishment and maintenance of hepatic glutathione stores, enhances the sulfation pathway of elimination and may directly reduce NAPQI back to acetaminophen[45–48] (See **Fig. 1**). NAC dramatically reduces the incidence of hepatotoxicity and progression to FHF when administered within the first 8–10 hours following an acute overdose. In patients who receive NAC within the first 8 hours after an acute overdose, the risk of hepatotoxicity is less than 5% whereas delays beyond 10 hours are associated with an increased risk of hepatic injury.[40–42,49,50] NAC should ideally be initiated within 8 hours of ingestion if the patient's APAP level plots above the treatment line (the 150 line) on the Rumack-Matthew nomogram. If an APAP level will not be available by 8 hours post ingestion, NAC should empirically be started pending the APAP level.

Patients with hepatic injury also benefit from NAC. This was demonstrated in several seminal papers in the early 1990s that showed improved transplant-free survival in patients with APAP-induced FHF.[51,52] The mechanism here is not the detoxification of NAPQI but rather enhanced recovery. Several different mechanisms seem to contribute to the efficacy of NAC in this setting. NAC improves hepatic perfusion and oxygen delivery and extraction in patients with APAP-induced FHF.[53] Other beneficial effects include scavenging of reactive oxygen and nitrogen species and improved mitochondrial energy production.[54,55] These beneficial effects of NAC do not seem to be unique to APAP hepatotoxicity.[56]

NAC is available both orally and intravenously. A 20-hour IV infusion of NAC has been widely used worldwide since this schedule was demonstrated effective by Prescott and colleagues[40] in the 1970s.[41,49] This regimen includes a loading dose of 150 mg/kg IV over 15 minutes followed by 50 mg/kg over the next 4 hours (rate of 12.5 mg/kg/h) and then 100 mg/kg over the next 16 hours (rate of 6.25 mg/kg/h). For patients weighing more than 100 kg, the US manufacturer of IV NAC recommends dosing equivalent to a 100 kg person (Cumberland Pharmaceuticals Inc. Professional Affairs, Nashville, TN, USA, 2011). The infusion is now more commonly given over 21 hours with the loading dose given over 60 minutes rather than 15 minutes to reduce the incidence of anaphylactoid reactions.

The standard oral course of NAC is a 140 mg/kg loading dose followed by 70 mg/kg orally every 4 hours for a total of 18 doses over 72 hours.[42] Although the two regimens are very different in duration and total dose, they are both very effective for the treatment of an acute APAP overdose (**Box 1**).[50,57] Given the disparity between the two regimens, other dosing schedules have been investigated. Shorter courses of oral NAC have been studied and seem to be safe and effective.[58–61] In the largest of these studies, NAC was discontinued after a minimum of 20 hours of treatment if a repeat APAP level was less than 10 µg/mL, and there was no increase in serum aminotransferases or international normalized ratio (INR) (ie, INR ≤1.3).[60] These abbreviated courses have not been rigorously investigated but suggest that a shorter duration of oral NAC is safe if the previously mentioned criteria are met, that is, no remaining APAP to be metabolized and no evidence of hepatic injury.

Box 1
Dosing of NAC

Oral NAC

    140 mg/kg loading dose, then 70 mg/kg orally every 4 hours for 18 total doses

    Repeat any dose vomited within 1 hour of administration.

IV NAC (Acetadote)

    Adults

    Loading dose: 150 mg/kg in 200 mL diluent over 1 hour, then 50 mg/kg in 500 mL diluent over 4 hours (12.5 mg/kg/h), then 100 mg/kg in 1000 mL diluent over 16 hours (6.25 mg/kg/h)

    For patient weight more than 100 kg, base the dose on 100 kg weight.

    Children

    Weight more than 20 kg to 40 kg or less: loading dose of 150 mg/kg into 100 mL diluent over 1 hour, then 50 mg/kg into 250 mL diluent over 4 hours, then 100 mg/kg into 500 mL diluent over 16 hours

    Weight less than 20 kg: loading dose of 150 mg/kg into 3 mL/kg diluent over 1 hour, then 50 mg/kg into 7 mL/kg diluent over 4 hours, then 100 mg/kg into 14 mL/kg diluent over 16 hours

    Acetadote is compatible with D5W (5% dextrose in water), 0.5NS (0.5% normal saline), and sterile water for injection.

An alternate IV regimen has also been investigated in patients with acute APAP overdose presenting within 24 hours of the overdose. This regimen consisted of 140 mg/kg NAC as a loading dose and then 70 mg/kg every 4 hours for 48 hours. This regimen was equally effective to the standard 72-hour oral and 20.25-hour IV courses.[62]

Whatever route of administration is selected, there are several very important aspects of management. Following an acute overdose, treatment should not be delayed beyond 8 hours after ingestion because of the dramatic protective effect when given within this time frame (**Box 2**).[41,42,50] Conversely, because of the benefit of NAC in patients with hepatotoxicity, NAC should be continued beyond the usual course of therapy in any patient with signs of liver injury.[52] Guidelines on when to

---

Box 2
Management of acute APAP overdose

1. Plot the APAP concentration onto the Rumack-Matthew nomogram. If the level will not return before 8 hours from the time of ingestion, begin NAC pending the level.

2. If the level plots above the 150 (μg/mL) treatment line, begin NAC.[a]

3. If NAC is administered IV, repeat the APAP level and measure serum AST and ALT before completion of NAC.

    a. May discontinue NAC if APAP level is less than 10 μg/mL and serum AST and ALT are not increased more than the reference range and increasing.

    b. If APAP is more than 10 μg/mL or either the serum AST or ALT are elevated, continue NAC until APAP is less than 10 μg/mL and the AST and ALT have peaked and are improving.

Abbreviations: ALT, alanine aminotransferase activity; AST, aspartate aminotransferase activity.
  [a] Consider treatment at the 100 μg/mL line (at 4 hours and parallel to the 150 line) if there is chronic alcoholism, prolonged fasting, pregnancy, or chronic isoniazid use.

discontinue NAC in this setting are not well defined but include aminotransferase activities that have peaked and are improving, a normal prothrombin time/INR (≤1.3), and no acidosis.

Treatment failures after the standard IV course of NAC have occurred after massive ingestions and after overdoses that included a co-ingestant that may slow GI motility, such as anticholinergic or opioid drugs. In these cases, either APAP was still present (and usually elevated) or signs of hepatic injury were evident at the completion of the 21-hour course of IV NAC.[63–66] These cases highlight the importance of assessing these same parameters (ie, a repeat APAP level as well as aminotransferase levels and an INR before discontinuing NAC in patients with a history of a large ingestion or one complicated by a co-ingestion). If APAP is still detectable or there are signs of hepatic injury, NAC should be continued until APAP is not detected and, if there were any signs of hepatic injury, these parameters are also improving. In this setting, the usual strategy is to continue NAC at a rate of 6.25 mg/kg/h (ie, the 16-hour bag).

For patients who present after RSTI, assessment should include a serum APAP level and aminotransferase activities, plus a prothrombin time/INR. A conservative definition of RSTI of APAP used by Daly and colleagues[67] was the ingestion of more than one dose of APAP over a period of more than 8 hours that results in more than 4 g ingested in a 24-hour period in an adult. In the study by Daley and colleagues, patients with a history of RSTI had an APAP level as well as serum transaminase levels measured on presentation. If either the APAP was more than 10 μg/mL or an aminotransferase was increased more than the normal range, NAC was started. NAC was continued until the APAP was less than 10 μg/mL and the transaminases had peaked and were either static or decreasing. With this strategy, the investigators found that no patient with a normal aspartate transaminase on presentation and an APAP less than 10 μg/mL developed hepatotoxicity. Another retrospective review of patients with RSTI found that all patients who progressed to hepatotoxicity, death, or transplant presented with an alanine transaminase of more than 200 IU/L.[68] The management described by Daley and colleagues is a very reasonable approach to patients seen with a history of repeated excess ingestion (**Box 3**). Clinical decision making in these more complicated cases can be aided by consultation with a regional poison center.

Tylenol ER contains immediate-release and sustained-release APAP. Delayed increases of the APAP concentration have been observed in some cases of Tylenol ER overdose, sometimes with an initial level plotting below and a second above the nomogram treatment line.[69,70] The clinical significance of line crossing is uncertain, as is the risk of hepatotoxicity in this situation.[71] In several reports, patients who were line crossers had ingested a large quantity of APAP (>35 g in 3 of 4 cases), which may have delayed the time to peak concentration. A reasonable and conservative

---

Box 3
Management of repeated supratherapeutic ingestion or time-unknown ingestion

1. Obtain serum APAP level and serum AST and ALT levels.

2. If APAP is less than 10 μg/mL and the AST and ALT are normal, no treatment is necessary.

3. If either the APAP level is detectable more than 10 μg/mL or either the AST or ALT are elevated more than the reference range and not otherwise explained, begin NAC treatment.

4. Continue NAC until APAP is less than 10 μg/mL and the AST and ALT have peaked and are improving and there are no other signs of hepatic dysfunction, including INR of 1.3 or less.

Abbreviations: ALT, alanine aminotransferase activity; AST, aspartate aminotransferase activity.

approach in this group is to obtain an initial APAP level between 4 and 8 hours and repeat this in 4 to 6 hours if the first level plots below the treatment line. If the second line is above the treatment line, NAC should be commenced. If the initial level is below the treatment line but the history suggests ingestion greater than 200 mg/kg, it would be reasonable to start NAC within the first 8 hours after ingestion pending a repeat APAP level. If the subsequent level is also below the treatment line, NAC can be discontinued.

IV APAP was approved for use in the United States in late 2010. It was first approved for use in France in 2001, and experience with overdose by this route is very limited. Most published reports of iatrogenic overdose are in infants. In one case, a 5-month-old child had 6-hour APAP level of 38 μg/mL after a tenfold dosing error (75 mg/kg). The next day, NAC was started because of increasing aminotransferase activity and an elevated INR. She recovered fully.[14] In several other cases of tenfold plus dosing errors, NAC was started early and no toxicity was reported.[14,72] Given the limited experience with this route of delivery, current expert opinion recommends the following approach to overdoses of IV APAP. Treatment with NAC should be initiated if either the parenteral dose of APAP exceeds 60 mg/kg or an APAP level plots above a 50 μg/mL line on the Rumack-Matthew nomogram (a line parallel to treatment line but at 50 μg/mL at 4 hours).[73] NAC should be continued until serum APAP is undetectable and there is no evidence of hepatic injury. This recommendation is very conservative and reflects the limited data available at this time regarding iatrogenic IV overdose.

Adverse effects associated with oral NAC are predominately GI with nausea and vomiting. These effects can be mitigated by pretreatment with an antiemetic.[74] Anaphylactoid reactions may be seen with IV NAC and are most likely to occur early during the loading dose, with an incidence as high as 15% to 20%. Although a randomized trial conducted in Australia found no difference in the incidence of anaphylactoid reactions when comparing a 15-minute to 1-hour infusion time for the loading dose, other investigators have reported a lower rate of anaphylactoid reactions with a 1-hour infusion.[75–77] In 2006, the manufacturer of Acetadote, the parenteral NAC formulation available in the United States, changed the recommended infusion time for the loading dose to 1 hour, increasing the total duration of therapy from 20.25 to 21.0 hours.

Anaphylactoid reactions occur more frequently in patients with lower acetaminophen levels. A study by Waring and colleagues[78] found a rate of anaphylactoid reactions of more than 20% in patients with an initial APAP level less than 150 μg/mL, whereas the incidence in patients with a level more than 200 μg/mL was less than 5%. NAC induces the release of histamine from basophils and mast cells, and in an in vitro model, higher APAP concentrations reduced the extent of NAC-induced histamine release.[79] Asthmatics may be at greater risk of adverse events with IV NAC.[80] Status asthmaticus with cardiac arrest and anoxic brain injury was reported in a patient with steroid-dependent asthma during the loading dose of NAC for APAP overdose.[81]

Minor anaphylactoid reactions, such as flushing or rash, can usually be managed with diphenhydramine. With more significant reactions, such as angioedema, hypotension, or wheezing, the infusion should be stopped and standard symptomatic therapy provided. The need for ongoing therapy with NAC should be reassessed and a switch to the oral route considered. If the IV route is considered necessary, the infusion can usually be resumed after about 1 hour at a slower rate.[78,82]

IV NAC administration to young children has resulted in dilutional hyponatremia and seizure from the free water load associated with the infusion.[83] The manufacturer of Acetadote has modified the instructions for the preparation of NAC for administration to young children because of this risk.[84] Massive overdose of NAC caused by dosing error has resulted in seizures, status epilepticus, intracranial hypertension, and cerebral edema.[85,86] The standard administration of NAC involving 3 bags of different concentrations over the 21-hour infusion is complicated and alternatives to this have been proposed.[87]

GI decontamination should also be considered. In volunteer studies, activated charcoal significantly reduced the absorption of APAP when given within 1 hour after ingestion. Although more modest, a reduction was still appreciated with administration at 2 hours after ingestion.[88] Even more delayed administration of activated charcoal may be beneficial in select cases of very large ingestions. In a group of patients with an APAP level above the 200 risk line and who received activated charcoal between 4 to 16 hours after an acute ingestion, fewer progressed to hepatotoxicity than a group that did not receive activated charcoal.[89] Contraindications to activated charcoal include a depressed level of consciousness, aspiration, uncontrolled vomiting, or co-ingestion of a corrosive or proconvulsant. Activated charcoal does not significantly interfere with the efficacy of oral NAC.[90]

ALCOHOL AND ACETAMINOPHEN

The interaction between APAP and ethanol is complex. Ethanol is a competitive substrate for CYP 2E1, the primary microsomal enzyme responsible for the metabolism of APAP to NAPQI. In rats, acute ethanol administration is hepatoprotective to a toxic dose of APAP.[91] A protective effect has also been observed in patients presenting within 24 hours of an acute APAP overdose. Hepatotoxicity occurred in 8% of patients who co-ingested ethanol compared with 23% of those who had not in a group of individuals with a presentation APAP level above the 200 line on the nomogram.[92]

Conversely, chronic ethanol administration to rats increases liver toxicity caused by APAP, with both upregulation of CYP 2E1 and glutathione depletion likely contributing. Both these effects are transient, lasting less than 1 day in rats.[93,94] Ethanol enhancement of CYP 2E1 is a result of both enzyme stabilization and increased synthesis of a new enzyme.[23] In humans, the maximal increase in NAPQI production after acute enzyme induction with ethanol occurs after 6 to 8 hours of abstinence and is short lived.[95] This finding suggests that there may be a brief window of increased risk in recently abstinent alcoholic patients who overdoses with APAP.

In a reanalysis of the US National Multicenter Open Study of Oral NAC for the Treatment of APAP Overdose, alcoholic patients in the higher-risk group, those with APAP levels plotting above the 200 line on the nomogram, were at an increased risk of progression to hepatotoxicity. In alcoholic patients with an APAP level plotting below the 200 line or those who received treatment with NAC within 8 hours, no increased risk was observed.[96] With respect to RSTI, Alhelail and colleagues,[68] in a retrospective series, found that alcoholic patients are at an increased risk of progression to hepatotoxicity. Makin and colleagues[97] did not find that alcoholic patients with hepatotoxicity fare any worse than nonalcoholic patients after admission to a liver unit.[98]

Are alcoholic patients at risk with therapeutic doses of APAP? Studies administering APAP at 4 g daily for up to 5 consecutive days in recently abstinent alcoholic patients found no evidence of hepatic injury.[99,100] Several comprehensive reviews have concluded that it is unlikely that at therapeutic doses of APAP there is any increased risk of hepatic injury in alcoholic patients.[22,101] Fasting may be a greater risk factor for hepatotoxicity with excessive repeated ingestion (>4 g daily). Fasting was a more common feature in a group of patients with APAP hepatotoxicity from repeated excessive use of 4 to 10 g daily than was chronic alcohol use. In patients who had ingested more than 10 g daily, both fasting and alcoholism were common. No cases of hepatotoxicity were associated with doses less than 4 g daily.[24]

TRANSPLANTATION

Transplantation can be life saving for those with FHF. The costs of transplantation and subsequent lifelong immunosuppression and the complications thereof are considerable. The challenge is to identify patients who are going to die of FHF from those who will spontaneously recover with supportive care. The most widely used prognostic criteria are those of King's College Hospital (KCH) (**Box 4**). These criteria were derived in the 1980s from a large cohort of patients with APAP hepatotoxicity. The criteria are either arterial pH less than 7.30 after fluid resuscitation or the combination of an INR greater than 6.5 plus serum creatinine greater than 3.4 mg/dL and grade III or IV encephalopathy (ie, marked somnolence, stupor, or coma).[102] These criteria, although not very sensitive, had a high specificity in identifying patients who would do poorly without a transplant. Less than 20% of those who met the KCH criteria survived spontaneously.[103] A modification to these criteria added blood lactate measured 2 to 3 days after acute overdose. A lactate level on day 2 to 3 greater than 3.5 mmol/L before adequate fluid resuscitation or greater than 3.0 mmol/L after patients have been adequately fluid resuscitated was predictive of death without transplant. This modification improved both the sensitivity and specificity of the KCH criteria.[104] More recently, a much lower specificity of the modified KCH criteria has been reported with increased survival in patients meeting the KCH criteria. This finding may reflect improvements in critical care and the medical management of FHF.[105]

Other prognostic criteria have been proposed. A serum phosphate of greater than 1.2 mmol/L at 48 to 96 hours after overdose was predictive of death.[106] Although this marker was very sensitive and specific in the original report, subsequent application of this marker to other series of APAP FHF have not duplicated this finding.[107,108]

The Model for End-Stage Liver Disease (MELD) score has been investigated with APAP hepatic injury. Components of the MELD score are INR, serum bilirubin, serum creatinine, and cause of liver injury. In a group of patients with APAP hepatotoxicity, a higher MELD score on admission to the intensive care unit (ICU) was associated with progression to encephalopathy, and an increase in the MELD score over the first day after the onset of hepatic encephalopathy was predictive of death. When compared with the KCH criteria, this tool performed no better.[109] The Acute Physiology and Chronic Health Evaluation (APACHE) II score has also been used to predict death from APAP hepatotoxicity. A score of more than 15 on admission to the ICU was a sensitive tool to predict patients likely to progress to FHF and was slightly more sensitive than the KCH criteria on the day of admission.[110] A score of more than 20 was associated with a lower transplant-free survival in the US Acute Liver Failure Study Group.[11]

A critical decision for clinicians is the decision to refer patients to a specialized liver unit. Criteria to consider in this decision include acidosis, renal insufficiency,

---

Box 4
KCH transplant criteria

Blood lactate concentration greater than 3.5 mmol/L before or greater than 3.0 mmol/L after fluid resuscitation

OR

Arterial blood pH less than 7.30 after fluid resuscitation

OR

Serum creatinine concentration greater than 3.2 mg/dL and INR greater than 6.5 and grade III or IV encephalopathy

a prothrombin time (PT) in seconds greater than the number of hours since the overdose, an INR greater than 5, hypoglycemia, or encephalopathy.[110] An increase in the INR from day 3 to 4 after overdose has also been associated with a poorer outcome.[111] An APACHE II score of more than 15 has also been suggested as a decision aid.[112]

LABORATORY

Increases in the INR early after APAP overdose may be seen that are not reflective of hepatocellular injury. An early increase in the INR seen at 12 to 16 hours after overdose seems to be the result of APAP interference in the production of active factor VII and is not reflective of hepatocellular injury. The effect is usually modest, with a mean increase to 1.36 in one series.[113] NAC has also been implicated as a cause of an early increase in the INR. Here too the increase observed was modest, to about 1.3.[114] This effect has been observed in patients receiving NAC without APAP present.[115] The important point is that a modest elevation in the INR early after an acute overdose and without other signs of liver injury should not be confused with an increasing INR after 24 hours suggestive of hepatic injury.

Colorimetric methods of measuring APAP are subject to interference by bilirubin. Depending on the specific instrument and method, this may occur at bilirubin levels as low as 10 mg/dL.[116,117] Microdialysis of the serum specimen before assay will correct this false-positive result.[117] Compared with other causes of acute liver failure, bilirubin levels more than 10 mg/dL are uncommon with APAP liver injury.[6]

SUMMARY

APAP toxicity is the most common cause of ALF in the United States.[6] With early recognition and prompt institution of NAC, serious toxicity can usually be mitigated or prevented following an acute overdose. Remember to obtain an appropriately timed APAP level and to start NAC within 8 hours of an acute overdose. With massive ingestions and polypharmacy overdose, there may be prolonged absorption of APAP with measurable levels of APAP still present at the completion of the standard course of IV NAC. NAC should not be discontinued until there is no further APAP to metabolize and any signs of liver injury are improving. In addition to the antidotal properties of early treatment with NAC to prevent the production of the toxic metabolite, NAC also is beneficial in the treatment of acetaminophen induced hepatic injury and should be used in patients with late presentation and signs of hepatic injury. Patients with FHF require expert management and are best served by transfer to a specialized liver unit with transplant capability.

REFERENCES

1. Temple AR, Lynch JM, Vena J, et al. Aminotransferase activities in healthy subjects receiving three-day dosing of 4, 6, or 8 grams per day of acetaminophen. Clin Toxicol (Phila) 2007;45(1):36–44.
2. FDA. Acetaminophen overdose and liver injury – background and options for reducing injury. Available at: http://www.fda.gov/downloads/AdvisoryCommittees/CommitteesMeetingMaterials/Drugs/DrugSafetyandRiskManagementAdvisoryCommittee/UCM164897.pdf. Accessed November 23, 2011.
3. Wysowski DK, Governale LA, Swann J. Trends in outpatient prescription drug use and related costs in the US: 1998-2003. Pharmacoeconomics 2006;24(3):233–6.

4. Prescott LF, Roscoe P, Wright N, et al. Plasma-paracetamol half-life and hepatic necrosis in patients with paracetamol overdosage. Lancet 1971;1(7698):519–22.
5. Bronstein AC, Spyker DA, Cantilena LR Jr, et al. 2009 Annual report of the American Association of Poison Control Centers' National Poison Data System (NPDS): 27th annual report. Clin Toxicol (Phila) 2010;48(10):979–1178.
6. Ostapowicz G, Fontana RJ, Schiødt FV, et al. Results of a prospective study of acute liver failure at 17 tertiary care centers in the United States. Ann Intern Med 2002;137(12):947–54.
7. FDA. Drug induced liver toxicity. Available at: http://www.fda.gov/Drugs/ScienceResearch/ResearchAreas/ucm071471.htm. Accessed October 8, 2011.
8. Davern TJ II, James LP, Hinson JA, et al. Measurement of serum acetaminophen-protein adducts in patients with acute liver failure. Gastroenterology 2006;130(3): 687–94.
9. Squires RH Jr, Shneider BL, Bucuvalas J, et al. Acute liver failure in children: the first 348 patients in the pediatric acute liver failure study group. J Pediatr 2006; 148(5):652–8.
10. Bond GR, Hite LK. Population-based incidence and outcome of acetaminophen poisoning by type of ingestion. Acad Emerg Med 1999;6(11):1115–20.
11. Larson AM, Polson J, Fontana RJ, et al. Acetaminophen-induced acute liver failure: results of a United States multicenter, prospective study. Hepatology 2005;42(6):1364–72.
12. Anon. Prescription Drug Products Containing Acetaminophen; Actions To Reduce Liver Injury From Unintentional Overdose. Federal Register 2011; 76(10):2691–7.
13. Available at: http://www.chpa-info.org/pressroom/05_05_11_PedAceConv.aspx. Accessed November 21, 2011.
14. Beringer RM, Thompson JP, Parry S, et al. Intravenous paracetamol overdose: two case reports and a change to national treatment guidelines. Arch Dis Child 2011;96(3):307–8.
15. Anon, editor. Tylenol professional product information. McNeil Consumer Healthcare, Division of McNEIL-PPC, Inc, Fort Washington, PA, 19034, USA; 2010.
16. Forrest JA, Clements JA, Prescott LF. Clinical pharmacokinetics of paracetamol. Clin Pharmacokinet 1982;7(2):93–107.
17. Prescott LF. Kinetics and metabolism of paracetamol and phenacetin. Br J Clin Pharmacol 1980;10(Suppl 2):291S–8S.
18. Gelotte CK, Auiler JF, Lynch JM, et al. Disposition of acetaminophen at 4, 6, and 8 g/day for 3 days in healthy young adults. Clin Pharmacol Ther 2007;81(6):840–8.
19. Mitchell JR, Jollow DJ, Potter WZ, et al. Acetaminophen-induced hepatic necrosis. IV. Protective role of glutathione. J Pharmacol Exp Ther 1973;187(1):211–7.
20. Jones DP, Lemasters JJ, Han D, et al. Mechanisms of pathogenesis in drug hepatotoxicity putting the stress on mitochondria. Mol Interv 2010;10(2):98–111.
21. Kaplowitz N, Shinohara M, Liu ZX, et al. How to protect against acetaminophen: don't ask for JUNK. Gastroenterology 2008;135(4):1047–51.
22. Prescott LF. Paracetamol, alcohol and the liver. Br J Clin Pharmacol 2000;49(4): 291–301.
23. Rumack BH. Acetaminophen hepatotoxicity: the first 35 years. J Toxicol Clin Toxicol 2002;40(1):3–20.
24. Whitcomb DC, Block GD. Association of acetaminophen hepatotoxicity with fasting and ethanol use. JAMA 1994;272(23):1845–50.
25. Prescott LF. Paracetamol overdosage. Pharmacological considerations and clinical management. Drugs 1983;25(3):290–314.

26. Bond GR, Krenzelok EP, Normann SA, et al. Acetaminophen ingestion in child-hood–cost and relative risk of alternative referral strategies. J Toxicol Clin Toxicol 1994;32(5):513–25.

27. Caravati EM. Unintentional acetaminophen ingestion in children and the potential for hepatotoxicity. J Toxicol Clin Toxicol 2000;38(3):291–6.

28. Mohler CR, Nordt SP, Williams SR, et al. Prospective evaluation of mild to moderate pediatric acetaminophen exposures. Ann Emerg Med 2000;35(3):239–44.

29. Watkins PB, Kaplowitz N, Slattery JT, et al. Aminotransferase elevations in healthy adults receiving 4 grams of acetaminophen daily: a randomized controlled trial. JAMA 2006;296(1):87–93.

30. Temple AR, Benson GD, Zinsenheim JR, et al. Multicenter, randomized, double-blind, active-controlled, parallel-group trial of the long-term (6-12 months) safety of acetaminophen in adult patients with osteoarthritis. Clin Ther 2006;28(2):222–35.

31. Dart RC, Bailey E. Does therapeutic use of acetaminophen cause acute liver failure? Pharmacotherapy 2007;27(9):1219–30.

32. Dart RC, Erdman AR, Olson KR, et al. Acetaminophen poisoning: an evidence-based consensus guideline for out-of-hospital management. Clin Toxicol (Phila) 2006;44(1):1–18.

33. Singer AJ, Carracio TR, Mofenson HC. The temporal profile of increased trans-aminase levels in patients with acetaminophen-induced liver dysfunction. Ann Emerg Med 1995;26(1):49–53.

34. Rumack BH, Matthew H. Acetaminophen poisoning and toxicity. Pediatrics 1975;55(6):871–6.

35. Waring WS, Jamie H, Leggett GE. Delayed onset of acute renal failure after significant paracetamol overdose: a case series. Hum Exp Toxicol 2010;29(1):63–8.

36. Jones AL, Prescott LF. Unusual complications of paracetamol poisoning. QJM 1997;90(3):161–8.

37. Wiegand TJ, Margaretten M, Olson KR. Massive acetaminophen ingestion with early metabolic acidosis and coma: treatment with IV NAC and continuous ve-novenous hemodiafiltration. Clin Toxicol (Phila) 2010;48(2):156–9.

38. Roth B, Woo O, Blanc P. Early metabolic acidosis and coma after acetamino-phen ingestion. Ann Emerg Med 1999;33(4):452–6.

39. Hodgman MJ, Horn JF, Stork CM, et al. Profound metabolic acidosis and oxo-prolinuria in an adult. J Med Toxicol 2007;3(3):119–24.

40. Prescott LF, Illingworth RN, Critchley JA, et al. Intravenous N-acetylcysteine: the treatment of choice for paracetamol poisoning. Br Med J 1979;2(6198):1097–100.

41. Prescott LF. Treatment of severe acetaminophen poisoning with intravenous acetylcysteine. Arch Intern Med 1981;141(3 Spec No):386–9.

42. Smilkstein MJ, Knapp GL, Kulig KW, et al. Efficacy of oral N-acetylcysteine in the treatment of acetaminophen overdose. Analysis of the national multicenter study (1976 to 1985). N Engl J Med 1988;319(24):1557–62.

43. Ashbourne JF, Olson KR, Khayam-Bashi H. Value of rapid screening for acet-aminophen in all patients with intentional drug overdose. Ann Emerg Med 1989;18(10):1035–8.

44. Dargan PI, Ladhani S, Jones AL. Measuring plasma paracetamol concentra-tions in all patients with drug overdose or altered consciousness: does it change outcome? Emerg Med J 2001;18(3):178–82.

45. Dahlin DC, Miwa GT, Lu AY, et al. N-acetyl-p-benzoquinone imine: a cytochrome P-450-mediated oxidation product of acetaminophen. Proc Natl Acad Sci U S A 1984;81(5):1327–31.

46. Lin JH, Levy G. Sulfate depletion after acetaminophen administration and replenishment by infusion of sodium sulfate or N-acetylcysteine in rats. Biochem Pharmacol 1981;30(19):2723–5.
47. Lauterburg BH, Corcoran GB, Mitchell JR. Mechanism of action of N-acetylcysteine in the protection against the hepatotoxicity of acetaminophen in rats in vivo. J Clin Invest 1983;71(4):980–91.
48. Slattery JT, Wilson JM, Kalhorn TF, et al. Dose-dependent pharmacokinetics of acetaminophen: evidence of glutathione depletion in humans. Clin Pharmacol Ther 1987;41(4):413–8.
49. Prescott LF, Park J, Ballantyne A, et al. Treatment of paracetamol (acetaminophen) poisoning with N-acetylcysteine. Lancet 1977;2(8035):432–4.
50. Buckley NA, Whyte IM, O'Connell DL, et al. Oral or intravenous N-acetylcysteine: which is the treatment of choice for acetaminophen (paracetamol) poisoning? J Toxicol Clin Toxicol 1999;37(6):759–67.
51. Harrison PM, Keays R, Bray GP, et al. Improved outcome of paracetamol-induced fulminant hepatic failure by late administration of acetylcysteine. Lancet 1990;335(8705):1572–3.
52. Keays R, Harrison PM, Wendon JA, et al. Intravenous acetylcysteine in paracetamol induced fulminant hepatic failure: a prospective controlled trial. BMJ 1991;303(6809):1026–9.
53. Harrison PM, Wendon JA, Gimson AE, et al. Improvement by acetylcysteine of hemodynamics and oxygen transport in fulminant hepatic failure. N Engl J Med 1991;324(26):1852–7.
54. Knight TR, Ho YS, Farhood A, et al. Peroxynitrite is a critical mediator of acetaminophen hepatotoxicity in murine livers: protection by glutathione. J Pharmacol Exp Ther 2002;303(2):468–75.
55. Saito C, Zwingmann C, Jaeschke H. Novel mechanisms of protection against acetaminophen hepatotoxicity in mice by glutathione and N-acetylcysteine. Hepatology 2010;51(1):246–54.
56. Lee WM, Hynan LS, Rossaro L, et al. Intravenous N-acetylcysteine improves transplant-free survival in early stage non-acetaminophen acute liver failure. Gastroenterology 2009;137(3):856–64, 864.e1.
57. Prescott L. Oral or intravenous N-acetylcysteine for acetaminophen poisoning? Ann Emerg Med 2005;45(4):409–13.
58. Betten DP, Cantrell FL, Thomas SC, et al. A prospective evaluation of shortened course oral N-acetylcysteine for the treatment of acute acetaminophen poisoning. Ann Emerg Med 2007;50(3):272–9.
59. Betten DP, Burner EE, Thomas SC, et al. A retrospective evaluation of shortened-duration oral N-acetylcysteine for the treatment of acetaminophen poisoning. J Med Toxicol 2009;5(4):183–90.
60. Woo OF, Mueller PD, Olson KR, et al. Shorter duration of oral N-acetylcysteine therapy for acute acetaminophen overdose. Ann Emerg Med 2000;35(4):363–8.
61. Yip L, Dart RC. A 20-hour treatment for acute acetaminophen overdose. N Engl J Med 2003;348(24):2471–2.
62. Smilkstein MJ, Bronstein AC, Linden C, et al. Acetaminophen overdose: a 48-hour intravenous N-acetylcysteine treatment protocol. Ann Emerg Med 1991; 20(10):1058–63.
63. Smith SW, Howland MA, Hoffman RS, et al. Acetaminophen overdose with altered acetaminophen pharmacokinetics and hepatotoxicity associated with premature cessation of intravenous N-acetylcysteine therapy. Ann Pharmacother 2008;42(9):1333–9.

64. Schwartz EA, Hayes BD, Sarmiento KF. Development of hepatic failure despite use of intravenous acetylcysteine after a massive ingestion of acetaminophen and diphenhydramine. Ann Emerg Med 2009;54(3):421–3.
65. Doyon S, Klein-Schwartz W. Hepatotoxicity despite early administration of intravenous N-acetylcysteine for acute acetaminophen overdose. Acad Emerg Med 2009;16(1):34–9.
66. Hendrickson RG, McKeown NJ, West PL, et al. Bactrian ("double hump") acetaminophen pharmacokinetics: a case series and review of the literature. J Med Toxicol 2010;6(3):337–44.
67. Daly FF, O'Malley GF, Heard K, et al. Prospective evaluation of repeated supratherapeutic acetaminophen (paracetamol) ingestion. Ann Emerg Med 2004; 44(4):393–8.
68. Alhelail MA, Hoppe JA, Rhyee SH, et al. Clinical course of repeated supratherapeutic ingestion of acetaminophen. Clin Toxicol (Phila) 2011;49(2):108–12.
69. Bizovi KE, Aks SE, Paloucek F, et al. Late increase in acetaminophen concentration after overdose of Tylenol extended relief. Ann Emerg Med 1996;28(5):549–51.
70. Cetaruk EW, Dart RC, Hurlbut KM, et al. Tylenol extended relief overdose. Ann Emerg Med 1997;30(1):104–8.
71. Dart RC, Green JL, Bogdan GM. The safety profile of sustained release paracetamol during therapeutic use and following overdose. Drug Saf 2005;28(11): 1045–56.
72. de la Pintiere A, Beuchee A, Betremieux PE. Intravenous propacetamol overdose in a term newborn. Arch Dis Child Fetal Neonatal Ed 2003;88(4):F351–2.
73. Gray T, Hoffman RS, Bateman DN. Intravenous paracetamol–an international perspective of toxicity. Clin Toxicol (Phila) 2011;49(3):150–2.
74. Wright RO, Anderson AC, Lesko SL, et al. Effect of metoclopramide dose on preventing emesis after oral administration of N-acetylcysteine for acetaminophen overdose. J Toxicol Clin Toxicol 1999;37(1):35–42.
75. Kao LW, Kirk MA, Furbee RB, et al. What is the rate of adverse events after oral N-acetylcysteine administered by the intravenous route to patients with suspected acetaminophen poisoning? Ann Emerg Med 2003;42(6):741–50.
76. Kerr F, Dawson A, Whyte IM, et al. The Australasian Clinical Toxicology Investigators Collaboration randomized trial of different loading infusion rates of N-acetylcysteine. Ann Emerg Med 2005;45(4):402–8.
77. Yip L, Dart RC, Hurlbut KM. Intravenous administration of oral N-acetylcysteine. Crit Care Med 1998;26(1):40–3.
78. Waring WS, Stephen AF, Robinson OD, et al. Lower incidence of anaphylactoid reactions to N-acetylcysteine in patients with high acetaminophen concentrations after overdose. Clin Toxicol (Phila) 2008;46(6):496–500.
79. Coulson J, Thompson JP. Paracetamol (acetaminophen) attenuates in vitro mast cell and peripheral blood mononucleocyte cell histamine release induced by N-acetylcysteine. Clin Toxicol (Phila) 2010;48(2):111–4.
80. Schmidt LE, Dalhoff K. Risk factors in the development of adverse reactions to N-acetylcysteine in patients with paracetamol poisoning. Br J Clin Pharmacol 2001;51(1):87–91.
81. Appelboam AV, Dargan PI, Knighton J. Fatal anaphylactoid reaction to N-acetylcysteine: caution in patients with asthma. Emerg Med J 2002;19(6):594–5.
82. Bailey B, McGuigan MA. Management of anaphylactoid reactions to intravenous N-acetylcysteine. Ann Emerg Med 1998;31(6):710–5.
83. Sung L, Simons JA, Dayneka NL. Dilution of intravenous N-acetylcysteine as a cause of hyponatremia. Pediatrics 1997;100(3 Pt 1):389–91.

84. Anon. In: Acetadote (acetylcysteine) injection package insert. Cumberland Pharmaceuticals, Inc; 2011.
85. Bailey B, Blais R, Letarte A. Status epilepticus after a massive intravenous N-acetylcysteine overdose leading to intracranial hypertension and death. Ann Emerg Med 2004;44(4):401–6.
86. Heard K, Schaeffer TH. Massive acetylcysteine overdose associated with cerebral edema and seizures. Clin Toxicol (Phila) 2011;49(5):423–5.
87. Johnson MT, McCammon CA, Mullins ME, et al. Evaluation of a simplified N-acetylcysteine dosing regimen for the treatment of acetaminophen toxicity. Ann Pharmacother 2011;45(6):713–20.
88. Christophersen AB, Levin D, Hoegberg LC, et al. Activated charcoal alone or after gastric lavage: a simulated large paracetamol intoxication. Br J Clin Pharmacol 2002;53(3):312–7.
89. Spiller HA, Winter ML, Klein-Schwartz W, et al. Efficacy of activated charcoal administered more than four hours after acetaminophen overdose. J Emerg Med 2006;30(1):1–5.
90. Spiller HA, Krenzelok EP, Grande GA, et al. A prospective evaluation of the effect of activated charcoal before oral N-acetylcysteine in acetaminophen overdose. Ann Emerg Med 1994;23(3):519–23.
91. Altomare E, Leo MA, Lieber CS. Interaction of acute ethanol administration with acetaminophen metabolism and toxicity in rats fed alcohol chronically. Alcohol Clin Exp Res 1984;8(4):405–8.
92. Waring WS, Stephen AF, Malkowska AM, et al. Acute ethanol coingestion confers a lower risk of hepatotoxicity after deliberate acetaminophen overdose. Acad Emerg Med 2008;15(1):54–8.
93. Zhao P, Kalhorn TF, Slattery JT. Selective mitochondrial glutathione depletion by ethanol enhances acetaminophen toxicity in rat liver. Hepatology 2002;36(2):326–35.
94. Zhao P, Slattery JT. Effects of ethanol dose and ethanol withdrawal on rat liver mitochondrial glutathione: implication of potentiated acetaminophen toxicity in alcoholics. Drug Metab Dispos 2002;30(12):1413–7.
95. Thummel KE, Slattery JT, Ro H, et al. Ethanol and production of the hepatotoxic metabolite of acetaminophen in healthy adults. Clin Pharmacol Ther 2000;67(6):591–9.
96. Smilkstein MJ, Rumack BH. Chronic ethanol use and acute acetaminophen overdose toxicity. Clin Toxicol (Phila) 1998;36(5):476.
97. Makin A, Williams R. Paracetamol hepatotoxicity and alcohol consumption in deliberate and accidental overdose. QJM 2000;93(6):341–9.
98. Makin AJ, Wendon J, Williams R. A 7-year experience of severe acetaminophen-induced hepatotoxicity (1987-1993). Gastroenterology 1995;109(6):1907–16.
99. Kuffner EK, Dart RC, Bogdan GM, et al. Effect of maximal daily doses of acetaminophen on the liver of alcoholic patients: a randomized, double-blind, placebo-controlled trial. Arch Intern Med 2001;161(18):2247–52.
100. Dart RC, Green JL, Kuffner EK, et al. The effects of paracetamol (acetaminophen) on hepatic tests in patients who chronically abuse alcohol - a randomized study. Aliment Pharmacol Ther 2010;32(3):478–86.
101. Dart RC, Kuffner EK, Rumack BH. Treatment of pain or fever with paracetamol (acetaminophen) in the alcoholic patient: a systematic review. Am J Ther 2000;7(2):123–34.
102. O'Grady JG, Alexander GJ, Hayllar KM, et al. Early indicators of prognosis in fulminant hepatic failure. Gastroenterology 1989;97(2):439–45.

103. Bernal W, Wendon J, Rela M, et al. Use and outcome of liver transplantation in acetaminophen-induced acute liver failure. Hepatology 1998;27(4): 1050–5.

104. Bernal W, Donaldson N, Wyncoll D, et al. Blood lactate as an early predictor of outcome in paracetamol-induced acute liver failure: a cohort study. Lancet 2002;359(9306):558–63.

105. Gow PJ, Warrilow S, Lontos S, et al. Time to review the selection criteria for transplantation in paracetamol-induced fulminant hepatic failure? Liver Transpl 2007;13(12):1762–3.

106. Schmidt LE, Dalhoff K. Serum phosphate is an early predictor of outcome in severe acetaminophen-induced hepatotoxicity. Hepatology 2002;36(3):659–65.

107. Bernal W, Wendon J. More on serum phosphate and prognosis of acute liver failure. Hepatology 2003;38(2):533–4.

108. Macquillan GC, Seyam MS, Nightingale P, et al. Blood lactate but not serum phosphate levels can predict patient outcome in fulminant hepatic failure. Liver Transpl 2005;11(9):1073–9.

109. Schmidt LE, Larsen FS. MELD score as a predictor of liver failure and death in patients with acetaminophen-induced liver injury. Hepatology 2007;45(3): 789–96.

110. Mitchell I, Bihari D, Chang R, et al. Earlier identification of patients at risk from acetaminophen-induced acute liver failure. Crit Care Med 1998;26(2):279–84.

111. Anand AC, Nightingale P, Neuberger JM. Early indicators of prognosis in fulminant hepatic failure: an assessment of the king's criteria. J Hepatol 1997;26(1): 62–8.

112. Bailey B, Amre DK, Gaudreault P. Fulminant hepatic failure secondary to acetaminophen poisoning: a systematic review and meta-analysis of prognostic criteria determining the need for liver transplantation. Crit Care Med 2003; 31(1):299–305.

113. Whyte IM, Buckley NA, Reith DM, et al. Acetaminophen causes an increased international normalized ratio by reducing functional factor VII. Ther Drug Monit 2000;22(6):742–8.

114. Schmidt LE, Knudsen TT, Dalhoff K, et al. Effect of acetylcysteine on prothrombin index in paracetamol poisoning without hepatocellular injury. Lancet 2002; 360(9340):1151–2.

115. Niemi TT, Munsterhjelm E, Poyhia R, et al. The effect of N-acetylcysteine on blood coagulation and platelet function in patients undergoing open repair of abdominal aortic aneurysm. Blood Coagul Fibrinolysis 2006;17(1):29–34.

116. Polson J, Wians FH Jr, Orsulak P, et al. False positive acetaminophen concentrations in patients with liver injury. Clin Chim Acta 2008;391(1–2):24–30.

117. Fong BM, Siu TS, Tam S. Persistently increased acetaminophen concentrations in a patient with acute liver failure. Clin Chem 2011;57(1):9–11.

Cocaine Intoxication

Janice L. Zimmerman, MD[a,b,*]

KEYWORDS

- Cocaine • Intracranial hemorrhage • Stroke • Chest pain
- Acute coronary syndrome • Rhabdomyolysis • Hyperthermia

KEY POINTS

- Cocaine is commonly abused by inhalation, nasal insufflation, and intravenous injection, resulting in many adverse effects that ensue from local anesthetic, vasoconstrictive, sympathomimetic, psychoactive, and prothrombotic mechanisms.
- Manifestations may include tachycardia, hypertension, hyperthermia, diaphoresis, tachypnea, mydriasis, euphoria, agitation, delirium, and psychosis.
- Knowledge of the spectrum of associated complications is essential to the clinical evaluation and management of cocaine intoxication.

Cocaine abuse and intoxication is a global problem leading to many medical complications that can result in significant morbidity and mortality. Current users of cocaine in the United States over the age of 12 years numbered 1.5 million in 2010, which is a decline from 2.4 million users in 2006.[1] In contrast, cocaine use is increasing in Europe, where it is second only to marijuana use. It is estimated that 4 million Europeans ages 15 to 64 used cocaine in 2009, with Spain, Italy, the United Kingdom, and Ireland having the highest prevalence.[2] Although cocaine abuse and intoxication is more common in young adults, older individuals are also affected. The rate of illicit drug use in the United States increased from 1.9% in 2002 to 4.1% in 2007 in the age group 50 to 59.[3] A recent review of patients ages 65 and older who had a drug screen performed in a suburban community hospital found 2.3% positive for cocaine.[4] These findings may represent continued drug use (aging of the baby boomer generation), new onset of use, or a return to use after a period of abstinence.

PHARMACOLOGY

Cocaine (benzoylmethylecgonine) is extracted from the leaves of the *Erythroxylon coca* plant by soaking leaves in organic solvents to form a thick paste sediment.

The author has nothing to disclose.
[a] Department of Medicine, Weill Cornell Medical College, New York, NY, USA; [b] Critical Care Division, Department of Medicine, The Methodist Hospital, Suite 1001, 6550 Fannin, Houston, TX 77030, USA
* Critical Care Division, Department of Medicine, The Methodist Hospital, Suite 1001, 6550 Fannin, Houston, TX 77030.
E-mail address: janicez@tmhs.org

The addition of hydrochloric acid to the paste results in the precipitation of cocaine hydrochloride salt. This water-soluble form of cocaine can be injected intravenously, snorted intranasally, or ingested orally. The hydrochloride salt of cocaine is converted into an alkaloid form that can be smoked by the addition of a base, such as sodium bicarbonate. This form of cocaine hardens to a rock-like state known as crack cocaine. The name is derived from the cracking noise made when the cocaine is heated. Most of the world supply of cocaine is produced in South America.

The time course of the physiologic effects of cocaine varies with the route of use, form of cocaine used, and concomitant use of other drugs.[5] The onset of effects occurs most rapidly with inhaled cocaine (3–5 seconds) followed by intravenous injection (10–60 seconds). The onset of effects is delayed with intranasal use (within 5 minutes) due to topical vasoconstriction. Conversely, the duration of effects is longest with intranasal cocaine use (60–90 minutes) and shortest with inhalation of crack cocaine (5–15 minutes). The short duration of effect with inhalation may lead to repetitive dosing to maintain desired effects.

Cocaine has a short half-life of 0.7 to 1.5 hours and is rapidly metabolized by plasma and liver cholinesterases to the major metabolites of benzoylecgonine and ecgonine methyl ester.[5] These water-soluble metabolites are excreted in the urine. The frequent concomitant use of cocaine and ethanol results in the hepatic formation of the active metabolite, cocaethylene, which has euphoric and sympathomimetic effects similar to cocaine but may also have greater toxicity.[6,7] The longer half-life of cocaethylene (2.5 hours) may prolong the euphoric effects of cocaine.

PATHOPHYSIOLOGY

Cocaine produces local anesthetic, vasoconstrictive and sympathomimetic effects.[5] Local anesthetic effects result from blockade of voltage-gated sodium channels in the neuronal membrane, resulting in inhibition of neural conduction. The vasoconstrictive effect of cocaine is primarily due to the stimulation of α-adrenergic receptors in arterial smooth muscle cells. Increased endothelin-1 and decreased nitric oxide blood concentrations may also contribute to cocaine's vasoconstrictive properties.[8] The major metabolites of cocaine, benzoylecgonine and ecgonine methyl ester, may persist in the body for more than 24 hours and contribute to delayed or recurrent coronary or cerebral vasoconstriction.

The major toxicities of cocaine use result from the sympathomimetic effects. Cocaine inhibits the presynaptic reuptake of biogenic amines, such as norepinephrine, dopamine, and serotonin, throughout the body, including the central nervous system (CNS). Systemic effects include an increase in heart rate and blood pressure with diffuse vasoconstriction. The CNS effects are most likely due to excess dopaminergic activity that produces profound euphoria and self-confidence at lower doses and agitation and delirium at higher doses.

Thrombogenic effects of cocaine have been ascribed to increases in plasminogen-activator inhibitor activity, platelet count, platelet activation, and platelet aggregation.[9] An inflammatory state characterized by elevated C-reactive protein, von Willebrand factor, and fibrinogen concentrations may also enhance thrombosis.[8]

DIAGNOSIS

Due to the short half-life of cocaine in the body, the presence of benzoylecgonine (half-life of approximately 6 hours) is used to detect cocaine exposure. For clinical purposes, urine is the most commonly used sample for detecting benzoylecgonine. After acute use of cocaine, urine testing is positive for 1 to 2 days. Chronic cocaine use may result in positive results for days to weeks after the last use.[10] No other drugs yield false-positive test results when benzoylecgonine urine assays are used. False-negative results could be obtained if testing is done too soon after cocaine use before metabolism to benzoylecgonine occurs.[5]

CLINICAL MANIFESTATIONS

Cocaine abusers may present for medical care with manifestations related to the acute sympathomimetic effects of cocaine or with manifestations related to complications resulting from cocaine use. Acute intoxication manifests with tachycardia, hypertension, and agitation. Additional physical examination findings often include mydriasis, diaphoresis, hyperthermia, and tachypnea. Any suspected cocaine user with agitation should have a core temperature measured to identify significant temperature elevations. Hypovolemia and hypotension are often present secondary to poor oral intake combined with exaggerated physical activity and exposure to high heat environments. The CNS effects of cocaine include agitation, paranoia, mania, and severe delirium. A depressed level of consciousness in a patient with acute cocaine use suggests a potential intracerebral catastrophe, significant systemic complication, or concomitant use of a sedating drug. Cocaine can affect all body systems and the clinical presentation may primarily result from organ toxicity. Major toxicities related to cocaine intoxication are discussed.

COCAINE TOXICITIES AND MANAGEMENT
Central Nervous System

Acute agitation is the most common presentation of cocaine intoxication in hospitals. Immediate intervention is often necessary to prevent self-injury or worsening of cocaine-related complications. The mainstay of treatment is sedation with benzodiazepines. Typically, lorazepam is administered intramuscularly or intravenously in doses of 2 mg and repeated until agitation is controlled. High doses may be needed but respiratory depression is uncommon. For rapid control of an agitated cocaine user, midazolam (5 mg) administered intramuscularly is effective.[11] Haloperidol is not used as a first-line drug because of its potential to lower the seizure threshold, which can add to the risk of seizures from cocaine.

Seizures due to cocaine use have been described since the use of the drug as a topical vasoconstrictor and local anesthetic. Cocaine lowers the seizure threshold with acute use and can precipitate new onset of seizure or exacerbate an existing seizure disorder. Focal seizures should prompt an evaluation for an intracerebral hemorrhage or infarction. Seizures are usually self-limited but multiple seizures should be treated with intravenous benzodiazepines. Status epilepticus can occur and treatment should follow standard protocols.[12,13] Refractory status epilepticus suggests severe CNS or metabolic complications.

Hemorrhagic and ischemic strokes associated with cocaine use are often devastating injuries. Hemorrhagic strokes may result from the acute elevation of blood pressure seen with acute cocaine intoxication. Patients with intracerebral hemorrhages related to cocaine have higher blood pressure on admission, more subcortical bleeds (basal ganglia, hypothalamus, and brainstem), and higher rates of intraventricular bleeding compared with spontaneous hemorrhages not related to cocaine.[14] Severe elevations of blood pressure due to cocaine are usually improved by the time a patient presents to the hospital. Guidelines for hemorrhagic stroke should be followed in this setting.[15] If blood pressure control is needed, nicardipine or labetalol is a reasonable option. CNS bleeding may also present as subarachnoid hemorrhage. The reported prevalence of vascular malformations as an underlying cause of subarachnoid hemorrhage has been variable.[14,16,17]

Ischemic strokes due to cocaine are thought to result from the cerebral vasoconstrictive effects and thrombogenic platelet effects.[18] Standard care for stroke victims is applicable to patients with cocaine associated ischemic strokes.[19]

Hyperthermia associated with cocaine abuse may result from central thermoregulatory dysfunction resulting in impaired heat dissipation and perception of heat stress coupled with the vasoconstrictive effects of vascular redistribution.[20] In addition, heat exposure and increased heat production due to agitation and motor activity contribute to the development of hyperthermia.[21] Patients presenting with hyperthermia associated with severe agitation and psychosis often have significant complications, such as disseminated intravascular coagulation, rhabdomyolysis, and multiple organ failure. Significant hyperthermia should be treated similarly to heat stroke with aggressive cooling techniques and control of agitation with benzodiazepines.[22]

Cardiovascular System

Acute coronary syndromes (myocardial ischemia and myocardial infarction [MI]) are among the most common toxicities of cocaine abuse.[23] Chest pain is the most frequent cocaine-related complaint in emergency departments. Adverse cardiovascular effects are independent of the amount of cocaine used, route of administration, or frequency of use. Ischemia is thought to result from increased myocardial oxygen demand caused by acute increases in heart rate, blood pressure, and contractility combined with decreases in myocardial oxygen supply potentially caused by coronary vasoconstriction.[24] The prothrombotic platelet effects of cocaine and the presence of coronary artery atherosclerosis may also be contributing factors. Cocaine-associated acute coronary syndrome (ACS) often occurs within the first few hours after cocaine exposure when cocaine concentrations are highest but may occur several hours to weeks after exposure. The effects of cocaine metabolites (benzoylecgonine and ecgonine methyl ester) are thought to contribute to delayed symptoms.[23]

Diagnosis of MI in cocaine abusers requires the measurement of cardiac-specific troponin. Creatine phosphokinase (CK) and CK-MB levels are less reliable due to elevations that may result from rhabdomyolysis. Electrocardiograms have limited diagnostic utility because abnormalities are common in cocaine users presenting with chest pain and early repolarization patterns may mimic ST segment elevation. A transient Brugada pattern on electrocardiogram likely results from the sodium channel effects of cocaine and must be distinguished from MI.[25,26]

Management of ACS in cocaine users is similar to management of other patients with ACS.[8] Aspirin should be administered as soon as possible when chest pain is thought to be ischemic. Nitroglycerin and benzodiazepines are recommended as primary therapy for ongoing chest pain.[27,28] Calcium channel blockers may be considered in patients with chest pain unresponsive to nitroglycerin and benzodiazepines.[8] Heparin use is recommended for unstable angina and MI in the absence of contraindications and percutaneous coronary intervention is preferred for reperfusion in ST-segment elevation MI. Evidence of myocardial necrosis has been associated with a high incidence of significant coronary disease in cocaine users and should prompt additional risk stratification and evaluation.[29] β-Blockers were often considered contraindicated in the management of ACS related to cocaine because of the potential for unopposed α-adrenergic–mediated vasoconstriction leading to elevated blood pressures. However, β-Blocker use was not found detrimental in 2 retrospective studies of patients with recent cocaine use and may be beneficial in some patients.[30,31] It is prudent to avoid the administration of a β-blocker in patients with evidence of an acute sympathomimetic syndrome. Current guidelines no longer recommend the routine use of intravenous β-blockers in ACS.[32,33]

Sinus tachycardia due to the sympathomimetic effects of cocaine is the most common presenting arrhythmia with acute cocaine intoxication. It usually responds to control of agitation with benzodiazepines. Supraventricular arrhythmias, such as atrial fibrillation, are usually self-limited but may also respond to benzodiazepines. Ventricular arrhythmias are less common and may be related to cocaine blockade of myocardial sodium channels leading to QRS and QT interval prolongation. Wide complex arrhythmias may respond to treatment with sodium bicarbonate.[34] Class IA antiarrhythmic drugs, such as procainamide, should be avoided.[23] Treatment of life-threatening arrhythmias should otherwise follow advanced life support guidelines.

The possibility of aortic dissection should also be considered in patients presenting with cocaine-associated chest pain. The incidence of aortic dissection associated with cocaine is low and is characterized by occurrence in patients with younger age, pre-existing hypertension, and black race. Descending dissections (type B) are more common in cocaine users than in similar patients without cocaine use.[35,36] The mechanism of injury is likely related to the sudden blood pressure elevation and tachycardia that create tremendous sheer forces on the aorta. Management of cocaine-associated aortic dissection should follow standard recommendations. Ascending dissections require urgent surgical repair, and blood pressure control and reduction of aortic sheer forces are indicated for descending dissections. Labetalol may be a reasonable option for blood pressure control for sustained hypertension in the cocaine user.[35]

Respiratory System

Pulmonary toxicities from abusing cocaine are less common than cardiovascular and CNS toxicities. Most pulmonary complications have been associated with inhaling cocaine. Barotrauma, including pneumomediastinum and pneumothorax, have been reported and may be due to cough triggered by inhalation or breath-holding maneuvers used to enhance the effects of inhaled cocaine. Large pneumothoraces may require tube thoracostomy but smaller pneumothoraces can be managed with supplemental oxygen, serial imaging, and monitoring for progression. Pneumomediastinum does not require specific therapy and these patients usually do not require hospitalization.

Bronchoconstriction has been experimentally shown to occur with inhaled cocaine and there are some reports of worsening of asthma due to cocaine.[37,38] Pulmonary infiltrates associated with cocaine use have sometimes been referred to as "crack lung." Although most infiltrates are transient, significant conditions, such as acute respiratory distress syndrome, can occur.[39] Noncardiogenic pulmonary edema due to cocaine use may be frequently associated with an alveolar hemorrhage component.[40] Hemoptysis alone may be a presenting complaint and usually resolves with avoidance of further cocaine exposure. Intravenous administration of cocaine contaminated with talc has been reported to cause granulomatous lung disease, but chronic inhalation may produce similar injury.[41] Pulmonary toxicities usually respond to supportive care and discontinuation of cocaine use. There is no evidence for the use of steroids in these conditions.

Musculoskeletal System

Muscle injury with cocaine abuse may result from several factors: direct myotoxic effect, ischemia from vasoconstriction and physical activity, and adulterants.[42] The possibility of rhabdomyolysis should be considered in any cocaine abuser with hyperthermia, seizure activity, agitation, or obtundation. Diagnosis is made by detection of elevated concentrations of CK in serum. Another helpful clue is the detection of blood in urine by dipstick in the absence of red blood cells on microscopic examination, which may indicate myoglobinuria. Initial CK concentrations may be normal (especially in hypovolemic patients) but repeat testing several hours after administration of intravenous fluids may reveal significant elevations.

It is prudent to initiate treatment of possible rhabdomyolysis in high-risk cocaine abusers pending laboratory results. The goal is to prevent renal tubular damage due to the nephrotoxic effects of myoglobin and hemoglobin decomposition products by providing aggressive intravenous hydration with crystalloids. Initial boluses of crystalloid (1–2 L or more) should be targeted to achieve hemodynamic stability and a euvolemic state. Continuous infusion of crystalloid is continued at 200 mL/h to 500 mL/h to achieve adequate urine output.[43,44] Routine use of intravenous bicarbonate and mannitol for rhabdomyolysis is not supported by available clinical data. Electrolytes should be monitored frequently to detect abnormalities, especially hyperkalemia. Severe cases of rhabdomyolysis may require early acute dialysis.

Gastrointestinal System

Cocaine intoxication can cause ischemic injury to the gastrointestinal (GI) tract and most cases tend to occur in younger individuals with no predisposing risks for ischemia. Ingested, intravenous, and inhaled cocaine have been associated with bowel ischemia, infarction, and perforation.[45–47] Most cases of GI ischemia involve segments of the small bowel, but ischemic colitis can also occur. Gastroduodenal perforations have also been described.[45] Proposed mechanisms for bowel ischemia include vasoconstriction and thrombosis of mesenteric vessels. Clinical presentation includes complaints of acute or chronic abdominal pain and bloody diarrhea. Peritoneal signs are often present on physical examination. Surgical exploration is often performed but nonoperative approaches with bowel rest and antibiotics may be appropriate in some patients. Preoperative angiography may be helpful to guide revascularization interventions by identifying occlusion of celiac or mesenteric vessels.

Renal System

Acute renal injury associated with cocaine use can be caused by vasoconstriction or thrombosis of renal vessels, rhabdomyolysis, severe hypertension, thrombotic microangiopathy, interstitial nephritis, and glomerulonephritis.[48] Renal infarction should be considered in cocaine abusers with significant persistent abdominal or flank pain with or without nausea, vomiting, and fever. Laboratory findings often include an elevated serum lactate dehydrogenase, proteinuria, and hematuria.[49,50] A predisposition to involve the right kidney may be related to the longer right renal artery.[49] Diagnostic modalities include imaging with CT and assessment of the renal vasculature with renal angiography. Management of renal infarction due to cocaine has included aspirin, anticoagulation, thrombolysis, thrombectomy, and supportive care.

Other Toxicities

Contamination of cocaine with other drugs or fillers can result in toxicities that are not directly related to the effects of cocaine. The presence of levamisole, an antihelminthic agent used in veterinary medicine, in cocaine supplies has been linked to the development of agranulocytosis.[51,52] Agranulocytosis resolves when drug use is discontinued. The presence of infectious complications may necessitate the use of filgrastim. Retiform purpura and skin necrosis secondary to thrombotic vasculopathy have also been linked to cocaine contaminated with levamisole.[53–55] Testing often reveals strongly positive perinuclear antineutrophil cytoplasmic antibodies and positive anticardiolipin immunoglobulin M antibodies. Management includes discontinuation of drug exposure and débridement of necrotic tissue in some cases. Methemoglobinemia has been reported after ingestion of cocaine contaminated with benzocaine.[56]

Cocaine Transport and Concealment

Cocaine as well as other illicit drugs may be ingested or inserted in the body for the purpose of transporting or concealing the drug. Body stuffing refers to the act of swallowing or hiding cocaine in body cavities to avoid detection and prosecution by authorities. These individuals are at risk of toxicities because the cocaine is either not wrapped or it is packaged in a manner that allows absorption in the GI tract. Body packing refers to the ingestion of larger quantities of cocaine for the purpose of drug smuggling. The risk of toxicity is low in these individuals because cocaine is precisely packaged to remain intact during passage through the GI tract.

Cocaine body stuffers are usually evaluated and managed in emergency departments. Mild signs of cocaine exposure, such as tachycardia, hypertension, and agitation, develop in most patients, but life-threatening toxicity (seizures, dysrhythmias, and cardiac arrest) can also occur.[57,58] Although activated charcoal is often administered, any beneficial effect on drug adsorption may be minimal due to the rapid absorption of cocaine from mucosal surfaces. Observation for 6 hours may be sufficient in asymptomatic body stuffers and those with minimal symptoms that resolve during the observation period.[59] Prolonged evidence of cocaine intoxication should raise the suspicion of ongoing absorption from a body site. Abdominal radiographs usually do not reveal packets in body stuffers, but some packets may be detected by CT scan. Patients with significant toxicities may require hospital or ICU admission and management.

Asymptomatic cocaine body packers can usually be managed conservatively until the packets have been eliminated.[60] An abdominal radiograph detects drug packets with a sensitivity of 85% to 90%, but CT scan is also frequently used for detection. Mild laxatives, such as lactulose or polyethylene glycol electrolyte lavage solution, can be administered to hasten elimination. Endoscopic retrieval is generally not recommended due to the risk of packet rupture. Surgical intervention is reserved for patients with evidence of obstruction or perforation of the GI tract, suspected packet rupture, or persistent significant cocaine toxicity.[60,61]

SUMMARY

Cocaine intoxication carries significant risk for medical complications requiring hospital care. Knowledge of the spectrum of toxicities associated with cocaine should prompt a thorough evaluation in patients suspected of acute or chronic cocaine use. Liberal use of benzodiazepines is warranted to control agitation and most major complications are managed similarly to patients without cocaine use along with supportive care. Referral for counseling should be considered for all cocaine users.

REFERENCES

1. Substance Abuse and Mental Health Services Administration. Results from the 2010 National Survey on Drug Use and Health: Summary of National Findings, NSDUH Series H-41, HHS Publication No. (SMA) 11-4658. Rockville (MD): Substance Abuse and Mental Health Services Administration; 2011.
2. European Monitoring Centre for Drugs and Drug addiction (EMCDDA). Annual Report 2011: the state of the drugs problem in Europe. Luxembourg (Europe): EMCDDA; 2011.

3. Gfroerer J, Penne M, Pemberton M, et al. Substance abuse treatment need among older adults in 2020: the impact of the aging baby-boom cohort. Drug Alcohol Depend 2003;69:127–35.
4. Chait R, Fahmy S, Caceres J. Cocaine abuse in older adults: an underscreened cohort. J Am Geriatr Soc 2010;58:391–2.
5. Goldstein RA, DesLauriers C, Burda AM. Cocaine: history, social implications, and toxicity—a review. Dis Mon 2009;55:6–38.
6. Brookoff D, Rotondo MF, Shaw LM, et al. Cocaethylene levels in patients who test positive for cocaine. Ann Emerg Med 1996;27:316–20.
7. Wilson LD, Jeromin J, Garvey L, et al. Cocaine, ethanol, and cocaethylene cardiotoxicity in an animal model of cocaine and ethanol abuse. Acad Emerg Med 2001;8:211–22.
8. McCord J, Jneid H, Hollander JE, et al. Management of cocaine-associated chest pain and myocardial infarction: a scientific statement from the American Heart Association Acute Cardiac Care Committee of the Council on Clinical Cardiology. Circulation 2008;117:1897–907.
9. Heesch CM, Wilhelm CR, Ristich J, et al. Cocaine activates platelets and increases the formation of circulating platelet containing microaggregates in humans. Heart 2000;83:688–95.
10. Burke WM, Ravi NV, Dhopesh V, et al. Prolonged presence of metabolite in urine after compulsive cocaine use. J Clin Psychiatry 1990;51:145–8.
11. Nobay F, Simon BC, Levitt A, et al. A prospective, double-blind, randomized trial of midazolam verus haloperidol versus lorazepam in the chemical restraint of violent and severely agitated patients. Acad Emerg Med 2004;11:744–9.
12. Marik PE, Varon J. The management of status epilepticus. Chest 2004;126:582–91.
13. Meierkord M, Boon P, Engelson B, et al. EFNS guideline on the management of status epilepticus. Eur J Neurol 2006;13:445–50.
14. Martin-Schild S, Albright KC, Hallevi H, et al. Intracerebral hemorrhages in cocaine users. Stroke 2010;41:680–4.
15. Krieger D, Mayberg M, Morgenstern L, et al. Guidelines for the management of spontaneous intracerebral hemorrhage in adults: 2007 update: a guideline from the American Heart Association/American Stroke Association Stroke Council, High Blood Pressure Research Council, and the Quality of Care and Outcomes in Research Interdisciplinary Working Group. Stroke 2007;38:2001–23.
16. Oyesiku NM, Colohan AR, Barrow DL, et al. Cocaine-induced aneurysmal rupture: an emergent negative factor in the natural history of intracranial aneurysms? Neurosurgery 1993;32:518–25.
17. Fessler RD, Esshaki CM, Stankewitz RC, et al. The neurovascular complications of cocaine. Surg Neurol 1997;47:339–45.
18. Kaufman MJ, Levin JM, Ross MH, et al. Cocaine-induced cerebral vasoconstriction detected in humans with magnetic resonance angiography. JAMA 1998;279:376–80.
19. Adams HP, del Zoppo G, Brass L, et al. Guidelines for the early management of adults with ischemic stroke, a guideline from the American Heart Association/American Stroke Association Council, Clinical Cardiology Council, Cardiovascular Radiology and Intervention Council, and the Atherosclerotic Peripheral Vascular Disease and Quality of Care Outcomes in Research Interdisciplinary Working Groups. Stroke 2007;38:1655–711.
20. Crandall CG, Vongpatanasin W, Victor RG. Mechanism of cocaine-induced hyperthermia in humans. Ann Intern Med 2002;136:785–91.

21. Marzuk PM, Tardiff K, Leon AC, et al. Ambient temperature and mortality from unintentional cocaine overdose. JAMA 1998;279:1795–800.
22. Bouchama A, Knochel JP. Heat stroke. N Engl J Med 2002;346:1978–88.
23. Lange RA, Hillis LD. Cardiovascular complications of cocaine use. N Engl J Med 2001;345:351–8.
24. Rezkalla SH, Kloner RA. Cocaine-induced myocardial infarction. Clin Med Res 2007;5:172–6.
25. Bebarta VS, Summers S. Brugada electrocardiographic pattern induced by cocaine toxicity. Ann Emerg Med 2007;49:827–9.
26. Robertson KE, Martin TN, Rae AP. Brugada-pattern ECG and cardiac arrest in cocaine toxicity: reading between the white lines. Heart 2010;96:643–4.
27. Honderick T, Williams D, Seaberg D, et al. A prospective, randomized, controlled trial of benzodiazepines and nitroglycerine or nitroglycerine alone in the treatment of cocaine-associated acute coronary syndromes. Am J Emerg Med 2003;21: 39–42.
28. Baumann BM, Perrone J, Hornig SE, et al. Randomized, double-blind, placebo-controlled trial of diazepam, nitroglycerin, or both for treatment of patients with potential cocaine-associated acute coronary syndromes. Acad Emerg Med 2000;7:878–85.
29. Kontos MC, Jesse RL, Tatum JL, et al. Coronary angiographic findings in patients with cocaine-associated chest pain. J Emerg Med 2003;24:9–13.
30. Dattilo PB, Halpern SM, Fearon K, et al. Beta-blockers are associated with reduced risk of myocardial infarction after cocaine use. Ann Emerg Med 2008; 51:117–25.
31. Rangel C, Shu RG, Lazar LD, et al. β-Blockers for chest pain associated with recent cocaine use. Arch Intern Med 2010;170:874–9.
32. Anderson JL, Adams CD, Antman EM, et al. ACC/AHA 2007 guidelines for the management of patients with unstable angina/non-ST-elevation myocardial infarction: a report of the American College of Cardiology/American Heart Association Task Force on Practice Guidelines. J Am Coll Cardiol 2007;50:e1–157.
33. O'Connor RE, Bossaert L, Arntz HR, et al. Part 9: Acute coronary syndromes, 2010 international consensus on cardiopulmonary resuscitation and emergency cardiovascular care science with treatment recommendations. Circulation 2010; 122(Suppl 2):S422–65.
34. Wood DM, Dargan PI, Hoffman RS. Management of cocaine-induced cardiac arrhythmias due to cardiac ion channel dysfunction. Clin Toxicol (Phila) 2009; 47:14–23.
35. Eagle KA, Isselbacher KM, DeSanctis RW. Cocaine-related aortic dissection in perspective. Circulation 2002;105:1529–30.
36. Hsue PY, Salinas CL, Bolger AF, et al. Acute aortic dissection related to crack cocaine. Circulation 2002;105:1592–5.
37. Tashkin DP, Kleerup EC, Koyal SN, et al. Acute effects of inhaled and i.v. cocaine on airway dynamics. Chest 1996;110:904–10.
38. Levine M, Iliercu ME, Margellos-Anast H, et al. The effects of cocaine and heroin use on intubation rates and hospital utilization with acute asthma exacerbations. Chest 2005;128:1951–7.
39. Ettinger NA, Albin RJ. A review of the respiratory effects of smoking cocaine. Am J Med 1989;87:664–8.
40. Forrester JM, Steele AW, Waldron JA, et al. Crack lung: an acute pulmonary syndrome with a spectrum of clinical and histopathologic findings. Am Rev Respir Dis 1990;142:462–7.

41. Oubeid M, Bickel JT, Ingram EA, et al. Pulmonary talc granulomatosis in a cocaine sniffer. Chest 1990;98:237–9.
42. Pagala M, Amaladevi B, Azad D, et al. Effect of cocaine on leakage of creatine kinase from isolated fast and slow muscles of rat. Life Sci 1993;52:751–6.
43. Richards JR. Rhabdomyolysis and drugs of abuse. J Emerg Med 2000;19:51–6.
44. Bosch X, Poch E, Grau JM. Rhabdomyolysis and acute kidney injury. N Engl J Med 2009;361:62–72.
45. Feliciano DV, Ojukwu JC, Rozycki GS, et al. The epidemic of cocaine-related juxtapyloric perforations. Ann Surg 1999;229:801–6.
46. Muniz AE, Evans T. Acute gastrointestinal manifestations associated with use of crack. Am J Emerg Med 2001;19:61–3.
47. Linder JD, Monkemuller KE, Raijman I, et al. Cocaine-associated ischemic colitis. South Med J 2000;93:909–13.
48. Nzerue CM, Hewan-Lowe K, Riley LJ. Cocaine and the kidney: a synthesis of pathophysiologic and clinical perspectives. Am J Kidney Dis 2000;35:783–95.
49. Bemanian S, Motallebi M, Nosrati SM. Cocaine-induced renal infarction: report of a case and review of the literature. BMC Nephrol 2005;6:10.
50. Madhrira MM, Mohan S, Markowitz GS, et al. Acute bilateral renal infarction secondary to cocaine-induced vasospasm. Kidney Int 2009;76:576–80.
51. CDC. Agranulocytosis associated with cocaine use—four states, March 2008-November 2009. MMWR Morb Mortal Wkly Rep 2009;58:1381–5.
52. Zhu NY, LeGatt DF, Turner AR. Agranulocytosis after consumption of cocaine adulterated with levamisole. Ann Intern Med 2009;150:287–9.
53. Bradford M, Rosenberg B, Moreno J. Bilateral necrosis of earlobes and cheeks: another complication of cocaine contaminated with levamisole. Ann Intern Med 2010;152:758–9.
54. Farhat EK, Muirhead TT, Chaffins ML, et al. Levamisole-induced cutaneous necrosis mimicking coagulopathy. Arch Dermatol 2010;146:1320–1.
55. Milman N, Smith CD. Cutaneous vasculopathy associated with cocaine use. Arthritis Care Res (Hoboken) 2011;63:1195–202.
56. Chakladar A, Willers JW, Perskokova E, et al. White powder, blue patient: Methaemoglobinemia associated with benzocaine-adulterated cocaine. Resuscitation 2010;81:138–9.
57. Sporer KA, Firestone J. Clinical course of crack cocaine body stuffers. Ann Emerg Med 1997;29:596–601.
58. June R, Aks SE, Keys N, et al. Medical outcome of cocaine bodystuffers. J Emerg Med 2000;18:221–4.
59. Moreira M, Buchanan J, Heard K. Validation of a 6-hour observation period for cocaine body stuffers. Am J Emerg Med 2011;29:299–303.
60. Traub SJ, Hoffman RS, Nelson LS. Body packing—the internal concealment of illicit drugs. N Engl J Med 2003;349:2519–26.
61. deBeer SA, Spiessens G, Mol W, et al. Surgery for body packing in the Caribbean: a retrospective study of 70 patients. World J Surg 2008;32:281–5.

Cardiac Glycoside Toxicity
More Than 200 Years and Counting

Salmaan Kanji, PharmD[a],*, Robert D. MacLean, PharmD[b]

KEYWORDS

- Digoxin • Digitoxin • Cardiac glycosides • Toxicity • Toxicology • Overdose
- Immunoglobulin fragments • Digoxin-specific antibody fragments

KEY POINTS

- Digitalis toxicity, regardless of the source, produces a toxidrome characterized by gastrointestinal, neurologic, electrolyte, and nonspecific cardiac manifestations.
- Chronic toxicity remains much more difficult to recognize compared with an acute presentation because of the nonspecific manifestations; therefore, serum glycoside levels are essential for diagnosis in this population.
- The mainstay of management continues to be rapid toxidrome identification followed by digoxin-specific antibody fragment therapy with supportive care.

Digitalis or cardiac glycosides have been used for medicinal purposes for more than 200 years, ever since Sir William Withering suggested that digitalis may be beneficial in patients with heart complaints in 1785.[1] Today, digoxin is the only cardiac glycoside commercially available for prescription in the United States, although digitoxin is also available internationally. Cardiac glycosides are, however, widely available in some botanic products and other naturally occurring substances (**Table 1**). Digitalis is still prescribed regularly for the management of atrial fibrillation and heart failure, although its clinical utility has been steadily decreasing and its narrow therapeutic index makes this drug a high risk for serious toxicity. Despite a relative decline in use over the last few decades, the prevalence of cases of toxicity has not paralleled the same trajectory.[2] In 2008, US poison control centers were called for 2632 cases involving digoxin toxicity, and 17 cases resulted in digoxin-related deaths.[3]

MECHANISM OF TOXICITY

Cardiac glycosides have separate mechanical and electrophysiological activity on the heart. Cardiac glycosides reversibly inhibit the sodium-potassium adenosine

Funding: None.
Financial disclosure, conflict of interest: The authors have nothing to disclose.
[a] Department of Pharmacy, The Ottawa Health Research Institute, The Ottawa Hospital, 501 Smyth Road, Ottawa, Ontario K1H 8L6, Canada; [b] Department of Pharmacy, The Ottawa Hospital, 501 Smyth Road, Ottawa, Ontario K1H 8L6, Canada
* Corresponding author.
E-mail address: Skanji@toh.on.ca

Crit Care Clin 28 (2012) 527–535
http://dx.doi.org/10.1016/j.ccc.2012.07.005

Table 1 Botanic sources of cardiac glycosides	
Common Name	Botanic Name
Foxglove	*Digitalis purpurea, Digitalis lanata*
Common oleander	*Nerium oleander*
Yellow oleander	*Thevetia peruviana*
Lily of the valley	*Convallaria majalis*
Red squill	*Urginea maritima*
Ouabain	*Strophanthus gratus*
Dogbane	*Apocynum cannabinum*
Wallflower	*Cheiranthus cheiri*
Milkweed	*Asclepias spp*
Mock azalea	*Menziesia ferruginea*
Pheasant's eye	*Adonis spp*
Star of Bethlehem	*Ornithogalum umbellatum*
Wintersweet, bushman's poison	*Carissa acokanthera*
Sea mango	*Cerbera manghas*
Frangipani	*Plumeria rubra*
King's crown	*Calotropis procera*
Rubber vine	*Cryptostegia grandiflora*

triphosphatase exchanger (Na-K-ATPase) in cardiac myocytes resulting in higher-than-normal intracellular concentrations of sodium. These high levels of intracellular sodium increase the resting membrane potential leading to the activation of voltage-gated calcium channels, which increase intracellular calcium concentrations. The net increase in intracellular calcium activates further calcium release from the sarcoplasmic reticulum and is responsible for increasing positive inotropy. From an electrophysiological perspective, the negative chronotropic activity of cardiac glycosides is largely attributed to increased vagal tone, which decreases the rate of sinoatrial node depolarization and increased refractory period of the atrioventricular node (AV). The result is a reduction in sinoatrial and AV conduction.

In toxicity, the influx of sodium increases phase IV depolarization, lowers the resting membrane potential threshold, and increases automaticity leading to its proarrhythmic potential. Although AV block and extrasystoles are the most common dysrhythmias seen with digoxin toxicity (and at therapeutic concentrations), this combination of suppression and excitation make almost *any* dysrhythmia possible.[4] Na-K-ATPase exchangers are not limited to cardiac myocytes, and systemic toxicity is commonly observed in addition to cardiac toxicity. Symptoms of toxicity may also manifest with a wide range of gastrointestinal, ocular, and neurologic symptoms.

THE CLINICAL TOXIDROME

The 3 most common scenarios resulting in cardiac glycoside toxicity are as follows: (1) intentional or accidental acute ingestion leading to acute toxicity, (2) systemic accumulation secondary to hepatic or renal dysfunction, and (3) systemic accumulation secondary to a drug interaction. The last 2 scenarios usually result in a slow progressive chronic toxicity as digoxin serum concentrations accumulate over time, which contrasts acute toxicity whereby serum levels are often very high on presentation.

In the second scenario, accumulation of digoxin in renal failure is a consequence of the kidneys being the primary route of elimination for digoxin. In the third scenario, the risk of drug interactions are numerous and significant because digoxin is metabolized to inactive metabolites via the cytochrome P450 system (isoenzyme 3A4) and is a substrate for the intestinal and renal drug transporter P-glycoprotein. Both acute and chronic presentations place patients at risk for life-threatening complications.

Cardiac manifestations of toxicity are the primary concern of both acute and chronic presentations of cardiac glycoside toxicity. Although any dysrhythmia is possible, certain aberrations are common, such as paroxysmal atrial tachycardia with conduction block, junctional tachycardia, and bidirectional ventricular tachycardia.[4] Death from digoxin overdose is usually a result of cardiovascular collapse. Neurologic symptoms (independent of those caused by circulatory collapse) can also be evident and include confusion, weakness, lethargy, delirium, and disorientation. Gastrointestinal problems, such as nausea, vomiting, and anorexia, are also common.

Acute Versus Chronic Presentation

Considerable overlap exists with respect to presenting signs and symptoms of cardiac glycoside toxicity, but the temporal aspects from a thorough history can help differentiate acute versus chronic exposure. With acute ingestion, patients often remain asymptomatic for several hours after ingestion because of the biphasic nature and large volume of distribution of digoxin. Digoxin has a 2-compartment model of distribution whereby the drug redistributes into the intracellular tissue compartment after peak plasma levels are obtained. With therapeutic dosing, peak plasma levels are obtained in 30 to 90 minutes, whereas peak tissue concentrations are delayed a further 30 to 60 minutes. In acute toxicity, this redistribution into the tissue compartment can take hours. Because clinical manifestations of toxicity are a result of tissue penetration, the cardiac, neurologic, ocular, and gastrointestinal effects are often delayed well beyond the time to peak serum concentrations. Therefore, serum levels within 6 hours may be highly variable and misleading in acute ingestions because they do not correlate with severity of toxicity.[5] Although the value of serum levels within 6 hours should not be used to predict the severity of illness or quantity of ingestion, it may still have diagnostic value in unknown overdoses or in situations when the reliability of the history is questionable.

Conversely, in chronic toxicity, the 2-compartment distribution of digoxin is irrelevant because presumably the pharmacokinetics of digoxin are already at a steady state. Patients who present with chronic digoxin toxicity usually seek medical attention because of an insidious onset of symptoms that have been occurring over a period of days to weeks. Gastrointestinal symptoms, such as nausea and vomiting, are usually less pronounced in chronic toxicity as compared with acute toxicity. Neurologic manifestations, such as lethargy, confusion, delirium, disorientation, and weakness, may be more prominent with chronic toxicity. Visual changes are more common with chronic toxicity and may include alterations in color vision, development of scotomata, or blindness.

Electrolyte Abnormalities

Hyperkalemia is a major manifestation of both acute and chronic cardiac glycoside toxicity and is a result of the inhibition of Na-K-ATPase and the subsequent increase in extracellular potassium. In acute toxicity, there is a strong correlation between degree of hyperkalemia and mortality from digoxin overdose. A landmark study published in 1973 of 91 patients with acute digitalis toxicity demonstrated a 100% mortality rate among patients presenting with potassium greater than 5.5 mEq/L (or 5.5 mmol/L) and a 100% survival rate in patients who presented with a serum potassium concentration less than 5 mEq/L. It is important to note that this study predates the availability of a digoxin-specific antibody antidote and excluded 24 patients with nondigitoxin ingestions or mild presenting symptoms.[6] This finding holds true for all cardiac glycosides regardless of the source. A more recent study has investigated the prognostic value of hyperkalemia in chronic digoxin toxicity and also found that hyperkalemia (defined as >5 mEq/L) was highly associated with mortality even after accounting for digoxin-specific antibody antidote administration.[7]

In chronic toxicity, hypokalemia is more worrisome. Hypokalemia, hypomagnesemia, and hypercalcemia have all been demonstrated to augment the toxicity of digoxin (even at therapeutic serum concentrations).[8] In this setting, these electrolyte abnormalities are usually a result of concomitant loop diuretic use for heart failure but could also be a result of persistent diarrhea or vomiting.

Serum Digoxin Measurements

Serum digoxin measurements are the key to differentiating digoxin toxicity from other sources of similar clinical presentation (eg, beta-adrenergic antagonist overdose, calcium channel antagonist overdose, sick sinus syndrome, hypothermia, hypothyroidism). The timing of blood sampling is an important consideration, especially for acute intoxications because levels within 6 hours of ingestion may be very high and precede clinical symptoms and electrophysiological aberrations. Serum concentrations after 6 hours are better correlated with the severity of toxicity. It is, however, important to recognize that even appropriately timed serum measurements do not always correlate well with toxicity because there are many case reports describing asymptomatic patients with highly toxic serum digoxin concentrations and patients with symptoms of toxicity despite therapeutic serum concentrations. In chronic toxicity, serum digoxin measurements are often only mildly elevated beyond the therapeutic range (0.8–2.0 ng/mL or 1.0–2.6 nmol/L). Although the standard radioimmunoassay used by most hospitals is specific for digoxin, cross-reactivity (although incomplete) does occur with digitoxin and naturally occurring sources of cardiac glycosides. In these instances, positive levels should be interpreted qualitatively rather than quantitatively.

APPROACH TO MANAGEMENT

A general approach to assessing and managing the intoxicated patient (ie, assessing and supporting airway, breathing, circulation) is beyond the scope of this review; guidance for management discussed herein focuses on therapies specific for cardiac glycoside toxicity.

Antidotes

Conventional treatment before digoxin-specific antibody fragments (DSFab) were limited to gastrointestinal decontamination and supportive measures. Digoxin antibodies were first used in humans to treat digitalis toxicity in 1976 but did not become widely available until the mid-1980s.[1] The digoxin-specific antibodies are produced in sheep and cleaved into antibody fragments via papain digestion. These fragments have the same affinity to digoxin as the complete antibody but are less immunogenic and the smaller size gives it a sevenfold greater volume of distribution.[9] Removing the immunogenic Fc component of the antibody has significantly reduced the risk of anaphylaxis that accompanies the systemic administration of foreign proteins.

Anaphylaxis has been reported in less than 1% of cases, and repeat administration has been done safely in case reports and postmarketing surveillance studies.[10,11]

The DSFab bind molecules of digoxin (and other cardiac glycosides) making them incapable of binding to Na-K-ATPase. The affinity of digoxin to DSFab is greater than the affinity of digoxin to Na-K-ATPase, resulting in a concentration gradient that promotes the progressive efflux of intracellular digoxin. Free serum digoxin concentrations drop to undetectable levels within minutes of administration, and cardiac manifestations of toxicity usually subside within 30 minutes. Hyperkalemia usually requires more time for redistribution and resolves within 2 to 6 hours.[12] DSFab bound to digoxin is eliminated renally, with an elimination half-life of 15 to 20 hours. The presence of renal failure will prolong the elimination half-life. The binding of digoxin to DSFab is reversible, and dissociation occurs necessitating additional doses of DSFab when symptoms of toxicity return (as late as 72–90 hours in severe renal dysfunction).

It is important to recognize that conventional serum digoxin assays cannot differentiate between unbound digoxin and digoxin bound to DSFab and, therefore, can result in clinically misleading elevations in serum digoxin concentration unless free unbound digoxin concentration can be measured.[13,14]

Efficacy of DSFab therapy has been established primarily via cohort studies and case series rather than randomized controlled trials. However, given the success described in the early cohort studies, a randomized trial to assess efficacy may be considered superfluous and unethical. The first published cohort study analyzed outcomes of 26 patients with severe digoxin or digitoxin toxicity who were given the DSFab antidote. Twenty-one of these 26 patients fully recovered.[15] In the second case series of 56 patients with severe digitalis toxicity (presenting with dysrhythmias or hyperkalemia) treated with DSFab, 53 patients had full recoveries.[16] In the largest published prospective cohort study 150 patients with severe digoxin toxicity enrolled from 21 US centers, 80% of patients had complete resolution of toxicity and 90% displayed some evidence of response to treatment. The median time to response was 19 minutes, and 75% of patients showed evidence of response within 60 minutes. Reported reasons for partial and nonresponse were exacerbations of underlying cardiac disease, dosing errors, and delays in treatment.[17]

Indications for DSFab administration are as follows: (1) life-threatening arrhythmia, such as ventricular tachycardia or fibrillation, asystole, complete heart block, Mobitz II heart block or symptomatic bradycardia; (2) evidence of end-organ dysfunction, such as renal failure or altered mental status; or (3) hyperkalemia (>5 to 5.5 mEq/L). These criteria are largely based on predictors of poor outcomes associated with acute digoxin toxicity. They do not take into account peak or presenting digoxin levels, although many centers recommend treatment for levels greater than 10 ng/mL (13 nmol/L) in acute ingestions or greater than 4 ng/mL (5.1 nmol/LL) in chronic toxicity. Others have suggested empiric dosing for ingestions of digoxin exceeding 10 mg in adults or 4 mg in a child.

Two commercially available DSFab products are available in the United States (Digibind and DigiFab). Both preparations are considered equivalent and interchangeable. A vial of Digibind contains 38 mg of DSFab, whereas a vial of DigiFab contains 40 mg of DSFab. A vial of either product will bind approximately 0.5 mg of digoxin. Dosing recommendations for patients with 6-hour or more serum digoxin levels, known amounts ingested, or neither are provided in **Fig. 1**. Despite the fact that the indications for use are largely based on acute ingestions, many patients with toxicity from chronic exposure will meet these criteria and may benefit from therapy with DSFab.[18] When considering the dose for chronic ingestions, steady-state digoxin

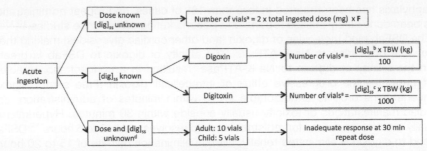

Fig. 1. Dosing recommendations for DSFab (Digibind or DigiFab). Infuse all doses over 30 minutes through a 0.22-μm filter. If cardiac arrest is imminent, give via slow intravenous push. [dig]$_{ss}$, serum digoxin concentration (nanogram per milliliter) at steady state; F, estimated bioavailability (if intravenous digoxin or digitoxin use 1, if digoxin tablets use 0.8); TBW, total body weight. [a] Round number of vials upward. [b] If measurement in nanomole per liter, multiply by 0.781. [c] If measurement in nanomole per liter, multiply by 0.765. [d] Ingestions of cardiac glycosides other than digoxin or digitoxin should be treated with empiric dosing recommendations.

concentrations are usually available and patients are more likely to have non–life-threatening symptoms. If this is the case, half of the calculated dose should be tried first to reduce the risk of unmasking the underlying cardiac disease (decompensated heart failure, atrial fibrillation with rapid ventricular rate). Postmarketing surveillance studies suggest that up to 25% of patients receiving DSFab will have posttreatment manifestations of their underlying disease.[11,19]

Gastrointestinal Decontamination

Patients who present to the emergency department within 2 hours of ingestion may benefit from gastrointestinal decontamination with activated charcoal.[20] The standard single dose is 50 g (1 g/kg for children) with or without the cathartic agent sorbitol. The role of charcoal in chronic toxicity is less well established. All cardiac glycosides undergo enterohepatic or enteroenteric recirculation to some extent making multiple-dose activated charcoal potentially worthwhile. The efficacy of this strategy has only been described in case reports and should only be considered if DSFab therapy is not available or in anuric renal failure.[21] Cholestyramine has also been reported as efficacious in case reports by binding digoxin in the lumen of the gastrointestinal tract undergoing enterohepatic recirculation.[22,23] Again, this should not be considered first-line therapy when DSFab therapy is available.

Augmenting Elimination

Extracorporeal elimination of digoxin via hemodialysis or hemoperfusion is not useful in the elimination of digoxin or digoxin-Fab fragment complexes. As stated before, multiple-dose activated charcoal or cholestyramine may be able to enhance elimination via enterohepatic recirculation. Others have advocated taking advantage of known drug interactions between digoxin and drugs that induce its metabolism, such as rifampicin. Rifampicin is a potent inducer of the cytochrome P450 isoenzymes 3A4 and 2C9. Digoxin is primarily metabolized via the isoenzyme 3A4, so combination therapy would theoretically enhance the metabolic capacity for digoxin. In one case report of a patient admitted to an institution where DSFab was not available, the half-life of digoxin was 26 hours when rifampicin was added as opposed to the predicted 36 to 48 hours without.[24] Another case report describes successful but incomplete removal of free digoxin and DSFab-digoxin complexes with plasma exchange.[25] Although this novel approach was effective in clearing the circulating drug, the volume of distribution is so large that the total removal represented less than 1% of the total drug ingested. It would seem that for plasma exchange to be worthy of consideration, it would have to be started before complete distribution of the drug (ie, within 6 hours of ingestion) or administered repeatedly (with repeated doses of DSFab) because the drug redistributes from the tissues to the circulation after each exchange.[26] The efficacy of these therapies has only been described in case reports and should only be considered in cases when DSFab are not available or patients present with severe renal dysfunction.

Managing Electrolyte Abnormalities

Hyperkalemia is the most common electrolyte abnormality observed in digoxin toxicity and is strongly associated with prognosis. However, treatment with traditional measures, such as insulin and dextrose, sodium bicarbonate, or ion-exchange resins, does not reduce the associated mortality.[6] Hyperkalemia usually resolves within hours of administration of DSFab as N-K-ATPase activity is restored and potassium is redistributed back into cells. Hypokalemia, on the other hand, has also been associated with worsening symptoms of digoxin toxicity, particularly in chronic toxicity when accompanied by hypomagnesemia in patients concomitantly taking loop diuretics. Potassium and magnesium replacement should be administered to these patients. Repletion of potassium is particularly important in patients with hypokalemia who are receiving DSFab because the antidote may further lower serum potassium concentrations.

Intravenous calcium has traditionally been considered contraindicated in digoxin overdose because hypercalcemia potentiates digoxin toxicity. This idea is based on studies of animal models whereby high levels of intracellular calcium could theoretically produce a noncontractile state because of the failure of diastolic relaxation as calcium binds to troponin C. This stone heart theory has been criticized because the animal models in which digoxin toxicity was potentiated by calcium administration only established this association at unrealistically high serum levels of calcium (>20 mg/dL or >5 mmol/L).[27] More recent animal studies using more realistic calcium dosing have not shown an association between calcium administration and worsening toxicity or death.[28] Recently, in a cohort of 159 patients with digoxin toxicity, 23 patients received intravenous calcium. In this cohort, calcium administration was not associated with malignant dysrhythmias or mortality.[29]

Managing Dysrhythmias

Because almost any dysrhythmia can be observed in cardiac glycoside toxicity, management depends on the nature of the dysrhythmia, the presence or absence of hemodynamic instability, and the presence or absence of electrolyte abnormalities. Hemodynamically stable bradyarrhythmias or tachyarrhythmias may be managed conservatively with close monitoring. DSFab is the treatment of choice and rapidly reverses cardiac manifestations of toxicity, hemodynamically stable or otherwise. Beta-adrenergic antagonists may be considered for supraventricular tachyarrhythmias with rapid ventricular response but may potentiate AV blockade, so short-acting agents, such as esmolol, are best. Calcium channel antagonists, such as verapamil or diltiazem, are contraindicated because they prevent renal excretion of digoxin via P-glycoprotein–mediated drug transport. Atropine may be considered a temporary adjunct to treatment with DSFab as is cardiac pacing, but pacing can theoretically lower the fibrillation threshold and induce ventricular dysrhythmias.

All hemodynamically unstable dysrhythmias respond best to DSFab therapy, but if this therapy is not available lidocaine (1.0–1.5 mg/kg followed by 1–4 mg/min) or phenytoin (up to 15–20 mg/kg loading dose) may be considered for ventricular tachycardia or fibrillation because they are the least likely to worsen AV conduction. Quinidine and procainamide are contraindicated in digoxin toxicity.

SUMMARY

Digoxin toxicity is still a common problem despite the relative decline in use over the last few decades. Traditional management included gastrointestinal decontamination and supportive measures, but the advent of an antidote in the form of DSFab has revolutionized the prognosis and management of cardiac glycoside toxicity from acute and chronic exposure. Before the availability of DSFab, only a minority of patients who presented with severe toxicity (dysrhythmias or severe hyperkalemia) survived, and now the converse is true. The considerable cost associated with this life-saving therapy, unfortunately, has limited its accessibility in some settings.

REFERENCES

1. Smith TW, Haber E, Yeatman L, et al. Reversal of advanced digoxin intoxication with Fab fragments of digoxin-specific antibodies. N Engl J Med 1976;294(15): 797–800.
2. Hussain Z, Swindle J, Hauptman PJ. Digoxin use and digoxin toxicity in the post-DIG trial era. J Card Fail 2006;12(5):343–6.
3. Bronstein AC, Spyker DA, Cantilena LR Jr, et al. 2008 annual report of the American Association of Poison Control Centers' National Poison Data System (NPDS): 26th annual report. Clin Toxicol (Phila) 2009;47(10):911–1084.
4. Ma G, Brady WJ, Pollack M, et al. Electrocardiographic manifestations: digitalis toxicity. J Emerg Med 2001;20(2):145–52.
5. Ng RH, Stempsey W, Statland BE. Biphasic profile in the elimination of digoxin from serum after a massive overdose. Clin Chem 1983;29(2):393–4.
6. Bismuth C, Gaultier M, Conso F, et al. Hyperkalemia in acute digitalis poisoning: prognostic significance and therapeutic implications. Clin Toxicol 1973;6(2): 153–62.
7. Manini AF, Nelson LS, Hoffman RS. Prognostic utility of serum potassium in chronic digoxin toxicity: a case-control study. Am J Cardiovasc Drugs 2011; 11(3):173–8.
8. Lip GY, Metcalfe MJ, Dunn FG. Diagnosis and treatment of digoxin toxicity. Postgrad Med J 1993;69(811):337–9.
9. Proudfoot AT. A star treatment for digoxin overdose? Br Med J (Clin Res Ed) 1986; 293(6548):642–3.
10. Bosse GM, Pope TM. Recurrent digoxin overdose and treatment with digoxin-specific Fab antibody fragments. J Emerg Med 1994;12(2):179–85.
11. Hickey AR, Wenger TL, Carpenter VP, et al. Digoxin immune Fab therapy in the management of digitalis intoxication: safety and efficacy results of an observational surveillance study. J Am Coll Cardiol 1991;17(3):590–8.
12. Wenger TL, Butler VP, Haber E, et al. Treatment of 63 severely digitalis-toxic patients with digoxin-specific antibody fragments. J Am Coll Cardiol 1985; 5(5 Suppl A):118A–23A.
13. George S, Braithwaite RA, Hughes EA. Digoxin measurements following plasma ultrafiltration in two patients with digoxin toxicity treated with specific Fab fragments. Ann Clin Biochem 1994;31(Pt 4):380–2.

14. Hursting MJ, Raisys VA, Opheim KE, et al. Determination of free digoxin concentrations in serum for monitoring Fab treatment of digoxin overdose. Clin Chem 1987;33(9):1652–5.
15. Smith TW, Butler VP, Haber E, et al. Treatment of life-threatening digitalis intoxication with digoxin-specific Fab antibody fragments: experience in 26 cases. N Engl J Med 1982;307(22):1357–62.
16. Smolarz A, Roesch E, Lenz E, et al. Digoxin specific antibody (Fab) fragments in 34 cases of severe digitalis intoxication. J Toxicol Clin Toxicol 1985;23(4–6): 327–40.
17. Antman EM, Wenger TL, Butler VP, et al. Treatment of 150 cases of life-threatening digitalis intoxication with digoxin-specific Fab antibody fragments. Final report of a multicenter study. Circulation 1990;81(6):1744–52.
18. Lapostolle F, Borron SW, Verdier C, et al. Assessment of digoxin antibody use in patients with elevated serum digoxin following chronic or acute exposure. Intensive Care Med 2008;34(8):1448–53.
19. Clark RF, Barton ED. Pitfalls in the administration of digoxin-specific Fab fragments. J Emerg Med 1994;12(2):233–4.
20. Pond S, Jacobs M, Marks J, et al. Treatment of digitoxin overdose with oral activated charcoal. Lancet 1981;318(8256):1177–8.
21. Critchley JA, Critchley LA. Digoxin toxicity in chronic renal failure: treatment by multiple dose activated charcoal intestinal dialysis. Hum Exp Toxicol 1997; 16(2):733–5.
22. Henderson RP, Solomon CP. Use of cholestyramine in the treatment of digoxin intoxication. Arch Intern Med 1988;148(3):745–6.
23. Rawashdeh NM, Al-Hadidi HF, Irshaid YM, et al. Gastrointestinal dialysis of digoxin using cholestyramine. Pharmacol Toxicol 1993;72(6):245–8.
24. Unal S, Bayrakci B, Yasar U, et al. Successful treatment of propafenone, digoxin and warfarin overdosage with plasma exchange therapy and rifampicin. Clin Drug Investig 2007;27(7):505–8.
25. Zdunek M, Mitra A, Mokrzycki MH. Plasma exchange for the removal of digoxin-specific antibody fragments in renal failure: timing is important for maximizing clearance. Am J Kidney Dis 2000;36(1):177–83.
26. Chillet P, Korach JM, Petitpas D, et al. Digoxin poisoning and anuric acute renal failure: efficiency of the treatment associating digoxin-specific antibodies (Fab) and plasma exchanges. Int J Artif Organs 2002;25(6):538–41.
27. Nola GT, Pope S, Harrison DC. Assessment of the synergistic relationship between serum calcium and digitalis. Am Heart J 1970;79(4):499–507.
28. Hack JB, Woody JH, Lewis DE, et al. The effect of calcium chloride in treating hyperkalemia due to acute digoxin toxicity in a porcine model. J Toxicol Clin Toxicol 2004;42(4):337–42.
29. Levine M, Nikkanen H, Pallin DJ. The effects of intravenous calcium in patients with digoxin toxicity. J Emerg Med 2011;40(1):41–6.

Carbon Monoxide Poisoning

Jorge A. Guzman, MD

KEYWORDS

- Carbon monoxide • Carboxyhemoglobin • Poisoning

KEY POINTS

- Carbon monoxide (CO) poisoning is the leading cause of death as a result of unintentional poisoning in the United States.
- Because of their higher metabolic rates, the cardiovascular and nervous systems are most frequently affected in severe intoxications.
- Diagnosis is made by prompt measurement of carboxyhemoglobin levels performed by spectrophotometric CO-oximetry (>3% in nonsmokers and >10% in smokers confirms CO exposure, but levels correlate poorly with the clinical picture).
- Treatment consists of the patient's removal from the source of exposure and the immediate administration of 100% supplemental oxygen in addition to aggressive supportive measures.

INTRODUCTION

Carbon monoxide (CO) poisoning is common. Unintentional, non–fire-related CO poisoning is responsible for approximately 15,000 emergency department (ED) visits and nearly 500 deaths annually in the United States.[1,2] CO is frequently unrecognized because the signs and symptoms are relatively nonspecific; consequently, the true incidence of CO poisoning remains unknown. Mortality rates range between 1% and 31%.[3]

EPIDEMIOLOGY

CO is an odorless, colorless gas that usually remains undetectable until exposure results in injury or death. CO poisoning occurs both as the result of routine domestic, occupational, and recreational activities and in the wake of large-scale disasters such as those caused by hurricanes,[4] floods,[5] and winter storms.[6,7]

Sources of CO include faulty furnaces, inadequate ventilation of flame-based heating sources, exposure to internal combustion engine exhaust (bus exhaust from attached garages, nearby roads, or parking areas can also be a source), and tobacco smoke.[8,9] Additionally, endogenous sources have been cited (eg, hemolytic anemia and sepsis), although they rarely reach concerning levels.[3,10]

Section of Critical Care, Respiratory Institute, Medical Intensive Care Unit, Cleveland Clinic, 9500 Euclid Avenue, G6-156, Cleveland, OH 44195, USA
E-mail address: guzmanj@ccf.org

Crit Care Clin 28 (2012) 537–548
http://dx.doi.org/10.1016/j.ccc.2012.07.007
0749-0704/12/$ – see front matter © 2012 Elsevier Inc. All rights reserved.

criticalcare.theclinics.com

It is estimated that each year in the United States at least 15,200 individuals seek medical attention in an ED or miss at least 1 day of work as a result of CO poisoning.[1,11] However, this estimate does not account for the full burden of illness because the toxic effects of CO exposure are nonspecific, easily misdiagnosed, and underreported; as a result, many people with mild exposure may not seek medical attention or may be treated in the field.

According to a recent report from the US Centers for Disease Control and Prevention using data from the Nation Poison Data System, there has been a steady decline in CO exposures during the past few years. Most victims of unintentional non–fire-related exposures were treated at a health care facility. However, a significant proportion (45.1%) were managed at the site of exposure with instructions received by telephone from poison center personnel.[2] CO exposures most frequently occurred among female victims, among those younger than 17 years, and during winter months, particularly in the Midwest region of the United States. In 2005, there were 24,891 CO-related hospitalizations nationwide: 17% were confirmed, 1% was probable, and 82% were suspected CO-poisoning cases. Of the confirmed cases (1.42/100,000 population), the highest hospitalization rates occurred among male victims, older adults (aged $\geq$85 years), and Midwestern US residents.[12]

MECHANISMS OF TOXICITY/PATHOPHYSIOLOGY

CO toxicity is the result of a combination of tissue hypoxia-ischemia secondary to carboxyhemoglobin (COHb) formation and direct CO-mediated damage at a cellular level (**Fig. 1**).

CO binds hemoglobin (Hb) to form COHb with an affinity that is more than 200 times greater than that of oxygen.[13,14] The amount of COHb formed depends on the duration of the exposure to CO, the concentration of CO in the inspired air, and alveolar ventilation. Additionally, bound CO ligand at any of the 4 oxygen-binding sites of Hb results in the complex having a greater affinity for oxygen at the remaining binding sites. Therefore, oxygen bound to COHb produces a complex that impairs the release of oxygen to peripheral tissues and causes a leftward shift in the oxygen-Hb dissociation curve.[3] The increased affinity for oxygen by the COHb complex is known as the Haldane effect.[15] The aforementioned effects of CO on the Hb complex ultimately cause a decrease in oxygen availability to the tissues with resultant tissue hypoxia.

CO also binds to heme-containing proteins other than Hb. The binding to cytochrome c oxidase impairs mitochondrial function, thereby worsening tissue hypoxia.[10,16] This disturbance in electron transport increases the production of reactive oxygen species and induces oxidative stress, which in turn worsens tissue hypoxia.[3,17] Additionally, CO binds myoglobin with an affinity 40 times greater than that for oxygen, and this high affinity is even more pronounced for cardiac myoglobin.[3] The high-affinity binding to myoglobin may further reduce oxygen availability to the myocardial cells and may be responsible for arrhythmias and cardiac dysfunction.[9,18]

Furthermore, CO binds to platelet hemoproteins, and the competition with intraplatelet nitric oxide (NO) increases NO release. Excess NO produces peroxynitritie, which further impairs mitochondrial function and worsens tissue hypoxia.[19,20]

Intravascularly, CO causes platelet-to-neutrophil aggregation and release of myeloperoxidase, proteases, and reactive oxygen species, leading to oxidative stress, lipid peroxidation, and apoptosis.[19,20] These effects seem to be more pronounced within the central nervous system, where NO-mediated vasodilatation and oxidative damage may explain the clinical syndrome of delayed neurologic damage.[9]

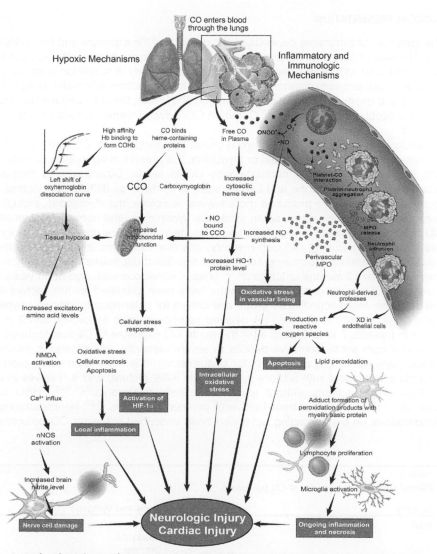

Fig. 1. Pathophysiology of CO poisoning. CO diffuses rapidly into the blood after entering through the lungs. CO causes hypoxia through the formation of COHb and a leftward shift of the oxyhemoglobin dissociation curve and the binding to heme-containing proteins, particularly cytochrome c oxidase and myoglobin. CO also causes inflammation by increasing cytosolic heme levels and the heme oxygenase-1 protein, resulting in increased intracellular oxidative stress. CO binds to platelet heme protein, causing the release of NO. Excess NO produces peroxynitrite (ONOO), which in turns impairs mitochondrial function and worsens tissue hypoxia. CO induces platelet-neutrophil aggregation and neutrophil degranulation; release of myeloperoxidase, proteases, and reactive oxygen species, which contribute to oxidative stress; lipid peroxidation; and apoptosis. The interaction of proteases with xanthine dehydrogenase in endothelial cells forms xanthine oxidase, which inhibits endogenous mechanisms against oxidative stress. Additionally, CO-induced hypoxia activates hypoxia-inducible factor 1a, which can stimulate either protective or injurious gene regulation depending on the CO dose and host factors. (*From* Weaver LK. Clinical practice. Carbon monoxide poisoning. N Engl J Med 2009;360(12):1217–25, Fig 1; with permission).

CLINICAL PRESENTATION

The spectrum of symptoms depends on the duration of the exposure and the levels of CO. The clinical effects of CO are diverse and symptoms are nonspecific and can be easily confused with other illnesses; therefore, a high index of suspicion is crucial for an appropriate and early diagnosis.[9,20] The severity ranges from mild flulike symptoms to coma and death. Because of their higher metabolic rate, the brain and the heart are most susceptible to CO toxicity.[21] Common CO-induced manifestations are listed in **Table 1**.

Headache is one of the most common presenting symptoms of CO poisoning. It is described as frontal, it can be dull or throbbing, it is present in up to 84% of victims, and its intensity does not correlate with COHb levels. Dizziness is a frequent companion of the headache and can be seen in as many as 92% of CO victims.[21] Increased CO exposure produces more severe neurologic manifestations, including confusion, syncope, seizures, acute strokelike syndromes, and coma.[9] Additionally, CO poisoning may result in neurologic sequelae, neurobehavioral changes, and cognitive impairment including reduced memory, attention disorders, impaired executive function, slow mental processing speed, and significant depression and anxiety that may persist for 12 months or longer.[22–24] Loss of consciousness, age of 36 years or older, and COHb levels of 25% or greater have been identified as risk factors for the development of cognitive sequelae and criteria for potential candidacy for hyperbaric oxygen (HBO) treatment.[25] A delayed neuropsychiatric syndrome (DNS) may occur in patients 7 to 240 days after the acute CO exposure.[26] Clinical features of DNS vary from subtle cognitive deficits to severe dementia, hallucinations, incontinence, parkinsonism, and other motor disturbances. It is more commonly seen in patients who present with a more symptomatic initial picture, and it resolves in up to 75% of the patients without additional specific treatments.[9,21,26,27] HBO has been used to prevent and treat DNS with contrasting results.[28,29] Neuropathologic abnormalities on brain imaging have also been described following CO poisoning,

Table 1 Clinical signs and symptoms of CO poisoning	
Severity	**Signs and Symptoms**
Mild	Fatigue, malaise Headache Dizziness Confusion, disorientation Blurred vision Nausea, vomiting
Moderate	Ataxia Syncope Tachypnea, dyspnea Palpitations, chest pain Rhabdomyolysis
Severe	Hypotension Cardiac arrhythmias Myocardial ischemia Coma Respiratory depression Noncardiogenic pulmonary edema Seizures

involving the basal ganglia (particularly globus pallidus lesions in cases of severe poisoning) and delayed atrophy of the corpus callosum.[22,30–32]

Cardiovascular effects of CO poisoning are common. Following acute exposure, tachycardia is frequently observed and considered a compensatory response to systemic hypoxia and cardiac dysfunction.[18] COHb, even at low levels, exacerbates myocardial ischemia, and cardiac necrosis can occur even in the absence of cardiac symptoms.[33] Conversely, elevations of cardiac biomarkers with normal coronary arteries are frequently observed in response to an acute CO exposure. Additionally, mild to moderate abnormalities in left ventricular function or structure have been described, and they have been correlated to the COHb level and the duration of the CO exposure.[34,35] Cardiac arrhythmias (either supraventricular or ventricular) have also been described and are likely secondary to CO-induced changes in cardiac conduction, cardiac ischemia, or myocardial cell hypoxia. In contrast to ventricular dysfunction, however, no correlation has been noted between COHb levels and electrocardiographic alterations.[18,34,36]

CO intoxication during pregnancy deserves particular attention because adverse fetal outcomes following accidental CO exposure have been reported.[37] Fetal tissues are more susceptible to hypoxia; furthermore, CO binds more tightly to fetal Hb and the elimination of CO by the fetus lags behind that of the mother.[9,38] As a consequence, low-level exposure, which may be inconsequential for the mother, can present greater risk for the fetus. Thus, prolonged oxygen therapy is necessary and HBO should be considered.

Rhadomyolysis and renal failure,[39–41] noncardiogenic pulmonary edema,[42] and cutaneous blisters[43,44] have also been described following an acute exposure to CO. On the other hand, the "cherry red" skin color classically attributed to CO poisoning is uncommon in clinical practice.[9,42]

DIAGNOSIS

Timely diagnosis of CO poisoning is critical, albeit challenging, because the clinical presentation is nonspecific and can mimic that of influenza or other viral illnesses. A high index of suspicion and consideration of the circumstances and environmental factors suggestive of exposure are therefore of paramount importance.[2,9,20,21] Source identification is important in cases of nonintentional poisoning to limit the risk to others. In the absence of exposure history, CO poisoning must be considered when 2 or more patients are similarly or simultaneously sick. Concomitant cyanide toxicity should be considered in patients with CO poisoning after smoke inhalation.

COHb levels should be promptly obtained in patients suspected of CO exposure. COHb levels depend on the magnitude of the exposure (ambient CO concentration and the duration of the exposure), alveolar ventilation, blood volume, and metabolic activity.[45] A COHb level greater than 3% in nonsmokers and greater than 10% in smokers confirms CO exposure; however, levels correlate poorly with the clinical picture.[20,46,47] COHb can be interchangeably monitored with use of arterial or venous blood samples.[48] Nonetheless, measurements should be performed with spectrophotometric CO-oximetry (a multiwavelength spectrophotometric method capable of separately quantifying COHb, oxyhemoglobin, and reduced Hb).[49,50] Unfortunately, COHb measurements are not always readily available (only half of acute care hospitals in a 4-state area were found to have the capability to measure COHb levels), and delays in treatment may occur.[51]

Pulse oximetry is unreliable in assessing oxygenation in CO-exposed patients because dual-wavelength spectrophotometry, the method used in most pulse oximeters, cannot distinguish between oxyhemoglobin and COHb. Pulse oximetry, therefore, overestimates arterial oxygenation in patients with severe CO poisoning. On the other hand, the difference in arterial saturation observed with pulse oximetry versus an in vitro assessment of oxyhemoglobin saturation (pulse oximetry gap) correlates with the COHb level and may be a cue to raise the suspicion of CO intoxication.[52–54] Newly available multiwavelength pulse CO-oximeters have not been reliable for quantifying COHb.[49,50]

As described, CO lowers the threshold for cardiac ischemia and predisposes to myocardial dysfunction and cardiac arrhythmias[18,34,36]; therefore, cardiac function must be closely monitored with the use of electrocardiography, echocardiography, and cardiac biomarkers. If results are abnormal, cardiology consultation is recommended.

Plasma biomarkers have not been found to be useful in correlating the severity of the exposure, the clinical course, or the development of late complications.[55] Conversely, a high blood lactate level on presentation was more frequently associated with altered mental status and high COHb levels and was independently associated with serious complications and the need for intensive care unit admission.[56]

Neuropsychological testing has been proposed to assess and quantify the degree of neurologic injury following CO exposure and the need for HBO[57,58]; however, this has limitations and is not widely used.[59] Neuroimaging, on the other hand, has been more broadly studied. Structural changes of the brain delineated by computed tomography, particularly bilateral globus pallidus low-density lesions and symmetric and diffuse hypodensity in the cerebral white matter, have been well described.[60–62] These lesions may appear several days after the CO exposure and may resolve with time. The clinical prognosis seems mostly associated with the severity of the cerebral white matter changes but not the size of the low-density abnormalities of the globus pallidus.[61] Nevertheless, patients with any kind of abnormal neuroimaging findings are more likely to have poorer long-term neurologic outcomes. Magnetic resonance imaging and functional (single-photon emission computed tomography) imaging are also used to assess CO-induced neurologic injuries but are less widely available.[9,30]

TREATMENT

Field treatment of the CO-poisoned patient consists of removal of the patient from the source of exposure, immediate administration of 100% high-flow supplemental oxygen, and transport to a hospital, where aggressive supportive measures, including airway and cardiovascular support, can be provided.[9,20,21] The administration of oxygen speeds the elimination of CO from the body. Without oxygen therapy, the elimination half-life of CO is 4 to 5 hours.[47,63] Supplementation with 100% oxygen via a tight-fitting mask at normal atmospheric pressure (NBO) decreases the half-life by approximately half,[47,64] whereas the use of hyperbaric oxygen (HBO) at 2.5 atm decreases it to less than 30 minutes.[47] NBO should be administered before laboratory confirmation when CO poisoning is suspected. Once the diagnosis is confirmed, oxygen therapy and observation must continue long enough to prevent delayed sequelae as COHb unloads.[65] Although there are no guidelines indicating the recommended duration of the NBO treatment, up to 24 hours for patients with minor neurologic symptoms and up to 72 hours for those with major neurologic symptoms have been proposed.[66]

HBO has been used for severe CO poisoning for decades; however, its indication remains controversial.[59,67–70] Proposed mechanisms by which HBO reduces tissue hypoxia are decreasing the elimination half-life of COHb, increasing the fraction of oxygen dissolved in plasma, preventing leukocyte-mediated inflammatory changes, improving mitochondrial oxidative processes, and decreasing cerebral edema by inducing vasoconstriction.[71] Despite the controversy, a significant number of patients receive HBO for CO poisoning in the United States.[68] Proponents of HBO recommend its use in patients presenting with severe neurologic or cardiovascular symptoms and very high COHb levels (>25%), citing reversal of neurologic injury or decreased incidence of DNS as a beneficial effect.[29,66] However, several randomized trials have failed to show any favorable effects.[72–74]

A recent clinical policy statement by the American College of Emergency Physicians concluded that HBO is a therapeutic option for CO-poisoned patients; however, its use could not be mandated. Furthermore, the American College of Emergency Physicians subcommittee failed to identify clinical variables, including COHb levels, that could identify a subgroup of poisoned patients for whom HBO would provide benefit or harm.[47] After recently evaluating 6 randomized controlled trials, authors of a Cochrane review concluded that existing evidence does not establish whether the administration of HBO for CO poisoning reduces the incidence of adverse neurologic outcomes.[70] Unfortunately, there is considerable heterogeneity among the trials reviewed; thus, the conclusions have to be carefully interpreted. The most apparent differences among these studies that may explain the contrasts in the observed outcomes after the use of HBO have been the duration of the CO exposure, the type of CO exposure (accidental or suicidal), the time interval between the exposure and the initiation of HBO therapy, the severity of the clinical presentation, the number and duration of treatments, the level of atmosphere absolute used, follow-up duration, and neurologic outcomes tracking.[71,74]

If a decision is made to provide HBO treatment, comatose patients with acute nonsuicidal CO poisoning and COHb greater than 25% may be the most suitable candidates. One HBO session at 2 atmosphere absolute initiated within 12 hours after the end of CO exposure may be the best approach.[66,74] The use of HBO in pregnant women deserves special mention. Pregnancy was an exclusion criterion in most of the randomized trials comparing HBO to NBO; thus, existing data are limited to small case reports.[75–77] Nevertheless, because of the potential benefit to the mother and the fetus and the difficulty of assessing intrauterine hypoxia, HBO should be considered when treating CO-poisoned pregnant women.[75,77]

No data exist on children younger than 15 years supporting the use of HBO in this population. Side effects of HBO include painful barotrauma (ears and sinuses) and, less commonly, oxygen toxicity, seizures, pulmonary edema, and decompression sickness.[9,45]

DISPOSITION/PREVENTION

No definitive guideline exists on how to triage patients with CO poisoning, although most patients can be managed in the ED because most symptoms improve with NBO. As a general approach, patients with minor symptoms should receive NBO in the ED until their COHb levels decrease to less than 10% and symptoms resolve. Patients with more severe or nonresolving symptoms, higher COHb levels, and major comorbidities should be hospitalized. Because many hospitals lack the ability to measure COHb,[51] clinicians practicing in such hospitals should consider the transfer of patients with severe intoxication to high-complexity medical centers with COHb-monitoring capabilities and access to HBO if needed.

CO poisoning can be entirely preventable by the correct installation, maintenance, and operation of combustion devices that may emit CO, combined with the appropriate use of home CO monitors, which are inexpensive and widely available.

Prevention strategies aimed at the general public are available from the US Environmental Protection Agency and the Centers for Disease Control and Prevention.[8,78]

SUMMARY

CO poisoning is common, potentially fatal, and frequently underdiagnosed because of its nonspecific clinical presentation. Immediate NBO with the highest possible fraction of inspired oxygen should be administered to patients with suspected poisoning, and aggressive supportive treatment should be promptly instituted. Diagnosis of CO exposure should be made by COHb measurement using multiwavelength spectrophotometry (CO-oximetry). The use of HBO is controversial and, if used, should be relegated for those patients presenting with severe symptoms, high COHb levels, or pregnancy. The source of CO should be identified and corrected.

REFERENCES

1. Centers for Disease Control and Prevention (CDC). Carbon monoxide–related deaths–United States, 1999-2004. MMWR Morb Mortal Wkly Rep 2007;56(50): 1309–12.
2. Centers for Disease Control and Prevention (CDC). Carbon monoxide exposures–United States, 2000-2009. MMWR Morb Mortal Wkly Rep 2011;60(30): 1014–7.
3. Omaye ST. Metabolic modulation of carbon monoxide toxicity. Toxicology 2002; 180(2):139–50.
4. Centers for Disease Control and Prevention (CDC). Carbon monoxide poisoning after hurricane Katrina–Alabama, Louisiana, and Mississippi, August-September 2005. MMWR Morb Mortal Wkly Rep 2005;54(39):996–8.
5. Centers for Disease Control and Prevention (CDC). Public health consequences of a flood disaster–Iowa, 1993. MMWR Morb Mortal Wkly Rep 1993;42(34):653–6.
6. Broder J, Mehrotra A, Tintinalli J. Injuries from the 2002 North Carolina ice storm, and strategies for prevention. Injury 2005;36(1):21–6.
7. Daley WR, Smith A, Paz-Argandona E, et al. An outbreak of carbon monoxide poisoning after a major ice storm in Maine. J Emerg Med 2000;18(1):87–93.
8. US Environmental Protection Agency. Carbon monoxide. An introduction to indoor air quality (IAQ). Available at: http://www.epa.gov/iaq/co.html#area. Accessed December 28, 2011.
9. Kao LW, Nanagas KA. Toxicity associated with carbon monoxide. Clin Lab Med 2006;26(1):99–125.
10. Bauer I, Pannen BH. Bench-to-bedside review: Carbon monoxide–from mitochondrial poisoning to therapeutic use. Crit Care 2009;13(4):220.
11. Centers for Disease Control, Prevention (CDC). Unintentional non-fire-related carbon monoxide exposures–United States, 2001-2003. MMWR Morb Mortal Wkly Rep 2005;54(2):36–9.
12. Iqbal S, Law HZ, Clower JH, et al. Hospital burden of unintentional carbon monoxide poisoning in the United States, 2007. Am J Emerg Med 2012;30(5): 657–64 [Epub 2011 May 12].
13. Haab P. The effect of carbon monoxide on respiration. Experientia 1990; 46(11–12):1202–6.
14. Hess W. Affinity of oxygen for hemoglobin–its significance under physiological and pathological conditions. Anaesthesist 1987;36(9):455–67.

15. Collier CR. Oxygen affinity of human blood in presence of carbon monoxide. J Appl Physiol 1976;40(3):487–90.
16. Alonso JR, Cardellach F, Lopez S, et al. Carbon monoxide specifically inhibits cytochrome c oxidase of human mitochondrial respiratory chain. Pharmacol Toxicol 2003;93(3):142–6.
17. Miro O, Cardellach F, Alonso JR, et al. Physiopathology of acute carbon monoxide poisoning. Med Clin (Barc) 2000;114(17):678.
18. Gandini C, Castoldi AF, Candura SM, et al. Carbon monoxide cardiotoxicity. J Toxicol Clin Toxicol 2001;39(1):35–44.
19. Thom SR, Bhopale VM, Han S, et al. Intravascular neutrophil activation due to carbon monoxide poisoning. Am J Respir Crit Care Med 2006;174(11):1239–48.
20. Weaver LK. Clinical practice. Carbon monoxide poisoning. N Engl J Med 2009; 360(12):1217–25.
21. Prockop LD, Chichkova RI. Carbon monoxide intoxication: an updated review. J Neurol Sci 2007;262(1–2):122–30.
22. Hopkins RO, Fearing MA, Weaver LK, et al. Basal ganglia lesions following carbon monoxide poisoning. Brain Inj 2006;20(3):273–81.
23. Jasper BW, Hopkins RO, Duker HV, et al. Affective outcome following carbon monoxide poisoning: a prospective longitudinal study. Cogn Behav Neurol 2005;18(2):127–34.
24. Bourgeois JA. Amnesia after carbon monoxide poisoning. Am J Psychiatry 2000; 157(11):1884–5.
25. Weaver LK, Valentine KJ, Hopkins RO. Carbon monoxide poisoning: risk factors for cognitive sequelae and the role of hyperbaric oxygen. Am J Respir Crit Care Med 2007;176(5):491–7.
26. Choi IS. Delayed neurologic sequelae in carbon monoxide intoxication. Arch Neurol 1983;40(7):433–5.
27. Bhatia R, Chacko F, Lal V, et al. Reversible delayed neuropsychiatric syndrome following acute carbon monoxide exposure. Indian J Occup Environ Med 2007; 11(2):80–2.
28. Gilmer B, Kilkenny J, Tomaszewski C, et al. Hyperbaric oxygen does not prevent neurologic sequelae after carbon monoxide poisoning. Acad Emerg Med 2002; 9(1):1–8.
29. Chang DC, Lee JT, Lo CP, et al. Hyperbaric oxygen ameliorates delayed neuropsychiatric syndrome of carbon monoxide poisoning. Undersea Hyperb Med 2010;37(1):23–33.
30. Hopkins RO, Woon FL. Neuroimaging, cognitive, and neurobehavioral outcomes following carbon monoxide poisoning. Behav Cogn Neurosci Rev 2006;5(3): 141–55.
31. Pulsipher DT, Hopkins RO, Weaver LK. Basal ganglia volumes following CO poisoning: a prospective longitudinal study. Undersea Hyperb Med 2006;33(4): 245–56.
32. Porter SS, Hopkins RO, Weaver LK, et al. Corpus callosum atrophy and neuropsychological outcome following carbon monoxide poisoning. Arch Clin Neuropsychol 2002;17(2):195–204.
33. Marius-Nunez AL. Myocardial infarction with normal coronary arteries after acute exposure to carbon monoxide. Chest 1990;97(2):491–4.
34. Kalay N, Ozdogru I, Cetinkaya Y, et al. Cardiovascular effects of carbon monoxide poisoning. Am J Cardiol 2007;99(3):322–4.
35. Chamberland DL, Wilson BD, Weaver LK. Transient cardiac dysfunction in acute carbon monoxide poisoning. Am J Med 2004;117(8):623–5.

36. Hanci V, Ayoglu H, Yurtlu S, et al. Effects of acute carbon monoxide poisoning on the P-wave and QT interval dispersions. Anadolu Kardiyol Derg 2011;11(1): 48–52.

37. Koren G, Sharav T, Pastuszak A, et al. A multicenter, prospective study of fetal outcome following accidental carbon monoxide poisoning in pregnancy. Reprod Toxicol 1991;5(5):397–403.

38. Margulies JL. Acute carbon monoxide poisoning during pregnancy. Am J Emerg Med 1986;4(6):516–9.

39. Florkowski CM, Rossi ML, Carey MP, et al. Rhabdomyolysis and acute renal failure following carbon monoxide poisoning: two case reports with muscle histopathology and enzyme activities. J Toxicol Clin Toxicol 1992;30(3): 443–54.

40. Jha R, Kher V, Kale SA, et al. Carbon monoxide poisoning: an unusual cause of acute renal failure. Ren Fail 1994;16(6):775–9.

41. Santos I, Amigo C. Rhabdomyolysis and carbon monoxide poisoning. An Med Interna 1998;15(7):397.

42. Thom SR. Smoke inhalation. Emerg Med Clin North Am 1989;7(2):371–87.

43. He H, Gao Y, Li C, et al. Cutaneous blistering secondary to acute carbon-monoxide intoxication. Clin Exp Dermatol 2007;32(1):129–31.

44. Torne R, Soyer HP, Leb G, et al. Skin lesions in carbon monoxide intoxication. Dermatologica 1991;183(3):212–5.

45. Weaver LK. Hyperbaric oxygen in the critically ill. Crit Care Med 2011;39(7): 1784–91.

46. Hampson NB, Hauff NM. Carboxyhemoglobin levels in carbon monoxide poisoning: do they correlate with the clinical picture? Am J Emerg Med 2008; 26(6):665–9.

47. Wolf SJ, Lavonas EJ, Sloan EP, et al. Clinical policy: critical issues in the management of adult patients presenting to the emergency department with acute carbon monoxide poisoning. Ann Emerg Med 2008;51(2):138–52.

48. Touger M, Gallagher EJ, Tyrell J. Relationship between venous and arterial carboxyhemoglobin levels in patients with suspected carbon monoxide poisoning. Ann Emerg Med 1995;25(4):481–3.

49. Touger M, Birnbaum A, Wang J, et al. Performance of the RAD-57 pulse CO-oximeter compared with standard laboratory carboxyhemoglobin measurement. Ann Emerg Med 2010;56(4):382–8.

50. Maisel WH, Lewis RJ. Noninvasive measurement of carboxyhemoglobin: how accurate is accurate enough? Ann Emerg Med 2010;56(4):389–91.

51. Hampson NB, Scott KL, Zmaeff JL. Carboxyhemoglobin measurement by hospitals: implications for the diagnosis of carbon monoxide poisoning. J Emerg Med 2006;31(1):13–6.

52. Hampson NB. Pulse oximetry in severe carbon monoxide poisoning. Chest 1998; 114(4):1036–41.

53. Bozeman WP, Myers RA, Barish RA. Confirmation of the pulse oximetry gap in carbon monoxide poisoning. Ann Emerg Med 1997;30(5):608–11.

54. Bozeman WP, Hampson NB. Pulse oximetry in CO poisoning-additional data. Chest 2000;117(1):295–6.

55. Thom SR, Bhopale VM, Milovanova TM, et al. Plasma biomarkers in carbon monoxide poisoning. Clin Toxicol (Phila) 2010;48(1):47–56.

56. Moon JM, Shin MH, Chun BJ. The value of initial lactate in patients with carbon monoxide intoxication: in the emergency department. Hum Exp Toxicol 2011; 30(8):836–43.

57. Messier LD, Myers RA. A neuropsychological screening battery for emergency assessment of carbon-monoxide-poisoned patients. J Clin Psychol 1991;47(5): 675–84.
58. Vieregge P, Klostermann W, Blumm RG, et al. Carbon monoxide poisoning: clinical, neurophysiological, and brain imaging observations in acute disease and follow-up. J Neurol 1989;236(8):478–81.
59. Seger D, Welch L. Carbon monoxide controversies: neuropsychologic testing, mechanism of toxicity, and hyperbaric oxygen. Ann Emerg Med 1994;24(2):242–8.
60. Klostermann W, Vieregge P, Bruckmann H. Carbon monoxide poisoning: the importance of computed and magnetic resonance tomographic cranial findings for the clinical picture and follow-up. Rofo 1993;159(4):361–7.
61. Miura T, Mitomo M, Kawai R, et al. CT of the brain in acute carbon monoxide intoxication: characteristic features and prognosis. AJNR Am J Neuroradiol 1985;6(5): 739–42.
62. Zeiss J, Brinker R. Role of contrast enhancement in cerebral CT of carbon monoxide poisoning. J Comput Assist Tomogr 1988;12(2):341–3.
63. Peterson JE, Stewart RD. Absorption and elimination of carbon monoxide by inactive young men. Arch Environ Health 1970;21(2):165–71.
64. Weaver LK, Howe S, Hopkins R, et al. Carboxyhemoglobin half-life in carbon monoxide-poisoned patients treated with 100% oxygen at atmospheric pressure. Chest 2000;117(3):801–8.
65. Varon J, Marik PE, Fromm RE Jr, et al. Carbon monoxide poisoning: a review for clinicians. J Emerg Med 1999;17(1):87–93.
66. Bentur Y. Hyperbaric oxygen for carbon monoxide poisoning. Toxicol Rev 2005; 24(3):153–4 [discussion: 159–60].
67. Buckley NA, Isbister GK, Stokes B, et al. Hyperbaric oxygen for carbon monoxide poisoning: a systematic review and critical analysis of the evidence. Toxicol Rev 2005;24(2):75–92.
68. Hampson NB, Little CE. Hyperbaric treatment of patients with carbon monoxide poisoning in the United States. Undersea Hyperb Med 2005;32(1):21–6.
69. Weaver LK, Hopkins RO, Larson-Lohr V. Carbon monoxide poisoning: a review of human outcome studies comparing normobaric oxygen with hyperbaric oxygen. Ann Emerg Med 1995;25(2):271–2.
70. Buckley NA, Juurlink DN, Isbister G, et al. Hyperbaric oxygen for carbon monoxide poisoning. Cochrane Database Syst Rev 2011;(4):CD002041.
71. Domachevsky L, Adir Y, Grupper M, et al. Hyperbaric oxygen in the treatment of carbon monoxide poisoning. Clin Toxicol (Phila) 2005;43(3):181–8.
72. Raphael JC, Elkharrat D, Jars-Guincestre MC, et al. Trial of normobaric and hyperbaric oxygen for acute carbon monoxide intoxication. Lancet 1989; 2(8660):414–9.
73. Scheinkestel CD, Bailey M, Myles PS, et al. Hyperbaric or normobaric oxygen for acute carbon monoxide poisoning: a randomized controlled clinical trial. Undersea Hyperb Med 2000;27(3):163–4.
74. Annane D, Chadda K, Gajdos P, et al. Hyperbaric oxygen therapy for acute domestic carbon monoxide poisoning: two randomized controlled trials. Intensive Care Med 2011;37(3):486–92.
75. Elkharrat D, Raphael JC, Korach JM, et al. Acute carbon monoxide intoxication and hyperbaric oxygen in pregnancy. Intensive Care Med 1991;17(5):289–92.
76. Brown DB, Mueller GL, Golich FC. Hyperbaric oxygen treatment for carbon monoxide poisoning in pregnancy: a case report. Aviat Space Environ Med 1992;63(11):1011–4.

77. Van Hoesen KB, Camporesi EM, Moon RE, et al. Should hyperbaric oxygen be used to treat the pregnant patient for acute carbon monoxide poisoning? A case report and literature review. JAMA 1989;261(7):1039–43.
78. Centers for Disease Control and Prevention. Carbon monoxide poisoning. Prevention guidance. You can prevent carbon monoxide exposure. Available at: http://www.cdc.gov/co/guidelines.htm. Accessed January 11, 2012.

Alcohol Withdrawal Syndrome

Richard W. Carlson, MD, PhD[a,b,c,]*, Nivedita N. Kumar, MD[d],
Edna Wong-Mckinstry, MD[e,f], Srikala Ayyagari, MD[g],
Nitin Puri, MD[h], Frank K. Jackson[a,k],
Shivaramaiah Shashikumar, MD[i,j]

KEYWORDS

- Alcohol withdrawal syndrome • Alcoholism • Intensive care
- Alcohol-related disease

KEY POINTS

- Alcohol abuse and the societal and economic costs of alcohol dependency are major problems in both the United States and throughout the world.
- In susceptible patients, alcohol withdrawal syndrome (AWS) is often precipitated by other medical or surgical disorders, and AWS can adversely affect the course of these underlying conditions.
- Although the mortality rate of AWS has decreased over the past few decades, significant risk for morbidity and death remain if conditions such as multiple trauma, severe sepsis, acute respiratory failure, and alcoholic liver disease complicate management.

Alcohol abuse and the societal and economic costs of alcohol dependency are major problems in both the United States and throughout the world.[1] More than 8 million Americans are dependent on alcohol; twice the number who abuse illicit drugs.[2] Alcohol abuse is associated with 85,000 deaths in the United States annually as well as additional morbidity and mortality related to accidents, suicides, family abuse, and other problems. The combined costs of alcohol abuse in the United States reach

The authors have no disclosures.
[a] Department of Medicine, Maricopa Medical Center, Phoenix, AZ 85008, USA; [b] Department of Internal Medicine, College of Medicine, University of Arizona, Phoenix, AZ, USA; [c] Department of Internal Medicine, Mayo Clinic College of Medicine, Scottsdale, AZ, USA; [d] Department of Medicine, Legacy Salmon Creek Medical Center, Vancouver, WA, USA; [e] Department of Medicine, University of Arizona, Tucson, AZ, USA; [f] Internal Medicine Department, College of Medicine, University of Arizona, 1501 North Campbell Avenue, Room 6408, Tucson, AZ 85724-5040, USA; [g] Department of Hospital Medicine, University of California San Diego School of Medicine, 200 West Arbor Drive, #8485, San Diego, CA 92103, USA; [h] Department of Internal Medicine, Inova Fairfax Hospital, Virginia Commonwealth University, Falls Church, VA, USA; [i] Department of Medicine, St John's Mercy Medical Center, St. Louis University, St Louis, MO, USA; [j] Mercy Critical Care Training Program, Critical Care Medicine, Saint Louis University, 621 South New Ballas Road, Suite 4006, Tower B, St Louis, MO 63141, USA; [k] Midwestern University, Glendale, Arizona
* Corresponding author. Department of Medicine, Maricopa Medical Center, 2nd Floor, 2601 Roosevelt, Phoenix, AZ 85008.
E-mail address: richardw_carlson@dmgaz.org

200 billion dollars each year.[3–6] Up to 40% of all emergency department patients have alcohol in their system, 10% of whom have blood alcohol levels above legal limits.[7] Once admitted, 8% of patients of general hospitals have been shown to exhibit signs and symptoms of the alcohol withdrawal syndrome (AWS), and the prevalence of these admissions to an intensive care unit (ICU) of inner-city public hospitals may exceed 20%.[8–11] Alcohol abuse directly or indirectly leads to acute and chronic conditions that affect all organ systems, and alcohol-use disorders are particularly common in critically ill patients.[10–15] In the susceptible patient AWS is often precipitated by other medical or surgical disorders with adverse effects on the course of both comorbid conditions and AWS.

This review of AWS focuses on the scope of the clinical problem, historical features, pathophysiology, clinical presentation, and approaches to therapy, with particular emphasis on severe AWS that requires ICU management.

SCOPE OF THE PROBLEM

All clinicians are likely to encounter AWS, especially those involved in emergency medicine, inpatient care, and ICU care. It has been estimated that 500,000 episodes of AWS require pharmacologic therapy each year in the United States.[2] Many patients with mild signs and symptoms can be managed as outpatients or referred to detoxification centers[16–23]; however, a significant number will present with more severe findings, often with comorbid psychiatric, medical, or surgical conditions, requiring evaluation and assessment in an emergency setting and hospital admission.[8,9,14,21–23]

For those admitted, a significant proportion may require ICU management. In a review of 279 episodes of severe AWS in a public hospital over an interval of more than 2 years, approximately one-third required ICU management.[24] Marik and colleagues[10,25] found that more than 20% of patients in an inner-city hospital required ICU admission, and Mostafa and colleagues[26] reported a similarly high percentage of admissions to an adult ICU for alcohol-associated problems. A high proportion of acute surgical, burn, and trauma patients will also exhibit signs and symptoms of AWS that have a significant impact on the management of their surgical problems.[12,26–29]

Disorders related to alcohol use have an unfavorable effect on the severity and outcome of a variety of medical and surgical conditions, particularly infections.[30–41]

MEDICAL AND SOCIAL HISTORICAL PERSPECTIVE

Alcohol abuse, including acute intoxication as well as AWS, no doubt has existed since the discovery of alcohol. Patrick McGovern of the University of Pennsylvania describes that in China 9000 years ago, stone-age inhabitants developed a mead from fermented honey and fruit with up to 10% alcohol content.[42] Brewing and wine making were common throughout much of the Greco-Roman world.[43] The Romans had a god of wine (Bacchus) and were more than familiar with both the acute effects of alcohol intoxication and the consequences of chronic use (**Fig. 1**).[44] The Latin term *morbis convivialis* was coined during this period to describe the harmful effects of wine as a result of excess partying.[45] Hippocrates described "anxiety, yawning, rigor" as consequences of drinking; problems which could be healed by drinking wine mixed with an equal portion of water.[46]

Adverse effects of alcohol were well known in the Middle Ages, as chronicled in 1314 by the famous physician John of Gaddesden (1280–1360) who was mentioned in *The Canterbury Tales*. "The adult must avoid immoderate drinking, because drunkenness is extremely harmful."[47] During the seventeenth century William Hogarth (1697–1764) vividly depicted the effects of excess alcohol in his paintings and

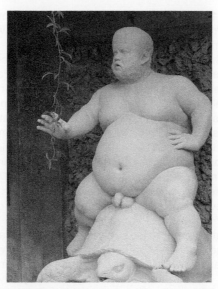

Fig. 1. Valerio Cioli's statue of Bacchus (*Fontana del Bacchino*), Roman god of wine, located in Boboli Gardens, Florence, Italy.

engravings such as *Beer Street* and *Gin Lane* (**Fig. 2**). Such works depict a period in which alcohol consumption by modern standards was excessive.[43,48,49] Continuing into the eighteenth century, alcohol abuse was common in Europe and was especially prevalent in Sweden. The term "chronic alcoholism," together with some of its medical complications, was described by the Swedish physician and temperance leader Magnus Huss (1807–1890).[50] His accounts of alcohol withdrawal included "tremors of the lips and tongue and sometimes of the whole body." Yet some 40 years earlier it was

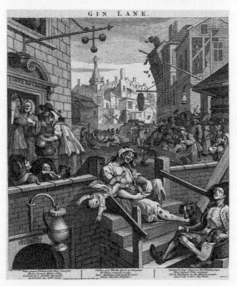

Fig. 2. William Hogarth's seventeenth-century etching *Gin Lane*.

Thomas Sutton (1767–1835) who coined the term delirium tremens from the Latin as "trembling delirium," followed by James Ware (1795–1864) who provided a more complete clinical description of AWS in 1836.[51,52]

During the nineteenth century many investigators wrote of alcohol abuse, and some succumbed to AWS themselves, as in the case of Edgar Allen Poe (1809–1849). In *Our Mutual Friend* and other novels, Charles Dickens (1812–1870) described many of the detrimental effects of alcoholism.[53] These and other writings and lectures of Victorian times depicted the evils of alcohol in Europe and the United States and helped foment the rise of the temperance movement, culminating in the founding of the Women's Christian Temperance Union (WCTU) in 1874 and ultimately the passage of the 18th Amendment to the Constitution, or Volstead Act, establishing prohibition in the United States in 1920. The "noble experiment" lasted until 1933. The effects on alcohol consumption and abuse during this period in the United States were often negligible. Instead, the era fostered illicit production, distribution, and use of alcohol, and the rise of organized crime.[54,55]

Throughout the twentieth century the subject of alcohol abuse was prevalent in literature and art, and some of the descriptions of alcoholism and withdrawal were accurate and insightful. A variety of artists, authors, actors, and prominent individuals have been associated with alcohol abuse, including O. Henry, Dylan Thomas, Eugene O'Neill, John Cheever, Raymond Chandler, and Tennessee Williams among many others.[56] In 1945 the Warner Brothers movie *Lost Weekend* tragically detailed the life of an alcoholic played by Ray Milland who is shown to suffer hallucinations and severe agitation. Other films and television dramas, such as *Days of Wine and Roses,* depicted the descent into alcoholism and withdrawal.

Although portrayals of the effects of alcohol abuse could be found in literature as well as films and television, public figures largely guarded their privacy regarding complications of alcoholism until Betty Ford (1918–2011), wife of President Gerald Ford, described her alcohol and drug addiction in 1987. Kitty Dukakis, the wife of a presidential candidate and Massachusetts governor, was hospitalized in 1989 with complications of alcohol abuse and withdrawal. In 1991 she published a memoir (*Now You Know*) describing her battle with alcohol. Both women were instrumental in subsequently fostering drug and alcohol treatment centers that now bear their names.

Acquisition of scientific as well as societal knowledge of AWS has been a slow and evolutionary process. In the first years of the eighteenth century the Scottish physician Thomas Trotter (1760–1832) was the first to characterize excessive drinking as a disease or medical condition.[57] Benjamin Rush (1746–1813), the physician-signer of the Declaration of Independence, identified alcoholism as a "loss of control" and used the term addiction in describing alcohol abuse. He is thought to have regarded alcoholism as a disease, recommending abstinence as the cure.[58]

The keen diagnostician and clinician, William Osler (1849–1919), made several crucial observations and comments regarding AWS and its management that were ahead of his time:

Delirium tremens (mania a pofu) is really only an incident in the history of chronic alcoholism, and results from the long-continued action of the poison on the brain…. A spree in a temperate person, no matter how prolonged, is rarely if ever followed by delirium tremens…. It sometimes develops in consequence of the sudden withdrawal of the alcohol…. At the onset of the attack the patient is restless and depressed and sleeps badly…. after a day or two the characteristic delirium sets in…the patient talks constantly and incoherently; he is incessantly in motion… hallucinations of sight and hearing develop…there is much muscular tremor…the pulse is soft and rapid…there is usually fever…the tremor persists for some days...by far the most common error is to overlook some local disease, such as pneumonia...or an accident as a fractured rib...in every instance a careful examination should be made, particularly of the lungs...should convulsions supervene, chloroform may be carefully administered... in the acute, violent alcoholic mania the hypodermic injection of apomorphia... is usually very effectual... withdrawal of the alcohol is the first essential... most effectively accomplished by placing the patient in an institution, in which he can be carefully watched during the trying period of the first week or ten days of abstention... for the sleeplessness the bromides or hyoscine may be employed... prolonged seclusion in a suitable institution is in reality the only effectual means of cure... in delirium tremens the patient should be confined to bed and carefully watched night and day... delirium tremens is a disease which in a large majority of cases runs a course very slightly influenced by medicine... the indications for treatment are to procure sleep.... Chloral is often of great service and may be given without hesitation... opium must be used cautiously....[59]

Over the past century, treatment of AWS has been facilitated by advances in pharmacology. The sedative, chloral hydrate, was available during the late 1800s, including illicit use as "knockout drops." As noted by Osler, the drug was used to control agitation and other signs and symptoms of AWS, and remained a standard approach to pharmacologic management of AWS for many years.[60-63] Chloral hydrate and its active metabolite, trichloroethanol, has been subsequently found to have barbiturate-like effects on γ-aminobutyric acid (GABA)-A receptors.[61,62] Paraldehyde was first introduced in clinical medicine in the 1880s but was not routinely given for treatment of delirium tremens until decades later. Paraldehyde can be administered orally, rectally, intravenously, or intramuscularly, although the latter route is painful and may lead to tissue necrosis and sterile abscesses. Because of its metabolism and excretion, paraldehyde can readily be detected on the breath. Wards for alcohol detoxification could easily be identified by their distinctive odor. Despite these limitations, paraldehyde was a standard agent in the management of AWS until the 1970s.[60,63-66]

The parent compound of barbiturates, barbituric acid, was first synthesized in the nineteenth century and spawned a variety of barbiturate products. Phenobarbital is one of the most common drugs of this class of sedatives, and remains a useful agent in the management of AWS.[67-69] A huge number of sedative, antiadrenergic, analgesic, antipsychotic, antihistaminic, anticonvulsant, and hypnotic agents, including phenothiazine heterocyclic compounds such as promazine and chlorpromazine, have been used in the treatment of AWS.[70-75] Since the early 1960s the benzodiazepines have become the most prescribed agents for AWS, although there is ongoing evaluation of agents that may be useful in the management of this syndrome. Magnesium, other electrolytes, and vitamins are also routinely supplemented. Techniques to identify and score severity of AWS and to titrate sedation have facilitated management.[76-86]

The recognition of alcohol-use disorders as disease entities as well as their clinical description dates from 1935 with the founding of Alcoholics Anonymous (AA), initially as the Oxford Group, with religious ties, but subsequently expanded with a more secular emphasis. AA famously developed the 12-step program that emphasizes abstinence.[54] The organization has had broad lay support, and has helped increase awareness of alcohol-use disorders and the concept that alcoholism is a clinical entity. Terminology has evolved and been refined over the past several decades, and scientifically based medical management of withdrawal and alcohol-use disorders can be traced to the mid-twentieth century. Treatment also has been facilitated by advances in the pharmacology of sedative agents.

Although organized detoxification and rehabilitation efforts could be found in the late 1940s with sites such as the Stella Maris Center in Cleveland, widespread availability of such centers are of more recent origin.[16–20,54]

Yet it was not until 1956 that the American Medical Association (AMA) declared alcoholism a disease, and eventually in 1971 the National Conference of Commissioners on Uniform State Laws adopted the Uniform Alcoholism and Intoxication Treatment Act. This Act led to the increase in prevalence and acceptance of detoxification programs. Following AA's promotion of alcohol abuse as a medical disorder, the publication of The Disease Concept of Alcoholism by E.M. Jellinek in 1960 was a powerful factor in the acceptance of this concept and the implementation of programs that offered specific medical management.[87–89] Jellinek (1890–1963), who originally trained as a plant physiologist, was a pioneering researcher at the Yale Center for Alcohol Studies and wrote extensively on the disease concept of alcohol abuse.

The AMA reaffirmed the classification of alcoholism as a disease in 1991 within both its psychiatric and medical sections. Since the late 1980s the US Supreme Court and the American Bar Association have affirmed that alcohol or drug dependence is a disease and that treatment and payment thereof is justified. The American Society of Addiction Medicine and the AMA have extensive policies regarding alcoholism, and the American Psychiatric Association recognizes both alcoholism and alcohol dependence. Other organizations, such as the American Hospital Association, the American Public Health Association, the National Association of Social Workers, and the American College of Physicians, recognize alcoholism as a disease. The National Institutes of Health includes the National Institute on Alcohol Abuse and Alcoholism (NIAAA), one of the major funding bodies for research on this topic in the United States. Throughout the United States, units such as the Betty Ford center and other acute-intervention sites for alcoholism are now prevalent. Acute treatment of alcohol withdrawal and subsequent rehabilitation efforts have now become a multidisciplinary activity.[18,89]

Although Osler clearly identified the relationship of withdrawal from alcohol and the syndrome we now know as AWS, this idea was not well established until the 1950s. Many clinicians believed that the syndrome accompanied ongoing heavy consumption of ethanol. However, Isabell and colleagues[90] demonstrated the relationship of cessation of drinking and the development of AWS symptomatology, especially withdrawal seizures. Victor and Adams confirmed these observations by showing that patients who lacked availability of alcohol developed tremulousness, hallucinations, seizures, and delirium.[91]

Since those pioneering studies, the neurochemical pathophysiology of AWS has been the subject of intense study, with identification of several mediators and alterations of neurotransmitter systems. This work has provided new options for pharmacologic management.

In concert with progress to unravel the mechanisms accounting for AWS, improvements in critical-care monitoring and care have improved the outlook for patients with severe AWS. Mortality of severe AWS, particularly delirium tremens, has decreased dramatically over the past few decades. Despite these advances, severe AWS remains a clinical challenge.

PATHOPHYSIOLOGY OF AWS

Until the middle of the twentieth century many physicians accepted the concept that signs and symptoms now regarded as AWS were related to the acute effects of alcohol or other factors. In 1953 Victor and Adams[91] observed "it is difficult to escape the conclusion that the clinical states under discussion depend for their production not only on the effects of prolonged exposure to alcohol, but temporally, on abstinence from the drug". Complementing and expanding on Victor's findings, Isabell and colleagues[90] demonstrated that "rum fits" and delirium could be induced by withholding alcohol after continuous administration to subjects. These and other ground-breaking observations led to the hypothesis stated by Sellers and Kalant[60] that AWS results from "acquired tolerance and physical dependence on ethanol with neurophysiologic alterations that offset the depressant effects of alcohol on neuronal excitability, impulse conduction and transmitter release." Subsequently there has been a watershed of biochemical, genetic, cellular, and subcellular studies on the genesis of AWS. Clinical and experimental work has demonstrated that although specific neurochemical adaptations appear crucial to the development of AWS, the process is multifactorial. Several avenues of research have yielded insights into the biology of AWS and potential avenues of treatment.

Sympathetic Stimulation and Adrenocortical Alterations

Characteristic features of AWS include tachycardia, diaphoresis, and hypertension, consistent with sympathetic hyperactivity. Studies by Carlsson, Perman, Klingman, Giacobini, and others documented that secretion and excretion of epinephrine and norepinephrine and their metabolites are increased after administration of alcohol.[92–106]

The increased catecholamine levels result from decreased inhibitory activity of $\alpha2$ receptors on presynaptic neurons. Accordingly, there is a general increase in autonomic activity over an interval of several days as patients progress to more severe stages of AWS (**Figs. 3** and **4**). These observations and experimental studies have led to clinical trials with β-adrenergic blocking agents as well as $\alpha2$ agonists, including clonidine and dexmedetomidine.[107–118] β-Adrenergic blocking agents have been helpful in treating tachycardia and hypertension, but delirium is a potential side effect of these drugs, and agitation, delirium, or seizures may not be adequately controlled by these agents.[115]

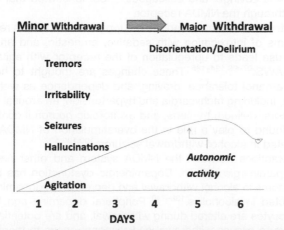

Fig. 3. Autonomic activity related to alcohol withdrawal signs and symptoms. (*Adapted from* Turner RC, Lichstein PR, Peden JG Jr, et al. Alcohol withdrawal syndromes: a review of pathophysiology, clinical presentation, and treatment. J Gen Intern Med 1989;4(5):432–44; with permission.)

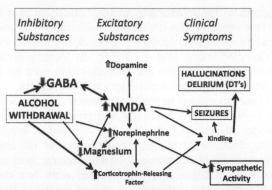

Fig. 4. Multifaceted pathogenesis of alcohol withdrawal syndrome. (*Data from* Glue P, Nutt D. Overexcitement and disinhibition: dynamic neurotransmitter interactions in alcohol withdrawal. Br J Psychiatry 1990;157:491–9.)

During the stress of withdrawal, increases in hydrocortisone and other adrenal hormones, as well as corticotropin-releasing factor (CRF), are observed.[119] CRF antagonists block some of the responses induced by withdrawal.[119–123] Therefore, alcohol inhibits sensitivity of the autonomic adrenergic system with consequent upregulation. When alcohol is stopped, central nervous system (CNS) and peripheral noradrenergic systems are activated.[92,118]

Glutamatergic Neurotransmitters

Glutamate is an important excitatory CNS neurotransmitter that affects *N*-methyl-D-aspartate (NMDA), metabotropic, and ionotropic receptors. Glutamate receptors are located on cell surfaces that are found on most neurons and some glial cells. The ionotropic receptors are ion channels that, on activation, lower neuronal cell membrane potential by transmembrane movement of cations such as sodium, potassium, and calcium. Calcium entry also affects other intracellular processes as a second messenger. In 1989 Lovinger and colleagues[124] demonstrated that alcohol directly inhibits ion flow through the NMDA receptor.

Acute administration of ethanol leads to a suppression of NMDA receptor function and the symptoms of intoxication with sedative, amnestic, and anxiolytic effects. Chronic alcohol use leads to upregulation of the receptor with agitation and other components of AWS.[97–99,124–135] These changes are thought to help explain the development of ethanol tolerance, craving, and dependence as well as withdrawal symptomatology, including tachycardia and hypertension; an arousal state that leads to seizures, tremors, delirium tremens, and excitotoxic neuronal death.[97] Homocysteine has been found to play a role in the overstimulation of NMDA receptors and has been implicated in alcohol-withdrawal seizures.[100,136,137]

There are interactions between the NMDA system and other neurotransmitters, including the dopaminergic system. Dopaminergic dysfunction has been related to depressive symptoms in alcohol withdrawal and decreases in dopamine D2 receptors have been detected in alcoholics.[138–140] Peripheral dopamine and NMDA-receptor activity in lymphocytes are altered during withdrawal, and are potential candidates as biological markers to assess withdrawal and responsiveness to therapy.[140] Not only has a relationship been found between delirium tremens and alcohol-related seizures to the dopamine transporter (DAT) gene, but other genes affecting dopamine metabolism have also been linked to withdrawal symptomatology.[121,138–143] Accordingly, multiple genes are thought to be involved in AWS, which affect dopamine, serotonin, NMDA, and opioidergic systems.

GABAergic Effects of Alcohol

The largest body of research and main approaches to management of AWS has been related to the effects of alcohol on GABA activity, a major neuroinhibitory system. The effects of alcohol on both the GABAergic system and NMDA are enhancing and complementary.[127] Since their introduction in 1958 with the drug chlordiazepoxide, the benzodiazepines, which have major GABA activity, have become the standard with which other sedatives are compared in the management of AWS.[115,143] The neurochemistry that accounts for these beneficial results has revealed that these drugs, as well as barbiturates, some anticonvulsants, anesthetics, endogenous neuro-steroids, and others, affect the inhibitory neurotransmitter GABA and the GABA-A subtype of GABA receptors that affect ligand-gated GABA-induced ionic currents.[144,145] When the GABA receptor is activated there is an influx of chloride ions through the postsynaptic membrane, causing an inhibition of transmission due to hyperpolarization of the nerve ending. There are at least 3 interacting parts of the postsynaptic receptor complex to which GABA combines: (1) the GABA-receptor sites, (2) a benzodiazepine site, and (3) a picrotoxinin site. Collectively these represent the benzodiazepine-GABA-receptor-ionophore complex.[95,146]

Alcohol increases the number of low-affinity GABA-receptor sites; during withdrawal, the affinity is decreased.[95] AWS is associated with blunting of GABA inhibition with resultant signs and symptoms of agitation, psychomotor activity, and the likelihood of seizures. Accordingly, development of drugs that affect the GABA-receptor system has been one of the primary therapeutic approaches to AWS.[13–24,115,118,144–150] These agents have included the benzodiazepines, barbiturates, baclofen, gabapentin clome-thiazole, pregablin, γ-hydroxybutyrate (GHB), valproic acid, tiagabine, vigabatrin, and others.[69,145,148,151–154]

Serotonin, Opioids, Nicotinic Cholinergic Receptors, and Electrolyte Disturbances

Other neurochemical systems have also been implicated in the pathogenesis of AWS. Alcohol stimulates the release of endogenous opioids, and this release is altered with the development of tolerance and withdrawal.[6] The observation that patients frequently have coexisting tobacco and alcohol abuse stimulated investigation on nicotinic cholinergic receptors.[154–156] Ethanol affects the activity of other gated ion channels, including serotonin (5-HT), and several 5-HT genes are associated with alcohol-use disorders.[121,157,158] Serotogenic factors may also have a facilitative role on dopamine pathways.[121] The array of mechanisms that involve genetic aspects of AWS is complex, but knowledge of these processes is expanding rapidly.[142]

Reductions of extracellular fluids, including blood volume, are commonly observed in AWS, and fluid repletion represents an important component of management.[159] Several electrolyte defects ensue during AWS and play a role in its pathogenesis. Since the 1950s hypomagnesemia has been identified as an important aspect of AWS and has been linked to the risk of seizures.[160] Magnesium interacts with NMDA and possibly other receptor systems, as well as a host of intracellular processes. Low magnesium levels are associated not only with seizures but also with cardiac arrhythmias.[161] Potassium, phosphate, and vitamin deficiencies, partic-ularly thiamine, may also contribute to the pathogenesis of AWS.

An integrated schema depicting the pathogenesis of AWS, including the GABA and NMDA receptor systems, electrolyte disturbances, and genetic and other factors was developed by Glue and Nutt[143] (see **Fig. 4**). Although other processes may also be involved, the schema illustrates the multifactorial nature of AWS and provides the clinician with a useful framework for understanding the syndrome.

CLINICAL FEATURES AND PRINCIPLES OF MANAGEMENT

After prolonged heavy intake of alcohol, AWS begins a few hours after cessation or decrease in consumption, associated with falling or absent blood alcohol levels. Admission blood alcohol assessments have been used as risk factors for development of AWS, although time from the last drink, delays in assessment, and other factors cloud the predictive value of such analyses.[162] As noted by Osler, intermittent or binge drinking does not lead to AWS. Although age may range from the 20s to those in their mid-70s, the typical patient is a middle-aged man. In the authors' review of 279 patients with AWS admitted to an inner-city hospital from 2005 to 2007, the mean age was 45 years and 91% were male.[24] These demographic findings have been remarkably similar over many decades.[10,27,75,78,107,111,163–168] Older patients are likely to have a more complex and potentially fatal course.[2,8,9,13–15,20,163–165,169–174] The youngest patient in the series was 23 years old; although it is uncommon to see patients in their early 20s because the syndrome develops only after several years of excessive drinking. A history of alcohol-use disorders is commonly obtained, and many patients will have had multiple prior episodes of AWS.[166,167]

Repeated bouts of AWS have been found to be a risk for a more severe course, described as the kindling effect or allostasis.[173–175] Other factors that may point to a more severe course of AWS are those with a greater maximum number of drinks in any 24-hour period, more withdrawal episodes, more nonmedical use of sedative-hypnotics, and other medical problems.[163,164,167,175,177] Approximately 10% of patients in the authors' series were documented to have at least 2 episodes of AWS during the 2.7-year interval of the study, although severity and course did not appear to be correlated with prior episodes.

The patient's psychiatric history must also be taken into account, as alcohol may induce various psychiatric problems including alcohol-induced mood or anxiety disorder, or alcohol-induced psychotic disorder. A variety of underlying psychiatric conditions may be present, such as antisocial personality disorder, other drug abuse or dependence, mania and schizophrenia, and bipolar I and major anxiety disorders.[167,177–179] Alcohol may therefore be taken in excess to offset psychiatric symptoms.

Patients are usually referred to inpatient facilities after initial evaluation in a detoxification center, or admitted to psychiatric, medical, or surgical units with a coexisting medical or surgical problem. In some instances, manifestations of AWS become apparent only after admission, as the syndrome is aggravated or precipitated by acute intercurrent medical, surgical, or psychological stresses. Alcohol-use disorder or withdrawal is well known to increase the morbidity and mortality of these conditions.[9,12,27–31,33,37–39,41] Risk factors for a protracted and severe course of AWS are shown in **Box 1**. The initial evaluation should determine if the signs and symptoms are related to AWS or another process and if other agents have been ingested. The clinician should assess the risk of progression to more advanced stages of AWS, perform a complete evaluation of the patient's clinical status, including comorbid conditions, and initiate management as needed. For patients who can be treated as an outpatient, referral to a rehabilitation program should be initiated.

Diagnostic criteria for alcohol withdrawal are defined within the *Diagnostic and Statistical Manual of Mental Disorders* of the American Psychiatric Association (**Box 2**). In general, the fully developed syndrome includes 4 progressively more

Box 1
Risk factors for severe course of AWS, including seizures and delirium

1. Prior episodes of AWS requiring detoxification, including seizures or delirium (kindling)

2. Grade 2 severity or higher on presentation (CIWA-Ar Score >10)

3. Advanced age

4. Acute or chronic comorbid conditions, including alcoholic liver disease, co-intoxications, trauma, infections, sepsis

5. Detectable blood alcohol level on admission

6. Use of "eye opener," high daily intake of alcohol, or number of drinking days/month

7. Abnormal liver function (serum aspartate aminotransferase activity >80 U/L)

8. Prior benzodiazepine use

9. Male sex

Abbreviation: CIWA-Ar, Clinical Institute of Withdrawal Assessment for Alcohol, revised.

severe levels or stages **(Table 1)**.[15,63,169–171,181,182,184,185] Some clinicians do not use the 4-tiered staging system, as patients may not progress sequentially and there is the potential for overlap. Nevertheless, the system provides a helpful approach to the clinical evolution and features of the syndrome.[171]

Box 2
Diagnostic criteria for alcohol withdrawal

A. Cessation of (or reduction in) alcohol use that has been heavy and prolonged

B. Two (or more) of the following developing within several hours to a few days after criterion A

　1. Autonomic hyperactivity (eg, sweating or pulse rate >100/min)

　2. Increased hand tremor

　3. Insomnia

　4. Nausea or vomiting

　5. Transient visual, tactile, or auditory hallucinations or illusions

　6. Psychomotor agitation

　7. Anxiety

　8. Grand mal seizures

C. The symptoms in criterion B cause clinically significant distress or impairment in social, occupational, or other important areas of functioning

D. The symptoms are not due to a general medical condition and are not accounted for by another mental disorder

Specify if with perceptual disturbances. This specifier may be noted in the rare instance when hallucinations with intact reality testing or auditory, visual, or tactile illusions occur in the absence of a delirium. Intact reality testing means that the person knows that the hallucinations are induced by the substance and do not represent external reality. When hallucinations occur in the absence of intact reality testing, a diagnosis of substance-induced psychomotor disorder, with hallucinations, should be considered.

From Diagnostic and statistical manual of mental disorders. 4th edition. Text revision. Washington, DC: American Psychiatric Association; 2000. p. 216; with permission.

Table 1
Stages of alcohol withdrawal syndrome

Stage	Onset	Signs and Symptoms
1	8+ h after cessation or reduction of alcohol intake	Mild tremulousness, nervousness, nausea; with or without tremor, tachycardia, hypertension
2	Approximately 24 h; may be up to 8 d	Marked tremors, diaphoresis, hyperactivity, insomnia. Lucid, but may have nightmares or illusions—may progress to hallucinations (visual, tactile, or auditory)
3	12–48 h	Similar to stage 2, plus tonic-clonic seizures—may be multiple; one-third progress to stage 4
4	Usually 3–5 d; may be delayed up to 12 d	Delirium tremens, typically with ongoing agitation, hyperactivity, global confusion; often with cardiovascular, respiratory, metabolic, and other abnormalities

Data from Behnke RH. Recognition and management of alcohol withdrawal syndrome. Hosp Pract 1976;11:79–84.

Within a few hours of abstinence the patient develops tremulousness, nervousness and, frequently, nausea and vomiting. This "hangover" interval or stage 1 may be the only manifestation, and most patients will not progress to more severe aspects of AWS. The patient may seek additional alcohol, such as a morning "eye opener" or "hair of the dog" to alleviate symptoms.

The Clinical Institute of Withdrawal Assessment for Alcohol (CIWA-Ar) scale is used to assess severity and progression of AWS (**Table 2**). The scale includes 10 items and requires patient participation. A score of less than 10 reflects mild AWS (stage 1). If there is no progression or complicating factors, pharmacologic management or admission is not required. The CIWA-Ar may be repeated after an interval of observation. Increases in the score reflect progression of AWS, and should prompt admission and management procedures. Another tool is the AWS scale, a simplified version of the CIWA-Ar that is shorter and easier to administer.[80] Neither of these scales has been validated for ICU patients, and scores are altered by pain, other medical or surgical issues, and the administration of sedation agents. Clinicians should exercise considerable caution when administering these screening tools. Hecksel and colleagues[183] found that the CIWA-Ar may be applied inappropriately to patients without confirmed history of alcohol abuse and limited communication abilities, resulting in erroneous data and potentially harmful management. CIWA-Ar scores greater than 10 require further evaluation and development of admission goals of therapy, including measures to abort progression, management of symptomatology, treatment of comorbid conditions and complications, and preparation of the patient for long-term rehabilitation (**Box 3**).[169,170,181,184,185]

Stage 2 typically develops within 24 to 48 hours; onset may be delayed by intercurrent problems or sedatives. Agitation, tremulousness, and hyperactivity are the most prominent features, and patients will exhibit tachycardia, hypertension, diaphoresis, and other manifestations of increased sympathetic activity plus a tremor of 6 to 8 cycles per second. The patient remains lucid and oriented, but insomnia can be a significant problem. The patient may attempt to climb out of bed, pull at catheters, or dislodge monitoring devices, and may require physical restraints; although at this juncture the subject will temporarily calm to requests by the bedside staff. Because of

Table 2
Clinical Institute Withdrawal Assessment for Alcohol, revised (CIWA-Ar)

Nausea-Vomiting: Ask: Do you feel sick to your stomach? Have you vomited? (Observation)
0. No nausea-vomiting
1. Mild nausea, no vomiting
2. –
3. –
4. Intermittent nausea with dry heaves
5. –
6. –
7. Constant nausea, frequent dry heaves

Visual Disturbances: Ask: Does light appear too bright? Is color different? Does it hurt your eyes? Are you seeing anything that is disturbing to you? Are you seeing things you know aren't there?
0. Not present
1. Very mild sensitivity
2. Mild sensitivity
3. Moderate sensitivity
4. Moderately severe hallucinations
5. Severe hallucinations
6. Extremely severe hallucinations
7. Continuous hallucinations

Paroxysmal Sweats: (Observation)
0. No sweat observed
1. –
2. –
3. –
4. Beads of sweat on forehead
5. –
6. –
7. Drenching sweats

Tactile Disturbances: Ask: Have you any itching, pins-needles sensations, any burning, any numbness or do you feel bugs crawling on or under your skin? (Observation)
0. None
1. Very Mild itching, pins-needles, burning-numbness
2. Mild itching, pins-needles, burning-numbness
3. Moderate itching, pins-needles, burning-numbness
4. Moderately severe hallucinations
5. Severe hallucinations
6. Extremely severe hallucinations
7. Continuous hallucinations

Agitation: (Observations)
0. Normal activity
1. Somewhat more than normal
2. –
3. –
4. Moderately fidgety, restless
5. –
6. –
7. Paces back-forth most of interview, constantly thrashes about

Auditory Disturbances: Ask: Are you more aware of sounds around you? Are they harsh? Do they frighten you? Are you hearing anything that is disturbing to you? Are you hearing things you know aren't there? (Observation)
0. Not present
1. Very mild harshness or ability to frighten
2. Mild harshness or ability to frighten
3. Moderate harshness or ability to frighten
4. Moderately severe hallucinations
5. Severe hallucinations
6. Extremely severe hallucinations
7. Continuous hallucinations

Headache, Fullness in Head: Ask: Does you head feel different? Does it feel like a band is around your head? (do not rate for dizziness or light-headedness)
0. Not present
1. Very mild
2. Mild
3. Moderate
4. Moderately severe
5. Severe
6. Very severe
7. Extremely severe

Orientation/Clouding of Sensorium: Ask: What day is today? What is this place?
0. Oriented and can do serial additions
1. Cannot do serial additions or uncertain regarding date
2. Disoriented for date by no more than 2 d
3. Disoriented for date by >2 calendar days
4. Disoriented for place and/or person

(continued on next page)

Table 2 (continued)	
Anxiety: Ask: Do you feel nervous? (Observation) 0. None 1. Mildly anxious 2. – 3. – 4. Moderately anxious, guarded, so anxiety is inferred 5. – 6. – 7. Equivalent to acute panic states	TOTAL CIWA-Ar SCORE: _____
Tremor: Extend arms, spread fingers apart (Observation) 0. None 1. Barely visible, but can feel 2. – 3. – 4. Moderate with arms extended 5. – 6. – 7. Severe, even with arms not extended	

Adapted from Sullivan JT, Sykora K, Schneiderman J, et al. Assessment of alcohol withdrawal: the revised clinical institute withdrawal assessment of alcohol scale (CIWA-Ar). Br J Addict 1989;84:1353–7; with permission.

progressive agitation and the need for pharmacologic management, hospital admission is indicated. The CIWA-Ar score is typically 10 to 18 or higher, corresponding to moderate to severe AWS. Kraemer and colleagues[164] documented that an initial CIWA-Ar score of more than 10 was statistically correlated with severe AWS. Scores of 15 to 18 or greater have been associated with significant risk of major complications if not treated.[115,118,164] In addition to trauma or other surgical conditions, comorbid medical disorders include pancreatitis, gastrointestinal hemorrhage, alcoholic ketoacidosis, and multiple cardiovascular disturbances, as well as infections, particularly pneumonia. Pneumonia and respiratory failure are the most common complications.[13–15,20,22,68,169,174]

Those with a protracted history of alcoholism may exhibit signs and symptoms of liver disease, including alcoholic hepatitis, jaundice, coagulopathy, and manifestations of portal hypertension. When hepatic encephalopathy coexists with AWS, diagnosis and management are more difficult. Both conditions are associated with seizures, but hepatic encephalopathy is characteristically a syndrome of CNS

Box 3
Alcohol withdrawal syndrome admission management goals
1. Monitor course of syndrome, ensuring patient safety
2. Use methods to abort progression and treat symptoms
3. Manage comorbid medical, surgical, toxicologic, and psychiatric problems
4. Anticipate need for intensive care monitoring and therapy
5. Ensure multidisciplinary approach to management, including preparation for rehabilitation

depression, whereas AWS is a state of general arousal. In contrast to AWS, hepatic encephalopathy involves endozepines or benzodiazepines of natural origin that act on the GABA-A receptor complex, resulting in increased inhibitory activity.[186,187] Other processes affecting mentation such as hypoglycemia, CNS trauma, bleeding or infection, or other intoxications should be excluded. Fluid losses and malnutrition, as well as electrolyte defects, including magnesium, should be anticipated. These defects require prompt therapeutic attention.[159–161,169,188–190] Rubeiz and colleagues[191] documented an association between mortality and hypomagnesemia in alcohol-abuse patients admitted to an ICU.

An initial laboratory panel should be obtained, including a complete blood count, serum glucose, electrolytes including magnesium, and renal function tests. Studies may also include serum calcium, phosphorus, liver function and coagulation studies, urine toxicology screen, blood alcohol level, and chest radiograph. Additional imaging as well as studies to detect gastrointestinal bleeding should be considered, plus a baseline electrocardiogram, cardiac biomarkers, lipase and creatine kinase activity, arterial blood gas, and sputum analysis with Gram stain and culture (**Box 4**).

Many institutions have protocols for AWS management that include vitamin supplementation, particularly thiamine. The development of Wernicke encephalopathy can be prevented by thiamine administration. Multivitamins given by "banana bag" intravenous (IV) infusions are routinely ordered, although controlled studies to assess the effectiveness of this practice are lacking. Nutritional support is an important concern, but the implementation of feeding may increase the risk of aspiration. If possible, enteral nutrition is preferred, but the selection of oral, nasogastric, nasoduodenal, or parenteral nutritional supplementation should be individualized.

For patients with stage 2 or higher, sequential CIWA-Ar evaluations should be supplemented with the results of agitation and sedation scoring studies, which may be used to titrate sedation. There are several agitation/sedation scales in wide use, although the Richmond Agitation Sedation Scale (RASS) is currently the most popular method (**Table 3**).[81–84]

Box 4
Admission studies for patients with moderate to severe alcohol withdrawal syndrome[a]

1. Complete blood cell count

2. Baseline metabolic panel with serum electrolytes (including magnesium), glucose, renal function tests

3. Blood alcohol, and urine and blood toxicology studies

4. Serum calcium, phosphate, lipase, CPK activity

5. Liver function tests, including INR and serum AST, ALT, bilirubin, ammonia

6. Chest radiograph

7. Electrocardiogram, cardiac biomarkers, echocardiogram

8. Urinalysis

9. Arterial blood gas analysis

10. Blood, urine, and sputum cultures

Abbreviations: ALT, alanine aminotransferase; AST, aspartate aminotransferase; CPK, creatine phosphokinase; INR, international normalized ratio.
[a] Laboratory, imaging, and clinical evaluations must be individualized.

Table 3
Richmond Agitation-Sedation Scale (RASS)

Score	Description	Definition
+4	Combative	Overtly combative, violent, risk to staff
+3	Very agitated	Pulls at tubes, aggressive
+2	Agitated	Frequent movements, dyssynchrony with ventilator
+1	Restless	Anxious, apprehensive
0	Alert, calm	
−1	Drowsy	Not fully alert, but awakens for >10 s with eye contact to voice
−2	Light sedation	Briefly (<10 s) awakens and makes eye contact to voice
−3	Moderate sedation	Any movement, but no eye contact to voice
−4	Deep sedation	No voice response, but movement to physical stimulation
−5	Unarousable	No response to voice or physical stimulation

Adapted from Sessler CN, Gosnell MS, Grap MJ, et al. The Richmond Agitation-Sedation Scale: validity and reliability in adult intensive care unit patients. Am J Resp Crit Care Med 2002;166(10):1338–44; with permission.

Advanced stage 2 is manifested by nightmares and disordered perception with visual, tactile or, occasionally, auditory hallucinations. An important distinguishing feature of alcohol-withdrawal hallucinations is that the patient remains lucid. The subject will recognize that the illusions are related to the withdrawal process, but the perceptions are nevertheless vivid and frequently frightening. A CIWA-Ar score of 20 or higher is typically recorded at this time, consistent with severe AWS.[118,164,171]

There should be a low threshold to transfer the patient to a critical care unit. Approximately one-third of patients in the study by Monte and colleagues,[174] and in the authors' review, required ICU care. Kraemer and colleagues[164] found that 24% of patients referred from a detoxification center met criteria for severe AWS and a higher level of care. Indications for transfer to an ICU include advanced stage 2 or greater AWS, requirement for intensive sedation and monitoring, respiratory failure, hemodynamic instability, and comorbid conditions such as trauma, gastrointestinal bleeding, acute CNS processes, or marked fluid and electrolyte and renal disorders (**Box 5**).

Stage 3 includes signs and symptoms of advanced stage 2 AWS, plus tonic-clonic (grand mal) seizures. Although seizures may develop at any time during the course, they may be recurrent, typically occur within 24 to 48 hours, and may affect up to one-third of hospitalized patients.[90,91,182] Seizures are more common in patients with a history of epilepsy.[192] Isolated AWS-related seizures do not require long-term

Box 5
Potential indications for ICU management

1. Advanced Stage 2 or greater alcohol withdrawal syndrome

2. Critical comorbid conditions including: trauma; severe sepsis; respiratory failure; acute respiratory distress syndrome; hemodynamic instability; gastrointestinal bleeding; hepatic failure; pancreatitis; rhabdomyolysis; co-intoxication; coagulopathies; acute CNS process; cardiac arrhythmias, ischemia, or congestive failure; severe fluid or electrolyte defects; renal failure; persistent fever; or complex acid-base defects

3. Escalating intravenous bolus or continuous-infusion sedation therapy

4. Persistent fever >39°C

anticonvulsant therapy and are inconsistently responsive to phenytoin.[193] Status epilepticus may occur but is relatively uncommon in AWS. A significant proportion of patients with seizures progress to stage 4 and are at increased risk for complications such as aspiration pneumonia and rhabdomyolysis.[64,170,194]

The most severe form of AWS is stage 4, alcohol-withdrawal delirium or delirium tremens.[60,63,64,182] Alcohol-withdrawal delirium is characterized by marked autonomic hyperactivity as well as global CNS clouding (**Box 6**). Delirium may be present on admission, particularly if there has been a delay in medical evaluation. However, in the typical course of AWS delirium tremens does not occur within the first 2 days.

Earlier reports suggested that fewer than 8% of hospitalized patients progress to delirium tremens.[64,65,91] Kraemer and colleagues[164] found 1% of patients with severe AWS developed delirium. Yet other studies have found that alcohol-withdrawal delirium may occur more frequently. Wojnar and colleagues[166] reported delirium in nearly all patients admitted to a Polish medical center over an interval of 14 years, usually with one or more accompanying somatic disorders. Concurrent acute medical illnesses were associated with delirium in 24% of admissions observed by Ferguson and colleagues.[163] These conditions may include infectious diseases, tachycardia at admission, a detectable blood alcohol level, and a history of seizures and previous episodes of delirium tremens.[176,195,196] In a Spanish study, alcohol-withdrawal delirium was present on admission in 43% of patients, with an additional 48% who subsequently progressed to delirium.[174] Foy and colleagues[8] reported a significant proportion of patients who developed delirium. In a review of AWS at 2 institutions, Daus and colleagues[190] reported 3% and 18% of subjects with delirium tremens, respectively. In the authors' review, 18% of patients admitted to an inner-city hospital with stage 2 or higher AWS developed delirium tremens. Accordingly, the prevalence of alcohol-withdrawal delirium varies considerably depending on the population studied.

Identification of delirium can be challenging for the clinician, particularly in the ICU setting. There are several delirium screening tools. The confusion assessment method for the intensive care unit (CAM-ICU) is widely used in critical care units and relies on scoring of at least 4 features by nurse, patient, and family: acute onset of mental status changes, inattention, disorganized thought, and altered level of consciousness.[86] Another tool is the symptom rating scale, which examines items such as temporal onset of symptoms, perceptual disturbances, hallucinations, delusions, psychomotor behavior, and mood lability.[197] The intensive care delirium screening checklist (ICDSC)

Box 6
Diagnostic criteria for substance (alcohol) withdrawal delirium

A. Disturbance of consciousness (ie, reduced clarity of awareness of the environment) with reduced ability to focus, sustain, or shift attention

B. A change in cognition (such as memory deficit, disorientation, language disturbance) or the development of a perceptual disturbance that is not better accounted for by a preexisting, established, or evolving dementia

C. The disturbance develops over a short period of time (usually hours to days) and tends to fluctuate during the course of the day

D. There is evidence from the history, physical examination, or laboratory findings that the symptoms in criteria A and B developed during, or shortly after, a withdrawal syndrome

Adapted from Diagnostic and statistical manual of mental disorders. 4th edition. Text revision. Washington, DC: American Psychiatric Association; 2000. p. 146; with permission.

is a third method, which has been shown to have good agreement with the CAM-ICU.[198]

Although widely used, the CAM-ICU has up to a 10% false-positive rate.[199] Furthermore, alcohol-withdrawal delirium is a hyperactive form of delirium, whereas the majority of other delirious ICU patients are likely to be older and manifest a mixed or hypoactive subtype of delirium.[199,200] The pathogenesis of delirium in the acute-care setting is multifactorial, but the pathogenesis of alcohol-withdrawal delirium may differ from other forms of delirium (also termed acute brain dysfunction) observed in the ICU, with implications for management. In contrast to GABA, NMDA, and other neurotransmitter alterations associated with alcohol-withdrawal delirium, cholinergic deficiency has been postulated to cause ICU delirium and cognitive defects, particularly in the elderly. Recently, the kynurenine-tryptophan pathway has also been implicated in acute brain dysfunction in critically ill patients.[201] Although benzodiazepines are one of the major pharmacologic approaches to management of delirium tremens, these drugs have been associated with an increased risk of delirium in ICU patients (**Table 4**).[199,200,202–207]

Management of patients with alcohol-withdrawal delirium is challenging and requires aggressive sedation that may lead to respiratory failure as well as other critical problems. Abraham and colleagues[208] studied the cardiorespiratory patterns of patients with severe delirium tremens and found increases in cardiac index, cardiac work, and oxygen delivery and consumption, consistent with a hyperdynamic cardiorespiratory status. Up to 50% of these patients develop pulmonary infections that may lead to severe sepsis, mandating goal-directed management with fluid loading as well as endotracheal intubation and mechanical ventilation.[12,14,15,68,166] In the series by Monte and colleagues,[174] 70% of patients admitted to the ICU required intubation and mechanical ventilation, with an increase in the odds ratio for death, particularly

Table 4
ICU delirium[a] versus alcohol-withdrawal delirium tremens

Feature	ICU Delirium[a]	Delirium Tremens
Predominate subtype of delirium	Mixed or hypoactive	Hyperactive
Age	Older	Middle age
Sex	No difference	Male predominance
Associated critical illness or respiratory failure	Usually	Sometimes
Prognosis	Adverse	Good
Duration	Variable; may progress to dementia	Days
Morbidity/mortality	Adverse association with presence of delirium	Related to comorbid conditions
Recurrence	Not expected	May have several Episodes of AWS or delirium tremens; ? kindling
Pathogenesis	Multifactorial ? Cholinergic ? Tryptophan	Multifactorial: GABA, NMDA, and so forth
Management	? Dexmedetomidine Avoid benzodiazepines	Multiple agents, especially benzodiazepines

[a] Also termed acute brain dysfunction during critical illness.

in the presence of pneumonia or chronic liver disease. De Wit and colleagues[41] found an increased risk of mechanical ventilation that was prolonged. One-half of ICU patients in the authors' series required intubation and mechanical ventilation with pneumonia as the major comorbid ICU condition; nearly identical to the findings of Gold and colleagues[68] for delirious patients who received one sedation protocol. An array of respiratory complications should be anticipated for patients with severe AWS and delirium.

Duration of AWS is proportional to severity. Patients with stage 1 recover within hours to a day or so and are usually treated as outpatients. Those with higher grades require hospitalization and have progressively longer and more complex lengths of stay. In the authors' review of 192 patients admitted to a ward, 83% had stage 2 AWS and 17% had stage 3 AWS. Hospital length of stay (LOS) for ward patients was 5.4 days whereas LOS for ICU patients was 12.5 days, of whom 57% had stage 4 AWS. Delirium usually persists for 3 to 5 days, although there are reports of patients remaining delirious for up to 2 weeks. The longest interval of delirium the authors observed was 11 days. Although delirium characteristically subsides within days, some patients require several weeks to return to baseline mental status.[180,182,209] A subgroup of patients develop protracted AWS.[210] Alterations of CNS dopamine outflow have been suggested as a mechanism for protracted craving, anhedonia, and dysphoric behavior.[152,210]

Sedation Pharmacology

A crucial aspect of management of AWS is the use of sedation to control agitation, abort the progression of signs and symptoms, and manage delirium. For most of the twentieth century chloral hydrate, paraldehyde, and various barbiturates were used for these purposes. Soon after the availability of benzodiazepines in the early 1960s, this class of sedatives became the standard with which other drugs have been compared. Although methodological flaws can be found in many of the trials that have assessed efficacy, the benzodiazepines have consistently shown superiority.[64,65,71,150,211–216] One of the most definitive controlled trials compared chlordiazepoxide with chlorpromazine, hydroxyzine, and thiamine.[72] Chlordiazepoxide helped abort the development of delirium and seizures, and was clearly the drug of choice. By contrast, chlorpromazine was associated with the highest incidence of these complications, confirming previous adverse results with a related compound, promazine.[214]

Most patients have mild to moderate AWS and can be managed with no drugs or oral medication. The "front-loading" approach uses high initial doses of medication such as 20 mg orally of diazepam or 100 mg of chlordiazepoxide, repeated every 2 to 3 hours for the first few hours. This method decreases AWS progression and the development of seizures.[149,215,217,218] A sedation level is reached quickly, and the prolonged effects of agents such as diazepam sustain the effect over several hours. A fixed-schedule treatment program has been shown to require larger total doses of drug and a longer duration of therapy.[217–220]

All benzodiazepines are potentially useful in the management of AWS, but there are significant differences in route of administration, onset of action, duration, cost, and metabolism.[219] Benzodiazepines are metabolized by the liver, but conjugation or oxidation processes lead to important pharmacokinetic differences. Chlordiazepoxide and diazepam undergo oxidation with an increase in half-life and the accumulation of active metabolites. Lorazepam is metabolized by glucuronidation, with an intermediate half-life and formation of inactive metabolites. Diazepam is more lipophilic, leading to early CNS distribution but also more rapid redistribution. In 3 studies that compared chlordiazepoxide, lorazepam, and diazepam, all were shown to have favorable qualities, but lorazepam was preferred because of its pharmacokinetic characteristics.[220–222] Chlordiazepoxide is generally administered orally, although it can be given parenterally. Diazepam and lorazepam can also be given parenterally, and lorazepam can be infused intravenously. The pharmacokinetics of IV diazepam in alcohol-withdrawal subjects appeared similar to those of normal controls, although some subjects had increased clearance suggesting enzyme induction or extrahepatic biotransformation, as well as alcohol or diazepam-induced tolerance.[223] Accordingly, dosing should be individualized and should use clinical end points. Another short-acting parenteral agent that may be given by IV infusion is midazolam. Difference in cost among these agents was an issue in the past, but current prices are similar, and lorazepam or midazolam are frequently infused for ICU sedation.[224–227] **Table 5** illustrates features of benzodiazepines commonly used for AWS.

A companion technique to front loading is symptom-triggered therapy given throughout the interval of AWS. Both methods use sequential CIWA-Ar and RASS or other scoring techniques to titrate dosing. Favorable results include decreases in total drug dosage and duration of AWS.[115,228,229] For patients with mild to moderately severe AWS, oral or parenteral therapy may be selected. However, for those with severe AWS, and especially delirium, symptom-triggered dosing requires frequent, often escalating doses of IV sedation to achieve target RASS scores. These patients have limited abilities to cooperate for CIWA-Ar scoring and should be in a monitored environment. Accordingly, the CIWA-Ar is not validated for ICU patients, and in this setting the RASS or other agitation-sedation scales becomes the primary mechanism to adjust dosage.[13,230] Patients who are extremely agitated and delirious therefore present significant challenges in reaching sedation goals. Dill[231] reported IV benzodiazepine doses of more than 2100 mg over a 24-hour interval to control symptoms of AWS, of whom 40% required intubation. In another study, patients defined as "resistant alcohol withdrawal" received more than 200 mg of diazepam equivalent over 3 hours to achieve goals of sedation and vital signs.[232] This group also experienced a high rate of respiratory failure requiring endotracheal intubation. There are other reports of the use of extremely high doses of benzodiazepines to achieve sedation goals in alcohol-withdrawal delirium.[233–235] Desensitization of GABA receptor sites

Table 5
Benzodiazepines used for alcohol withdrawal syndrome

Name (Brand)	Routes of Administration	Comment	Dosage	Half-Life (h)
Chlordiazepoxide (Librium)	Oral, IM, or IV	Long-acting metabolites	25–100 mg every 1–4 h	5–15
Diazepam (Valium)	Oral, IM or IV, or by IV infusion	Early-onset but long-acting metabolites (hepatic oxidation)	5–20+ mg oral, IV, or by slow IV infusion	30–60
Lorazepam (Ativan)	Oral, IM or IV, or by IV infusion	Intermediate half-life (hepatic glucuronidation)	1–4+ mg IM or IV, or by IV infusion	10–20
Midazolam (Versed)	IV or IM, or by IV infusion	Rapid metabolism (hepatic hydroxylation)	1–4+ mg IV or IM, or by IV infusion	2

Abbreviations: IM, intramuscular; IV, intravenous.

or decreasing the number of sites have been postulated as possible mechanisms for the requirement of such huge doses in this setting.[236–238]

Several approaches may be selected to sedate severely agitated delirious patients, including transition to IV infusion of sedation agents, escalating bolus doses of benzodiazepines or barbiturates, or use of adjunctive rescue medications given by IV infusion (**Box 7**). Spies and colleagues[22] reported that the choice of sedating agents for IV infusion in trauma patients with AWS affected the duration of mechanical ventilation as well as the incidence of pneumonia and respiratory failure. Selection of a benzodiazepine-clonidine cocktail reduced the frequency of pneumonia and shortened the duration of mechanical ventilation. In a follow-up study, 90% of surgical ICU patients who received continuous-infusion therapy required intubation and mechanical ventilation, in comparison with 65% of those with bolus therapy.[228] There was also a reduction in ICU LOS for the bolus-treated group. Gold and colleagues[68] successfully used progressively larger bolus doses of sedatives that led to a reduction in the need for mechanical ventilation from 47% to 22% for delirious patients. However, other investigators have reported difficulties in reaching sedation goals for severely agitated patients. In the study by Monte and colleagues,[174] 78% of patients were transferred to the ICU because of uncontrollable agitation, despite a combination of fixed dosage and symptom-adjusted therapy with a variety of agents. More than 75% required intubation, and pneumonia and respiratory failure were statistically associated with a fatal outcome. The authors found that delirious ICU patients for whom agitation was ultimately controlled by IV infusion of benzodiazepines after unsuccessful bolus dosing required significantly higher mean 24-hour benzodiazepine dosage (244 vs 101 mg/d, $P<.05$). Those who reached sedation goals by bolus dosing experienced shorter ICU and hospital LOS (ICU: 3.1 vs 7.5 days, hospital: 6.4 vs 13.8 days; both $P<.05$) and lower requirements for intubation and mechanical ventilation (13% vs 61%, $P<.05$). However, it is likely that patients who responded to bolus therapy had less severe agitation. Accordingly, for some patients conversion from bolus to IV infusion benzodiazepines may be considered if sedation goals are not met. Patients who require large doses of sedatives by infusion may be more severely agitated and are very likely to experience a stormy, protracted course that includes respiratory failure.

A third option for patients who require very high doses of sedatives is to institute rescue therapy that includes ongoing bolus or infusion medication, supplemented with propofol or dexmedetomidine. Propofol (2,6-diisopropylphenol) is an IV hypnotic agent formulated in a lipid emulsion and having both GABA-A activity and inhibitory properties on NMDA receptors.[239] When propofol is given by continuous infusion, endotracheal intubation and mechanical ventilation are required. The agent may be administered in conjunction with a benzodiazepine such as lorazepam or midazolam.

Box 7
Options to achieve sedation goals for severely agitated delirious patients[a]

1. Progressively larger IV bolus doses of benzodiazepines or barbiturates

2. Titrated IV infusion of benzodiazepines

3. Addition of IV rescue therapy to #1 or #2

    a. Propofol

    b. Dexmedetomidine

[a] All methods are associated with substantial risk of respiratory failure.

Hypotension or bradycardia may develop, and high infusion rates have been associated with the propofol infusion syndrome.[240] There are several reports of the use of propofol for refractory agitation associated with delirium tremens.[241–244] Another option is infusion of dexmedetomidine.[114,244] Dexmedetomidine is an $\alpha2$ agonist that was developed as an ICU sedative. The drug has CNS and spinal activity that is substantially more potent than that of clonidine. Infusions may be associated with bradycardia and hypotension. Dexmedetomidine is routinely used for IV sedation of critically ill patients, and has been associated with a lower incidence of ICU delirium than infusion of lorazepam.[205,225,245]

For severely agitated patients the addition of propofol or dexmedetomidine to benzodiazepines or barbiturates might allow achievement of sedation goals with a benzodiazepine-sparing effect as well as facilitating sedation holidays and ventilator-weaning efforts. However, additional studies are needed to determine the appropriate roles of propofol and dexmedetomidine in the management of severe agitation and AWS delirium. In the interim, the clinician must be prepared to use progressively higher bolus doses of sedatives, or convert to IV infusion therapy that may include rescue medications. All patients with severe agitation who receive aggressive sedation protocols are at substantial risk of respiratory complications.

Although benzodiazepines are overwhelmingly the most frequently used class of drugs for AWS, other agents with GABA activity also have efficacy. Phenobarbital has been used in front loading as well as symptom-adjusted therapy with results similar to benzodiazepines.[69,246] Phenobarbital has a long half-life and a narrow therapeutic window, which complicates dosage titration. In addition, respiratory depression is a potential complication. If phenobarbital is used, the patient should be observed in a monitored environment.

A variety of other medications that have activity on the GABA system have been evaluated. Clomethiazole is available in Europe as a sedative-hypnotic that enhances neurotransmission at GABA-A receptors. It also inhibits the enzyme alcohol dehydrogenase, slowing elimination of alcohol. Significant alterations in the pharmacokinetics of this agent may occur in the presence of liver disease, resulting in oversedation. In the study by Spies and colleagues,[22] those who received chlormethiazole experienced a longer duration of mechanical ventilation and a higher incidence of pneumonia.

Baclofen is a stereoselective GABA receptor agonist that has been shown to reduce AWS signs and symptoms including the CIWA-Ar score. Limited controlled trials have been conducted with baclofen. Another potential problem with baclofen is that it may lower the seizure threshold.[153,247] Other medications with GABA activity include gabapentin, pregabalin, GHB, tiagabine, valproic acid, and vigabatrin. GHB performed favorably in comparison with clomethiazole for AWS in an open-label trial of ICU patients, with decreases in CIWA-Ar scores and improvement in symptomatology.[248] Gabapentin in high doses was comparable with lorazepam for treatment of outpatients with CIWA-Ar scores of less than 10.[249] In another recent outpatient study, pregabalin was found to be safe and more effective than tiapride or lorazepam.[152] Accordingly, the role of other agents that affect the GABA system is evolving.[144] Valproate has been found to be helpful in mild to moderate AWS, appears to reduce the risk of seizures, and is frequently used as a postdetoxification relapse-prevention agent.[145,250–252] Carbamazepine is a tricyclic anticonvulsant that has been widely used in Europe for patients with mild to moderate AWS. The drug may help prevent AWS-induced seizures and retard the kindling effect.[2,115,250,253] Phenytoin has shown limited effectiveness in the management of alcohol-withdrawal seizures and is not indicated in the management of AWS.[193,254,255]

There are numerous reports of using β-adrenergic blocking agents and α agonists in AWS. β-Blocking agents may be helpful as adjuncts for patients with tremor, tachycardia, cardiac arrhythmias, hypertension, and craving.[2,75,107,256] However, β-blocking agents may increase the risk of delirium and are not recommended as monotherapy. Clonidine is an α agonist that reduces severity of withdrawal symptoms in mild to moderate AWS.[257,258] This drug has been used in combination therapy with agents such as benzodiazepines.[27] Since the availability of dexmedetomidine, several reports have supported its complementary role in treating severe AWS. Dexmedetomidine has been used primarily as rescue therapy for patients who have failed high-dose benzodiazepine or other agents.[114,244]

Neuroleptic agents, including phenothiazines and butyrophenones such as haloperidol, have been used to treat delirium, although with less effectiveness than benzodiazepines.[259] These agents prolong the QT interval and lower the seizure threshold, and haloperidol has been shown to enhance alcohol-withdrawal seizures in animal models.[260] Nevertheless, intermittent IV doses of haloperidol may be considered in delirious, agitated patients.[60] Infusions of haloperidol and chlormethiazole in intensive care trauma patients led to more respiratory complications.[22] As noted earlier, promazine and chlorpromazine performed poorly against benzodiazepines and were associated with significant complications.[60,72] Accordingly, phenothiazines are not recommended because of the risk of seizures, effects of thermoregulation, and the potential for hemodynamic instability.[169,170] Similarly, antihistamines are not indicated because of their anticholinergic effects.

Several antiglutamatergic strategies for alcohol withdrawal have emerged over the past few years, but they have not achieved first-line status. Nevertheless, several potential candidates with NMDA-receptor antagonists, especially NR2B subunit-selective agents, are under investigation for pharmacotherapy to treat alcohol withdrawal and alcohol dependence.[131] NMDA-receptor antagonist drugs may therefore be helpful in suppressing alcohol-withdrawal symptoms.[135,261] Preliminary studies on patients with mild AWS, comparing agents with NMDA activity such as lamotrigine, memantine, and topiramate with diazepam and placebo have supported the efficacy of this approach.[134]

A recurring strategy to abort or manage AWS is the use of alcohol. Subjects who perceive the development of withdrawal symptoms frequently resort to drinking to prevent progression of withdrawal. The phenomenon has been observed repeatedly, and is a component of the CAGE screening test for unhealthy alcohol use.[3,262] Acutely elevating the blood alcohol level may alter GABA, NMDA, and other neurotransmitter alterations and blunt or reverse the progression of AWS. However, controlled trials that compare ethanol with other drugs, such as benzodiazepines, are lacking, and reviews of AWS management have consistently not recommended this approach.[13,20,115,118,181,184,185] Nevertheless, some practitioners prescribe alcoholic beverages or infuse ethanol to patients for this purpose. Hansbrough and colleagues[263] reported that IV alcohol prevented withdrawal in 22 burns patients, using infusion rates of 0.03 to 0.06 mg/kg per hour, which yielded blood alcohol levels of 2 to 8 mg/dL. Specific criteria for identification and severity of AWS were not given, but the investigators concluded that the infusions prevented signs of withdrawal during and subsequent to the ethanol infusions. Predominately in the surgical literature there have been several case reports and series attesting to the efficacy of alcohol therapy.[264–267] A retrospective review followed by a prospective study of surgical patients who received alcohol prophylaxis demonstrated significant variation in dosage, duration, and indications for ethanol therapy; although the investigators reported that this approach led to a reduced rate of withdrawal symptoms and shorter duration of treatment, and increased the referral of patients to substance abuse management.[267] However, Weinberg and colleagues[268] compared IV ethanol with diazepam for alcohol-withdrawal prophylaxis in critically ill trauma patients, and found no advantage of alcohol and considerable variation in sedation-agitation scores for those who received alcohol. Use of ethanol infusions is also complicated by alcohol's inconsistent pharmacokinetic profile as well as substantial difficulties assessing ethanol elimination rate, its narrow therapeutic window, the high failure rate of IV ethanol prophylaxis, and the risk of extravasation injury and organ damage.[115,269–273] Accordingly, most authorities do not recommend the use of alcohol for the prevention or treatment of AWS.

Analgesia is infrequently mentioned in the management of AWS, yet many patients with comorbid conditions require pain management. Pain treated only with sedative agents may lead to signs and symptoms that suggest worsening severity of AWS, prompting higher doses of sedating agents and difficulties assessing the course of withdrawal. The assessment of pain, particularly in the intubated, sedated ICU patient, is imperfect. Nevertheless, if pain is believed to contribute to the patient's clinical status, intermittent IV bolus doses or infusions of agents such as morphine or fentanyl should be considered on an individual basis.

SUMMARY

Fortunately, most patients experience mild signs and symptoms of AWS and have a benign course. For those with severe withdrawal there has been a marked decrease in mortality over the past few decades, which has been achieved by improvements in identification and management of withdrawal as well as advances in supportive therapy, especially intensive care. Prognosis is best if there are no other acute medical problems. However, significant morbidity and death are risks if conditions such as multiple trauma, severe sepsis, pneumonia, and acute respiratory failure, as well as alcoholic liver disease, complicate management. Accordingly, severe AWS with delirium presents challenges to the critical care practitioner. Benzodiazepines are currently the pharmacologic agents of choice for the treatment of AWS, although studies of newer drugs may result in advances in sedation therapy. Optimal therapy for alcohol withdrawal requires an interdisciplinary, coordinated approach with use of outpatient, inpatient, and rehabilitation services.

ACKNOWLEDGMENTS

The authors are indebted to the medical libraries of Maricopa Medical Center and Banner Dell E. Webb Medical Center, and to Judy Hodgkins.

REFERENCES

1. Rehm J, Mathers C, Popova S, et al. Global burden of disease and injury and economic costs attributable to alcohol use and alcohol-use disorders. Lancet 2009;373(9682):2223–33.
2. Kosten TR, O'Connor PG. Management of drug and alcohol withdrawal. N Engl J Med 2003;348(18):1786–95.
3. Saitz R. Unhealthy alcohol use. N Engl J Med 2005;352(6):596–607.
4. 10th special report to the US Congress on alcohol and health. US Dept of Health & Human Services; 2000.
5. Harwood HJ. Updating estimates of the economic costs of alcohol abuse in the United States: estimates, update methods & data. Lewin Group for the National

Institute on Alcohol Abuse & Alcoholism; 2000. Available at: http://www.niaaa. nih.gov. Accessed March 29, 2012.

6. Gold MS. Alcohol, alcohol abuse and alcohol dependence. #651. Sacramento (CA): CME Resource; 2003.

7. Holt S, Stewart IC, Dixon JM, et al. Alcohol and the emergency service patient. Br Med J 1980;281(6241):638–40.

8. Foy A, Kay J, Taylor A. The course of alcohol withdrawal in a general hospital. QJM 1997;90(4):253–61.

9. Foy A, Kay J. The incidence of alcohol-related problems and the risk of alcohol withdrawal in a general hospital population. Drug Alcohol Rev 1995;14(1):49–54.

10. Marik P, Mohedin B. Alcohol-related admissions to an inner city hospital intensive care unit. Alcohol Alcohol 1996;31(4):393–6.

11. Baldwin WA, Rosenfeld BA, Breslow MJ, et al. Substance abuse related admissions to an adult intensive care unit. Chest 1993;103(1):21–5.

12. de Wit M, Jones DG, Sessler CN, et al. Alcohol-use disorders in the critically ill patient. Chest 2010;138(4):994–1003.

13. Sarff MC, Gold JA. Alcohol withdrawal syndromes in the intensive care unit. Crit Care Med 2010;38S:S494–501.

14. Moss M, Burnham EL. Alcohol abuse in the critically ill patient. Lancet 2006; 368(9554):2231–42.

15. Al-Sanouri I, Dikin M, Soubani AO. Critical care aspects of alcohol abuse. South Med J 2005;98(3):372–81.

16. Manwell LB, Fleming MF, Johnson K, et al. Tobacco, alcohol and drug use in a primary care sample: 90-day prevalence and associated factors. J Addict Dis 1998;17(1):67–81.

17. Hayashida MA, Alterman AI, McLellan AT, et al. Comparative effectiveness and cost of inpatient and outpatient detoxification of patients with mild-to-moderate alcohol withdrawal syndrome. N Engl J Med 1989;320(6):358–65.

18. Soyka M, Horak M. Outpatient alcohol detoxification; implementation efficacy and outcome effectiveness of a model project. Eur Addict Res 2004;10(4): 180–7.

19. Soyka M, Schmidt S. Outpatient alcoholism treatment—24-month outcome and predictors of outcome. Subst Abuse Treat Prev Policy 2009;4:15–23.

20. Hoffman RS, Weinhouse GI. Management of moderate and severe alcohol withdrawal syndromes. In: Traub SJ, Grayzel J, editors. UpToDate. Waltham (MA): UpToDate; 2011. Available at: http://www.uptodate.com. Accessed March 29, 2012.

21. Soderstrom CA, Trifillis AL, Shankar BS, et al. Marijuana and alcohol use among 1023 trauma patients. A prospective study. Arch Surg 1988;123(6):733–7.

22. Spies CD, Dubisz N, Neumann T, et al. Therapy of alcohol withdrawal syndrome in intensive care unit patients following trauma: results of prospective randomized trial. Crit Care Med 1996;24(3):414–22.

23. Field CA, Classen CA, O'Keefe G. Association of alcohol use and other high-risk behaviors among trauma patients. J Trauma 2001;50(1):13–9.

24. Srivatsav M, Wong-McKinstry ES, Ayagari S, et al. Review of respiratory complications in alcohol withdrawal syndrome at a public hospital. Crit Care Med 2008; 36(12):SA69.

25. Baldwin WA, Rosenfeld BA, Breslow MJ, et al. Substance abuse related admissions to an adult intensive care unit. Chest 1993;103(1):21–5.

26. Mostafa SM, Murthy BV. Alcohol-associated admissions to an adult intensive care unit: an audit. Eur J Anaesthesiol 2002;19(3):193–6.

27. Rootman DB, Mustard R, Kalia VB, et al. Increased incidence of complications in trauma patients cointoxicated with alcohol and other drugs. J Trauma 2007; 62(3):755–8.

28. Spies CD, Nemer B, Neurmann T, et al. Intercurrent complications in chronic alcoholic men admitted to the intensive care unit following trauma. Intensive Care Med 1996;22(4):286–93.

29. Silver GM, Albright JM, Schermer CR, et al. Adverse clinical outcomes associated with elevated blood alcohol levels at the time of burn injury. J Burn Care Res 2008;29(5):784–9.

30. Diaz LE, Montero A, Gonzalez-Gross M, et al. Influence of alcohol consumption on immunologic status: a review. Eur J Clin Nutr 2002;56(Suppl 3):S50–3.

31. Fernández-Solá J, Junqué A, Estruch R, et al. High alcohol intake as a risk and prognostic factor for community acquired pneumonia. Arch Intern Med 1995; 155(15):1649–54.

32. Ruiz M, Ewig S, Torres A, et al. Severe community-acquired pneumonia. Risk factors and follow-up epidemiology. Am J Respir Crit Care Med 1999;160(3):923–9.

33. Saitz R, Ghali WA, Moskowitz MA. The impact of alcohol-related diagnoses on pneumonia outcomes. Arch Intern Med 1997;157(13):1446–52.

34. Hudson LD, Milberg JA, Anardi D, et al. Clinical risks for development of the acute respiratory distress syndrome. Am J Respir Crit Care Med 1995; 151(2 Pt 1):293–301.

35. Happel KI, Nelson S. Alcohol, immunosuppression, and the lung. Proc Am Thorac Soc 2005;2(5):428–32.

36. Pavia CS, La Mothe M, Kavanaugh M. Influence of alcohol on antimicrobial immunity. Biomed Pharmacother 2004;58(2):84–9.

37. Szabo G. Consequences of alcohol consumption on host defense. Alcohol Alcohol 1999;34(6):830–41.

38. O'Brien JM, Lu B, Ali NA, et al. Alcohol dependence is independently associated with sepsis, septic shock and hospital mortality among adult intensive care patients. Crit Care Med 2007;35(2):345–50.

39. Gacouin A, Legay F, Camus C, et al. At-risk drinkers are at higher risk to acquire a bacterial infection during an intensive care unit stay than abstinent or moderate drinkers. Crit Care Med 2008;36(6):1735–41.

40. Guarneri JJ, Laurenzi GA. Effect of alcohol on the mobilization of alveolar macrophages. J Lab Clin Med 1968;72(1):40–51.

41. de Wit M, Best AM, Gennings C, et al. Alcohol use disorders increase the risk for mechanical ventilation in medical patients. Alcohol Clin Exp Res 2007;31(7): 1224–30.

42. McGovern PE. Uncorking the past: the quest for wine, beer and other alcoholic beverages. Berkeley (CA): University of California Press; 2009.

43. Standage T. A history of the world in six glasses. New York: Walker & Co; 2005.

44. Martin D. When to say when: wine and drunkenness in ancient Rome [MA dissertation]. Columbia (MO): University of Missouri; 2010.

45. Lennox WG. Alcohol and epilepsy. Q J Stud Alcohol 1941;11(1):1–11.

46. Adams F. The genuine works of Hippocrates. New York: William Wood & Co; 1886.

47. Lennox WG. John of Gaddesden on epilepsy. Ann Med Hist 1939;1:283–307.

48. Smyth A. Introduction. In: Smyth A, editor. A pleasing sinne: drink and conviviality in 17th century England. Cambridge (United Kingdom): Brewer DS; 2004. p. xviii.

49. Earnshaw S. The pub in literature: England's altered state. Manchester (United Kingdom): Manchester University Press; 2000.

50. Huss M. Alcoholismus chronicus. Eller chronisk alkoholssjukdom; ett bidrag till dyskrasiernas kännedom. Enligt egen och andras efarenhet. Stockholm (Sweden): Beckman; 1851. p. 1849–51. [in Swedish].

51. Sutton T. Tracts on delirium tremens, on peritonitis and some other internal inflammatory affections, and on the gout. London: James Moyes for Thomas Underwood; 1813.

52. Ware J. Remarks on the history and treatment of delirium tremens. Med Commun Mass Med Soc 1836;5:136–94 cited by Cutshall BJ. The Saunders-Sutton syndrome: an analysis of delirium tremens. Q J Stud Alcohol 1965;26(3):423–8.

53. Dickens C. Our mutual friend. In: Poole A, editor. New York: Penguin; 1997.

54. Griffith E. Alcohol: the world's favorite drug. New York: Thomas Dunne Books; 2000. p. 73–92.

55. Peterson V, Nisenholz B, Robinson G. A nation under the influence: America's addiction to alcohol. Boston: Pearson Education; 2003.

56. Djos MG. Writing under the influence: alcoholism and the alcoholic perception from Hemingway to Berryman. New York: Palgrave-MacMillan; 2010.

57. Trotter T. An essay medical, philosophical, and chemical, on drunkenness and its effects on the human body. London; 1988. (Facsimile of the 1804 London edition and based on the thesis presented to Edinburgh University in 1788). Wikipedia, The Free Encyclopedia, Wikimedia Foundation. Accessed March 29, 2012.

58. Rush B. An inquiry into the effects of ardents spirits upon the human body and mind: with an account of the means to preventing, and of the remedies for curing them. Philadelphia: Thomas Dobson; 1808.

59. Osler W. The principles and practice of medicine. New York: D Appleton & Co; 1895. p. 1057–71.

60. Sellers EM, Kalant H. Alcohol intoxication and withdrawal. N Engl J Med 1976; 294(14):757–62.

61. Charney DS, Mihic SJ, Harris RA. Hypnotics and sedatives. In: Brunton LL, Lazo JS, Parker KL, editors. Goodman & Gillman's pharmacological basis of therapeutics. 11th edition. New York: McGraw Hill; 2006. p. 402, 420–1.

62. Lovinger DM, Zimmerman SA, Levitin M, et al. Trichlorethanol potentiates synaptic transmission mediated by gamma-aminobutyric acid$_A$ receptors in hippocampal neurons. J Pharmacol Exp Ther 1993;264(3):1097–103.

63. Victor M. Treatment of alcoholic intoxication and the withdrawal syndrome. Psychosom Med 1966;28(4):636–48.

64. Thompson WL, Johnson AD, Maddrey WL, et al. Diazepam and paraldehyde for treatment of severe delirium tremens. A controlled trial. Ann Intern Med 1975; 82(2):175–80.

65. Sainsbury MJ. The management of delirium tremens. Med J Aust 1975;1(1):15–6.

66. Hart WT. A comparison of promazine and paraldehyde in 175 cases of alcohol withdrawal. Am J Psychiatry 1961;118(4):323–7.

67. Lopez-Munoz F, Ucha-Udabe R, Alamo C. The history of barbiturates a century after their clinical introduction. Neuropsychiatr Dis Treat 2005;1(4):329–43.

68. Gold JA, Rimal B, Nolan A, et al. A strategy of escalating doses of benzodiazepines and phenobarbital administration reduces the need for mechanical ventilation in delirium tremens. Crit Care Med 2007;35(3):724–30.

69. Hendey GW, Dery RA, Barnes RL, et al. A prospective, randomized trial of phenobarbital versus benzodiazepines for acute alcohol withdrawal. Am J Emerg Med 2011;29(4):382–5.

70. Sereny G, Kalant H. Comparative clinical evaluation of chlordiazepoxide and promazine in treatment of alcohol-withdrawal syndrome. Br Med J 1965;1(5427):92–7.

71. Greenblatt DJ, Greenblatt M. Which drug for alcohol withdrawal? J Clin Pharmacol 1972;12(11):429–31.

72. Kaim SC, Klett CJ, Rothfeld B. Treatment of the acute alcohol withdrawal state: a comparison of four drugs. Am J Psychiatry 1969;125(12):1640–6.

73. Knott DH, Beard JD. Diagnosis and therapy of acute withdrawal from alcohol. Curr Psychiatr Ther 1970;10:145–50.

74. Greenblatt DJ, Shader RI. Rational use of psychotropic drugs II. Antianxiety agents. Am J Health Syst Pharm 1974;31:1077–80.

75. Kraus ML, Gottlieb LD, Horwitz RI, et al. Randomized clinical trial of atenolol in patients with alcohol withdrawal. N Engl J Med 1985;313(15):905–9.

76. Buchsbaum DG, Buchanan RG, Centor RM, et al. Screening for alcohol abuse using CAGE scores and likelihood ratios. Ann Intern Med 1991;115(10):774–7.

77. Bush B, Shaw S, Cleary P, et al. Screening for alcohol abuse using the CAGE questionnaire. Am J Med 1987;82(2):231–5.

78. Shaw JM, Kolesar GS, Sellers EM, et al. Development of optimal treatment tactics for alcohol withdrawal. I. Assessment and effectiveness of supportive care. J Clin Psychopharmacol 1981;1(6):382–7.

79. Sullivan JT, Sykora M, Schneiderman J, et al. Assessment of alcohol withdrawal: the revised clinical institute withdrawal assessment for alcohol scale (CIWA-Ar). Br J Addict 1989;84(11):1353–7.

80. Wetterling T, Kanitz R-D, Besters B, et al. A new rating scale for the assessment of the alcohol-withdrawal syndrome (AWS scale). Alcohol Alcohol 1997;32(6): 753–60.

81. Ramsay MA, Savege TM, Simpson BR, et al. Controlled sedation with alphax-alone-alphadolone. Br Med J 1974;2(5920):656–74.

82. Sessler CN, Gosnell MS, Grap MJ, et al. The Richmond Agitation-Sedation Scale: validity and reliability in adult intensive care unit patients. Am J Respir Crit Care Med 2002;166(10):1338–44.

83. Simmons LE, Riker RR, Prato S, et al. Assessing sedation during intensive care unit mechanical ventilation with the bispectral index and the sedation-agitation scale. Crit Care Med 1999;27(8):1499–504.

84. Riker RR, Picard JT, Frasher GL. Prospective evaluation of the sedation-agitation scale for adult critically ill patients. Crit Care Med 1999;27(7):1325–9.

85. American Psychiatric Association. Diagnostic and statistical manual of mental disorders. 4th edition (text revision). Washington, DC: American Psychiatric Association; 2000.

86. Ely EW, Margolin R, Francis J, et al. Evaluation of delirium in critically ill patients: validation of the confusion assessment method for the intensive care unit (CAM-ICU). Crit Care Med 2001;29(7):1370–9.

87. Jellinek EM. The disease concept of alcoholism. New Haven (CT): Hillhouse; 1960.

88. Booth BM, Blow FC, Ludke RL, et al. Utilization of acute inpatient services for alcohol detoxification. J Ment Health Adm 1996;23(4):366–74.

89. Zacharias S, Rodriguez-Garcia A, Honz N, et al. Development of an alcohol withdrawal clinical pathway: an interdisciplinary process. J Nurs Care Qual 1998;12(3):9–18.

90. Isabell H, Fraser HF, Wikler A, et al. An experimental study of the etiology of "rum fits" and delirium tremens. Q J Stud Alcohol 1955;16(1):1–33.

91. Victor M, Adams RD. The effect of alcohol on the nervous system. Res Publ Assoc Res Nerv Ment Dis 1953;32:526–73.

92. Carlsson C, Häggendal J. Arterial noradrenaline levels after ethanol withdrawal. Lancet 1967;2(7521):889.

93. Perman ES. The effect of ethyl alcohol on the secretion from the adrenal medulla in man. Acta Physiol Scand 1958;44(3–4):241–7.
94. Krystal JH, Staley J, Mason G, et al. Gamma-aminobutyric acid type A receptors and alcoholism: intoxication, dependence, vulnerability and treatment. Arch Gen Psychiatry 2006;63(9):957–68.
95. Ticku MK, Burch TP, Davis WC. The interactions of ethanol with the benzodiazepine-GABA receptor-ionophore complex. Pharmacol Biochem Behav 1983;18(S1):15–8.
96. Buck KJ, Hahner L, Sikela J, et al. Chronic ethanol treatment alters brain levels of gamma-aminobutyric acid a receptor subunit mRNAs: relationship to genetic differences in ethanol withdrawal seizure severity. J Neurochem 1991;57(4):1452–5.
97. Tsai G, Coyle JT. The role of glutamatergic neurotransmission in the pathophysiology of alcoholism. Annu Rev Med 1998;49(1):173–84.
98. Biermann T, Reulbach U, Lenz B, et al. N-methyl-D-aspartate 2b receptor subtype (NR2B) promoter methylation in patients during alcohol withdrawal. J Neural Transm 2009;116(5):615–22.
99. Haugbøl SR, Ebert B, Ulrichsen J. Upregulation of glutamate receptor subtypes during alcohol withdrawal in rats. Alcohol Alcohol 2005;40(2):89–95.
100. Lutz UC. Alterations of homocysteine metabolism among alcohol dependent patients—clinical, pathobiochemical and genetic aspects. Curr Drug Abuse Rev 2008;1(1):47–55.
101. Giacobini E, Izikowitz S, Wegman A. Urinary norepinephrine and epinephrine excretion in delirium tremens. Arch Gen Psychiatry 1960;3:289–96.
102. Klingman GI, Goodall M. Urinary epinephrine and levarternol excretion during acute sublethal alcohol intoxication in dogs. J Pharmacol Exp Ther 1957; 121(3):313–8.
103. Sjoquist B, Borg S, Kvande H. Catecholamine derived compounds in urine and cerebrospinal fluid from alcoholics during and after long-standing intoxication. Subst Alcohol Actions Misuse 1981;2(10):63–72.
104. Hawley RJ, Major LF, Schulman EA, et al. CSF levels of norepinephrine during alcohol withdrawal. Arch Neurol 1981;38(5):289–92.
105. Hawley RJ, Major LF, Schulman EA. Cerebrospinal fluid 3-methoxy-4-hydroxy-phenylglycol and norepinephrine levels in alcohol withdrawal. Correlates with clinical signs. Arch Gen Psychiatry 1985;42(11):1056–62.
106. Borg S, Czarnecka A, Kvande H, et al. Clinical conditions and concentrations of MOPEG in the cerebrospinal fluid and urine of male alcoholic patients during withdrawal. Alcohol Clin Exp Res 1983;7(4):411–5.
107. Sellers EM, Zilm DH, Degani NC. Comparative efficacy of propranolol and chlordiazepoxide in alcohol withdrawal. J Stud Alcohol 1977;38(11): 2096–108.
108. Manhem P, Nilsson LH, Moberg A, et al. Alcohol withdrawal: effects of clonidine treatment on sympathetic activity, the renin-aldosterone system and clinical symptoms. Alcohol Clin Exp Res 1985;9(3):238–43.
109. Romero C, Bugedo G, Bruhn A, et al. Experiencia preliminar del tratamiento con dexmedetomidine del estado confusional e hiperadrenergia en la unidad de cuidados intensivos. Rev Esp Anestesiol Reanim 2002;49(8):403–6 [in Spanish].
110. Baumgartner GR, Rowen RC. Transdermal clonidine versus chlorodiazepoxide in alcohol withdrawal: a randomized controlled clinical trial. South Med J 1991;84(3):312–21.
111. Baumgartner GR, Rowen RC. Clonidine vs chlordiazepoxide in the management of the acute alcohol withdrawal syndrome. Arch Intern Med 1987;147(7):1223–6.

112. Yam PCI, Forbes A, Kox WJ. Clonidine in the treatment of alcohol withdrawal in the intensive care unit. Br J Anaesth 1992;68(1):106–8.

113. Baddigam K, Russo P, Russo J, et al. Dexmedetomidine in the treatment of withdrawal syndromes in cardiothoracic surgery patients. J Intensive Care Med 2005;20(2):118–23.

114. Rovasalo A, Tohmo H, Aantaa R, et al. Dexmedetomidine as an adjuvant in the treatment of alcohol withdrawal delirium: a case report. Gen Hosp Psychiatry 2006;28(4):362–3.

115. Mayo-Smith MF. Pharmacological management of alcohol withdrawal: a meta-analysis and evidence-based practice guideline. JAMA 1997;278(2):144–51.

116. Zilm DH, Jacob MS, MacLeod SM, et al. Propranolol and chlordiazepoxide effects on cardiac arrhythmias during alcohol withdrawal. Alcohol Clin Exp Res 1980;4(4):400–5.

117. Worner TM. Propranolol versus diazepam in the management of the alcohol withdrawal syndrome: double-blind controlled trial. Am J Drug Alcohol Abuse 1994;20(1):115–24.

118. Mayo-Smith MF. Management of alcohol intoxication and withdrawal. In: Ries RK, Fiellin DA, Miller SC, et al, editors. Principles of addiction medicine. 4th edition. Philadelphia: Lippincott Williams & Wilkins; 2009. p. 559–72.

119. Pich EM, Lorang M, Yeganeh M, et al. Increase of extracellular corticotropin-releasing factor-like immunoreactivity levels in the amygdala of awake rats during restraint stress and ethanol withdrawal as measured by microdialysis. J Neurosci 1995;15(8):5439–47.

120. Rassnick S, Heinrichs SG, Britton KT, et al. Microinjection of corticotropin-releasing factor antagonist into the central nucleus of the amygdala reverses anxiogenic-like effects of ethanol withdrawal. Brain Res 1993;605(1):25–32.

121. De Witte P, Pinto E, Ansseau M, et al. Alcohol and withdrawal: from animal research to clinical issues. Neurosci Behav Rev 2003;27(3):189–97.

122. Bannan LT, Potter JF, Beevers DG, et al. Effect of alcohol withdrawal on blood pressure, plasma rennin activity, aldosterone, cortisol and dopamine beta-hydroxylase. Clin Sci 1984;66(6):659–63.

123. Mendelson JH, Stein S. Serum cortisol levels in alcoholic and nonalcoholic subjects during experimentally induced ethanol intoxication. Psychosom Med 1966;28(4):616–26.

124. Lovinger DM, White G, Weight FF. Ethanol inhibits NMDA-activated ion current in hippocampal neurons. Science 1989;243(4899):1721–4.

125. Kumari M, Ticku MK. Regulation of NMDA receptors by alcohol. Prog Drug Res 2000;54:152–89.

126. Gonzales RA, Jaworski JN. Alcohol and glutamate. Alcohol Health Res World 1997;2(2):120–7.

127. Davis KM, Wu JY. Role of glutamatergic and GABAergic systems in alcoholism. J Biomed Sci 2001;8(1):7–19.

128. Tsai GE, Gastfriend DR, Coyle JT. The glutamatergic basis of human alcoholism. Am J Psychiatry 1995;152(3):332–40.

129. Tsai GE, Ragan P, Chang R, et al. Increased glutamatergic neurotransmission and oxidative stress after alcohol withdrawal. Am J Psychiatry 1998;155(6):726–32.

130. Blevins T, Mirshahi T, Woodward JJ. Increased agonist and antagonist sensitivity of N-methyl-D-aspartate stimulated calcium flux in cultured neurons following chronic ethanol exposure. Neurosci Lett 1995;2002(3):214–8.

131. Nagy J. Renaissance of NMDA receptor antagonists: do they have a role in the pharmacotherapy for alcoholism? Drugs 2004;7(4):339–50.

132. Hoffman PL, Grant KA, Snell LD, et al. NMDA receptors: role in ethanol withdrawal seizures. Ann N Y Acad Sci 1992;654:52–60.
133. Grant KA, Valverius P, Hudspith M, et al. Ethanol withdrawal seizures and the NMDA receptor complex. Eur J Pharmacol 1990;176(3):289–96.
134. Krupitsky EM, Rudenko AA, Burakov AM, et al. Antiglutamatergic strategies for ethanol detoxification: comparison with placebo and diazepam. Alcohol Clin Exp Res 2007;31(4):604–11.
135. Krystal JH, Petrakis IL, Krupisky E, et al. NMDA receptor antagonism and the ethanol intoxication signal: from alcoholism risk to pharmacotherapy. Ann N Y Acad Sci 2003;1003:176–84.
136. Bleich S, Degner D, Bandelow B, et al. Plasma homocysteine is a predictor of alcohol withdrawal seizures. Neuroreport 2000;11(12):2749–52.
137. Bleich S, Degner D, Sperline W, et al. Homocysteine as a neurotoxin in chronic alcoholism. Prog Neuropsychopharmacol Biol Psychiatry 2004;28(3):453–64.
138. Volkow ND, Wang G-J, Marynard L, et al. Effects of alcohol detoxification on dopamine D2 receptors in alcoholics: a preliminary study. Psychiatry Res 2002;116(3):163–72.
139. Seeman P, Tallerico T, Ko F. Alcohol-withdrawn animals have a prolonged increase in dopamine D2 high receptors, reversed by general anesthesia: relation to relapse? Synapse 2004;52(2):77–83.
140. Biermann T, Bonsch D, Reulbach U, et al. Dopamine and N-methyl-D-aspartate receptor expression in peripheral blood of patients undergoing alcohol withdrawal. J Neural Transm 2007;114(8):1081–4.
141. Gorwood P, Limosin F, Batel P, et al. The A9 allele of the dopamine transporter gene is associated with delirium tremens and alcohol-withdrawal seizure. Biol Psychiatry 2003;53(1):85–92.
142. Schmidt LG, Sander T. Genetics of alcohol withdrawal. Eur Psychiatry 2000; 15(2):135–9.
143. Glue P, Nutt D. Overexcitement and disinhibition: dynamic neurotransmitter interactions in alcohol withdrawal. Br J Psychiatry 1990;157:491–9.
144. López-Muñoz L, Alamo C, García-García P. The discovery of chlordiazepoxide and the clinical introduction of benzodiazepines: half a century of anxiolytic drugs. J Anxiety Disord 2011;25(4):554–62.
145. Caputo F, Bernardi M. Medications acting on the GABA system in the treatment of alcoholic patients. Curr Pharm Des 2010;16(19):2118–25.
146. Enoch MA. The role of GABA_A receptors in the development of alcoholism. Pharmacol Biochem Behav 2008;90(1):95–104.
147. Olsen RW. GABA-benzodiazepine-barbiturate receptor interactions. J Neurochem 1981;37(1):1–13.
148. Amato L, Minozzi AL, Vecchi S, et al. Benzodiazepines for alcohol withdrawal [review]. Cochrane Database Syst Rev 2010;(3):1–111:CD005063.
149. Saitz R, O'Malley SS. Pharmacotherapies for alcohol abuse: withdrawal and treatment. Med Clin North Am 1997;81(4):881–907.
150. Holbrook AM, Crowther R, Lotter A, et al. Meta-analysis of benzodiazepine use in the treatment of acute alcohol withdrawal. CMAJ 1999;160(5):649–79.
151. Legio L, Kenna GA, Swift RM. New developments for the pharmacological treatment of alcohol withdrawal: A focus on non-benzodiazepine GABAergic medications. Prog Neuropsychopharmacol Biol Psychiatry 2008;32(5):1106–17.
152. Martinotti G, de Nicola M, Frustaci A, et al. Pregabalin, tiapride and lorazepam in alcohol withdrawal syndrome: a multi-centre, randomized single-blind comparison trial. Addiction 2010;105(2):288–99.

153. Liu J, Wang L. Baclofen for alcohol withdrawal [review]. Cochrane Database Syst Rev 2011;(1):1–17:CD008502.

154. Tabakoff B, Hoffman PL. Neurobiology of alcohol. In: Galanter M, Kleber HD, editors. Textbook of substance abuse treatment. 3rd edition. Washington, DC: American Psychiatric Publishing; 2004.

155. Yu D, Zhang L, Eisele JL, et al. Ethanol inhibition of nicotinic acetylcholine type alpha 7 receptors involves the amino-terminal domain of the receptor. Mol Pharmacol 1996;50(4):1010–6.

156. Zuo Y, Kuryatov A, Lindstrom JM, et al. Alcohol modulation of neuronal nicotinic acetylcholine receptors in alpha subunit dependent. Alcohol Clin Exp Res 2002; 26(6):779–84.

157. Schucket MA. Vulnerability factors for alcoholism. In: Davis KL, Charney D, Coyle JT, et al, editors. Neuropsychopharmacology: the 5th generation of progress. Philadelphia: Lippincott Williams & Wilkins; 2002.

158. Barr CS, Newman TK, Lindell S, et al. Interaction between the serotonin transporter gene variation and rearing condition in alcohol preference and consumption in female primates. Arch Gen Psychiatry 2004;61(11):1146–52.

159. Elisaf M, Merkouropoulos M, Tsianos EV, et al. Acid-base and electrolyte abnormalities in alcoholic patients. Miner Electrolyte Metab 1994;20(5):274–81.

160. Flink EB, Stutzman FL, Anderson AR, et al. Magnesium deficiency after prolonged parenteral fluid administration and after chronic alcoholism complicated by delirium tremens. J Lab Clin Med 1954;43(2):169–83.

161. Victor M. The role of hypomagnesemia and respiratory alkalosis in the genesis of alcohol-withdrawal symptoms. Ann N Y Acad Sci 1973;215:235–48.

162. Vinson DC, Menezes M. Admission alcohol level: a predictor of the course of alcohol withdrawal. J Fam Pract 1991;33(2):161–7.

163. Ferguson JA, Suelzer CJ, Eckert GJ, et al. Risk factors for delirium tremens development. J Gen Intern Med 1996;11(7):410–4.

164. Kraemer KL, Mayo-Smith MF, Calkins DR. Independent clinical correlates of severe alcohol withdrawal. Subst Abus 2003;24(4):197–209.

165. Feuerlein W, Reiser E. Parameters affecting the course and results of delirium tremens treatment. Acta Psychiatr Scand Suppl 1986;s329(73):120–3.

166. Wojnar M, Bizon Z, Wasilewski D. The role of somatic disorders and physical injury in the development and course of alcohol withdrawal delirium. Alcohol Clin Exp Res 1999;23(2):209–13.

167. Schuckit MA, Tipp JE, Reich T, et al. The histories of withdrawal convulsions and delirium tremens in 1648 alcohol dependent subjects. Addiction 1995;90(10): 1335–47.

168. Sullivan JT. Benzodiazepine requirements during alcohol withdrawal syndrome: clinical implications of using a standardized withdrawal scale. J Clin Psychopharmacol 1991;11(5):291–5.

169. Turner RC, Lichstein PR, Peden JG Jr, et al. Alcohol withdrawal syndromes: a review of pathophysiology, clinical presentation, and treatment. J Gen Intern Med 1989;4(5):432–44.

170. Brown CG. The alcohol withdrawal syndrome. Ann Emerg Med 1982;11(5):276–80.

171. Carlson RW, Keske B, Cortez A. Alcohol withdrawal syndrome: alleviating symptoms, preventing progression. J Crit Illn 1998;13(5):311–7.

172. Smothers BA, Yahr HT. Alcohol use disorder and illicit drug use in admissions to general hospitals in the United States. Am J Addict 2005;14(3):256–67.

173. Ballenger JC, Post RM. Kindling as a model for alcohol withdrawal syndromes. Br J Psychiatry 1978;133:1–14.

174. Monte R, Rabunal R, Casariego E, et al. Clinical aspects: analysis of the factors determining survival of alcoholic withdrawal syndrome patients in a general hospital. Alcohol Alcohol 2010;45(2):151–8.

175. Booth BM, Blow FC. The kindling hypothesis: further evidence from a US national study of alcoholic men. Alcohol Alcohol 1993;28(5):593–8.

176. Wright T, Myrick H, Henderson S, et al. Risk factors for delirium tremens: a retrospective chart review. Am J Addict 2006;15(3):213–9.

177. Breese GR, Sinha R, Heilig M. Chronic alcohol neuroadaptation and stress contribute to susceptibility for alcohol craving and relapse. Pharmacol Ther 2011;129(2):149–71.

178. Helzer JE, Pryzbeck TR. The co-occurrence of alcoholism with other psychiatric disorders in the general population and its impact on treatment. J Stud Alcohol 1988;49(3):219–24.

179. Ramsay A, Vredenbrugh J, Gallagher RM. Recognition of alcoholism among patients with psychiatric problems in a family practice clinic. J Fam Pract 1983;17(5):829–32.

180. deRoux A, Cavalcanti M, Marcos MA, et al. Impact of alcohol abuse in the etiology and severity of community-acquired pneumonia. Chest 2006;129(5): 1219–25.

181. Chang PH, Steinberg MB. Alcohol withdrawal. Med Clin North Am 2001;85(5): 1191–212.

182. Behnke RH. Recognition and management of alcohol withdrawal syndrome. Hosp Pract 1976;11(11):79–84.

183. Hecksel KA, Bostwick JM, Jaeger TM, et al. Inappropriate use of symptom-triggered therapy for alcohol withdrawal in the general hospital. Mayo Clin Proc 2008;83(3):274–9.

184. Carlson RW, Raj J. Alcohol withdrawal syndrome. In: Kruse JA, Fink MP, Carlson RW, editors. Saunders manual of critical care. Philadelphia: Elsevier Science; 2003. p. 240–3.

185. Carlson RW, Cortez A, Keske B. Alcohol withdrawal syndrome: clinical problems. Houston (TX): Snow Tiger Medical Data Base; 1999.

186. Ahaboucha S, Butterworth RF. Role of endogenous benzodiazepine ligands and their GABA-A-associated receptors in hepatic encephalopathy. Metab Brain Dis 2005;20(4):425–37.

187. Bismuth M, Funakoshi N, Cadranel JF, et al. Hepatic encephalopathy: from pathophysiology to therapeutic management. Eur J Gastroenterol Hepatol 2011; 23(1):9–22.

188. Shane SR, Flink EB. Magnesium deficiency in alcohol addiction and withdrawal. Magnes Trace Elem 1991;10(2–4):263–8.

189. Flink EB. Magnesium deficiency in alcoholism. Alcohol Clin Exp Res 1986;10(6): 590–4.

190. Daus AT, Freeman WM, Wilson J, et al. Clinical experience with 781 cases of alcoholism evaluated and treated on an inpatient basis by various methods. Int J Addict 1985;20(4):643–50.

191. Rubeiz GJ, Thill-Baharozian M, Hardie D, et al. Association of hypomagnesemia and mortality in acutely ill medical patients. Crit Care Med 1993;21(2):203–9.

192. Yeh H-S, Dhopesh V, Maany I. Seizures during detoxification. J Gen Intern Med 1992;7(1):123.

193. Alldredge BK, Lowenstein DH, Simon RP. Placebo-controlled trial of intravenous diphenylhydrantoin for short-term treatment of alcohol withdrawal seizures. Am J Med 1989;87(6):645–8.

194. Thompson WL. Management of alcohol withdrawal syndromes. Arch Intern Med 1978;138(2):278–83.
195. Schuckit MA. Alcohol-related disorders. In: Sadock BJ, Sadock VA, Ruiz P, editors. Comprehensive textbook of psychiatry. 9th edition. Philadelphia: Lippincott; 2009.
196. Palmstierna T. A model for predicting alcohol withdrawal delirium. Psychiatr Serv 2001;52(6):820–3.
197. Trzepacz PT, Baker RW, Greenhouse J. A symptom rating scale for delirium. Psychiatry Res 1988;23(1):89–97.
198. Bergeron N, Dubois MJ, Durmont M, et al. Intensive care delirium screening checklist: evaluation of a new screening tool. Intensive Care Med 2001;27(5): 859–64.
199. Maldonado JR. Delirium in the acute care setting: characteristics, diagnosis and treatment. Crit Care Clin 2008;24(4):657–722.
200. Meagher DJ, Trzepacz PT. Motoric subtypes of delirium. Semin Clin Neuropsychiatry 2000;5(2):75–85.
201. Adams Wilson JR, Morandi A, Girard TD, et al. The association of the kynurenine pathway of tryptophan metabolism with acute brain dysfunction during critical illness. Crit Care Med 2012;40(3):835–41.
202. Girard TD, Jackson JC, Pandharipande PP, et al. Delirium as a predictor of long-term cognitive impairment in survivors of critical illness. Crit Care Med 2010; 38(7):1513–20.
203. Meagher DJ, O'Hanlon D, O'Mahony E, et al. Relationship between symptoms and motoric subtype of delirium. J Neuropsychiatry Clin Neurosci 2000;12(1): 51–6.
204. Pandharipande PP, Shintani A, Peterson J, et al. Lorazepam is an independent risk factor for transitioning to delirium in intensive care unit patients. Anesthesiology 2006;104(1):21–6.
205. Pandharipande PP, Pun BT, Herr DT, et al. Effect of sedation with dexmedetomidine vs lorazepam on acute brain dysfunction in mechanically ventilated patients: the MENDS randomized controlled trial. JAMA 2007;298(22):2644–53.
206. Tune LE, Bylsma FW. Benzodiazepine-induced and anticholinergic-induced delirium in the elderly. Int Psychogeriatr 1991;3(2):397–408.
207. Hshieh TT, Fong TG, Marcantonio ER, et al. Cholinergic deficiency hypothesis in delirium: a synthesis of current evidence. J Gerontol A Biol Sci Med Sci 2008; 63(7):764–72.
208. Abraham E, Shoemaker WC, McCartney SF. Cardiorespiratory patterns in severe delirium tremens. Arch Intern Med 1985;145(6):1057–9.
209. Trevisan LA, Boutros N, Petrakis IL, et al. Complications of alcohol withdrawal: pathophysiological insights. Alcohol Health Res World 1998;22(1):61–6.
210. Bonnet U, Specka M, Hamzavl-Abed R, et al. Severe protracted alcohol withdrawal syndrome: prevalence and pharmacological treatment at an inpatient detoxification unit—a naturalistic study. Pharmacopsychiatry 2009; 42(2):76–8.
211. Favazza AR, Martin P. Chemotherapy of delirium tremens: a survey of physicians' preferences. Am J Psychiatry 1974;131(9):1031–3.
212. Moskowitz G, Chalmers TC, Sacks HS, et al. Deficiencies of clinical trials of alcohol withdrawal. Alcohol Clin Exp Res 1983;7(1):42–4.
213. Amato L, Minozzi S, Davoli M. Efficacy and safety of pharmacological interventions for the treatment of the alcohol withdrawal syndrome. Cochrane Database Syst Rev 2011;15(6):1–25.

214. Golberrt TM, Sanz CJ, Rose HD, et al. Comparative evaluation of treatments of alcohol withdrawal syndromes. JAMA 1967;201(2):99–102.
215. Sellers EM, Naranjo CA, Harrison M, et al. Diazepam loading: simplified treatment of alcohol withdrawal. Clin Pharmacol Ther 1983;34:822–6.
216. Weaver MF, Hoffman HJ, Johnson RE. Alcohol withdrawal pharmacotherapy for inpatients with medical comorbidity. J Addict Dis 2006;25(2):17–24.
217. Daeppen JB, Gache P, Landry U, et al. Symptom-triggered vs fixed-schedule doses of benzodiazepine for alcohol withdrawal: a randomized treatment trial. Arch Intern Med 2002;162(10):1117–21.
218. Saitz R, Mayo-Smith MF, Roberts MS, et al. Individualized treatment for alcohol withdrawal. JAMA 1994;272(7):519–23.
219. Bird RD, Makela EH. Alcohol withdrawal: what is the benzodiazepine of choice? Ann Pharmacother 1994;28(1):67–71.
220. Miller WC Jr, McCurdy L. A double-blind comparison of the efficacy and safety of lorazepam and diazepam in the treatment of the acute alcohol withdrawal syndrome. Clin Ther 1984;6(3):364–71.
221. Ritson B, Chick J. Comparison of two benzodiazepines in the treatment of alcohol withdrawal: effects on symptoms and cognitive recovery. Drug Alcohol Depend 1986;18(4):329–34.
222. Solomon J, Rouch LA, Koepke HH. Double-blind comparison of lorazepam and chlordiazepoxide in the treatment of the acute alcohol abstinence syndrome. Clin Ther 1983;6(1):52–8.
223. Sellers EM, Sandor P, Giles HG, et al. Diazepam pharmacokinetics after intravenous administration in alcohol withdrawal. Br J Clin Pharmacol 1983;15(1):125–7.
224. Malacrida R, Fritz ME, Suter PM, et al. Pharmacokinetics of midazolam administered by continuous intravenous infusion to intensive care patients. Crit Care Med 1992;20(8):1123–6.
225. Riker RR, Shehabi Y, Bokesch PM, et al. Dexmedetomidine vs midazolam for sedation of critically ill patients. JAMA 2009;301(5):489–99.
226. Kollef MH, Levy NT, Ahrens TS, et al. The use of continuous IV sedation is associated with prolongation of mechanical ventilation. Chest 1998;114(2):541–8.
227. Maze M, Scarfini C, Cavaliere F. New agents for sedation in the intensive care unit. Crit Care Clin 2001;17(4):881–97.
228. Spies CD, Otter HE, Hiske B, et al. Alcohol withdrawal severity is decreased by symptom-oriented adjusted bolus therapy in the ICU. Intensive Care Med 2003;29(12):2230–8.
229. Reoux JP, Miller K. Routine hospital alcohol detoxification practice compared to symptom triggered management with an objective withdrawal scale (CIWA-Ar). Am J Addict 2009;9(2):135–44.
230. Kahan S, Petersen K, Krimsley J. Impact of severe delirium tremens (DT) on postoperative-traumatic recovery with the application of the CIWA-Ar. Crit Care Med 2010;38(12):793.
231. Dill C. High-dose intravenous benzodiazepine. Acad Emerg Med 2000;7(3):308–10.
232. Hack JB, Hoffman RS, Nelson LS. Resistant alcohol withdrawal: does an unexpectedly large sedative requirement identify these patients early? J Med Toxicol 2006;2(2):55–60.
233. Nolop KP, Natow A. Unprecedented sedative requirements during delirium tremens. Crit Care Med 1985;13(4):246–7.

234. Wolf KM, Shaughnessy AF, Middleton DB. Prolonged delirium tremens requiring massive doses of medication. J Am Board Fam Pract 1993;6(5):502–4.
235. Woo E, Greenblatt DJ. Massive benzodiazepine requirements during alcohol withdrawal. Am J Psychiatry 1979;136(6):821–3.
236. Volicer L, Biagioni TM. Effect of ethanol administration and withdrawal on benzodiazepine receptor binding in the rat brain. Neuropharmacology 1982;21(7):283–6.
237. Morrow AL, Suzdak PD, Karanian JW, et al. Chronic ethanol administration alters gamma-aminobutyric acid, pentobarbital and ethanol-mediated ^{36}Cl-uptake in cerebral cortical synaptoneurosomes. J Pharmacol Exp Ther 1988;246(1):158–64.
238. Nutt D, Adinoff B, Linnoila M. Benzodiazepines in the treatment of alcoholism. Recent Dev Alcohol 1989;7:283–313.
239. Marik PE. Propofol: therapeutic indications and side-effects. Curr Pharm Des 2004;10(29):3639–49.
240. Vasile B, Rasulo F, Candiani A, et al. The pathophysiology of the propofol infusion syndrome: a simple name for a complex syndrome. Intensive Care Med 2003;29(9):1417–25.
241. McCowan C, Marik P. Refractory delirium tremens: a case series. Crit Care Med 2000;28(6):1781–4.
242. Coomes TR, Smith SW. Successful use of propofol in refractory delirium tremens. Ann Emerg Med 1997;30(6):825–8.
243. Crippen DW. Strategies for managing delirium tremens in the ICU. J Crit Illn 1997;12(3):140–9.
244. Darrouj J, Puri N, Prince E, et al. Dexmedetomidine infusion as adjunctive therapy to benzodiazepines for acute alcohol withdrawal. Ann Pharmacother 2008;42(11):1703–5.
245. Coursin DB, Coursin DB, Maccioli GA. Dexmedetomidine. Curr Opin Crit Care 2001;7(4):221–6.
246. Michaelsen IH, Anderson JE, Fink-Jensen A, et al. Phenobarbital versus diazepam for delirium tremens—a retrospective study. Dan Med Bull 2010;57(8):A4169.
247. Addolorato G, Leggio L, Abenavoli L, et al. Baclofen in the treatment of alcohol withdrawal syndrome: a comparative study vs diazepam. Am J Med 2006;119(3):276.e13–8.
248. Elsing C, Stremmel WS, Grenda U, et al. Gamma-hydroxybutyric acid versus clomethiazole for the treatment of alcohol withdrawal syndrome in a medical intensive care unit: an open, single-center randomized study. Am J Drug Alcohol Abuse 2009;35(3):189–92.
249. Myrick H, Malcolm R, Randall PK, et al. A double-blind trial of gabapentin versus lorazepam in the treatment of alcohol withdrawal. Alcohol Clin Exp Res 2009;33(9):1582–8.
250. Ait-Daoud N, Malcolm RJ Jr, Johnson BA. An overview of medications for treatment of alcohol withdrawal and alcohol dependence with an emphasis on the use of older and newer anticonvulsants. Addict Behav 2006;31(9):1628–49.
251. Longo LP, Campbell T, Hubatch S. Divalproex sodium (Depakote) for alcohol withdrawal and relapse prevention. J Addict Dis 2002;21(2):55–64.
252. Malcolm R, Myrick H, Brady KT, et al. Update on anticonvulsants for the treatment of alcohol withdrawal. Am J Addict 2001;10(Suppl):116–23.
253. Romach MK, Sellers EM. Management of the alcohol withdrawal syndrome. Annu Rev Med 1991;42(1):323–40.

254. Sampliner R, Iber FL. Diphenylhydantoin control of alcohol withdrawal seizures. JAMA 1974;230(10):1430–2.
255. Rathlev NK, D'Onofrio G, Fish SS, et al. The lack of efficacy of phenytoin in the prevention of recurrent alcohol-related seizures. Ann Emerg Med 1994;23(3): 513–8.
256. Jacob MS, Zilm DH, MacLeod SM, et al. Propranolol associated confused states during alcohol withdrawal. J Clin Psychopharmacol 1983;3(3):185–7.
257. Wilkins AJ, Jenkins WJ, Steiner JA. Efficacy of clonidine in treatment of alcohol withdrawal state. Psychopharmacology 1983;81(1):78–80.
258. Robinson BJ, Robinson GM, Maling TJ, et al. Is clonidine useful in the treatment of alcohol withdrawal? Alcohol Clin Exp Res 1989;13(1):95–8.
259. Palestine M, Alatorre E. Control of acute alcoholic withdrawal symptoms: a comparative study of haloperidol and chlordiazepoxide. Curr Ther Res Clin Exp 1976;20(3):289–99.
260. Blum K, Eubanks JD, Wallace JE, et al. Enhancement of alcohol-withdrawal convulsions in mice by haloperidol. Clin Toxicol 1976;9(3):427–34.
261. Krupitsky EM, Neznanova O, Masalov D, et al. Effect of memantine on cue-induced alcohol craving in recovering alcohol-dependent patients. Am J Psychiatry 2007;164(3):519–23.
262. Mayfield D, McLeod G, Hall P. The CAGE questionnaire: validation of a new alcoholism screening instrument. Am J Psychiatry 1974;131(10):1121–3.
263. Hansbrough JF, Zapata-Sirvent RL, Carroll WJ, et al. Administration of intravenous alcohol for prevention of withdrawal in alcoholic burn patients. Am J Surg 1984;148(2):266–9.
264. Craft PP, Foil MB, Cunningham PR, et al. Intravenous ethanol for alcohol detoxification in trauma patients. South Med J 1994;87(1):47–54.
265. Rosenblaum M, McCarty T. Alcohol prescription by surgeons in the prevention and treatment of delirium tremens: historic and current practice. Gen Hosp Psychiatry 2002;24(4):257–9.
266. Lineaweaver WC. Massive doses of midazolam infusion for delirium tremens. Crit Care Med 1989;17(6):597.
267. Dissanaike S, Halldorsson A, Frezza EE, et al. An ethanol protocol to prevent alcohol withdrawal syndrome. J Am Coll Surg 2006;203(2):186–91.
268. Weinberg JA, Magnotti LJ, Fischer PE, et al. Comparison of intravenous ethanol versus diazepam for alcohol withdrawal prophylaxis in the trauma ICU: results of a randomized trial. J Trauma 2008;64(1):99–104.
269. Wilkens L, Ruschulte H, Ruckoldt H, et al. Standard calculation of ethanol elimination rate is not sufficient to provide ethanol substitution therapy in the postoperative course of alcohol-dependent patients. Intensive Care Med 1998;24(5): 459–63.
270. Eggers V, Tio J, Neumann T, et al. Blood alcohol concentration for monitoring ethanol treatment to prevent alcohol withdrawal in the intensive care unit. Intensive Care Med 2002;28(10):1475–82.
271. Hodges B, Mazur JE. Intravenous ethanol for the treatment of alcohol withdrawal syndrome in critically ill patients. Pharmacotherapy 2004;24(11):1578–85.
272. Muller CA, Hein J. Ethanol for the treatment of alcohol withdrawal symptoms: a questionable approach. Neurologist 2010;16(3):211.
273. Fleming M, Mihic SJ, Harris RA. Ethanol. In: Brunton LL, Lazo JS, Parker KL, editors. Goodman & Gillman's the pharmacological basis of therapeutics. 11th edition. New York: McGraw Hill; 2006. p. 591–601.

Miscellaneous Central Nervous System Intoxicants

Matthew W. Hedge, MD

KEYWORDS

- Central nervous system • Intoxicants • Therapeutic drugs • Overdose

KEY POINTS

- Many toxic ingestions can be managed solely with good supportive care.
- Overdoses often involve central nervous system depressants in which, once a secure airway is obtained, the rest of the management often revolves around waiting for metabolism and excretion of the drugs in question.
- Early and aggressive supportive care, particularly airway protection and appropriate ventilatory support, will limit the potential complications and facilitate control in the unstable patient.
- Toxin-induced seizures should be controlled with GABAergic drugs such as benzodiazepines, barbiturates, or propofol.
- Methods of enhancing elimination (eg, multidose activated charcoal, hemodialysis, or charcoal hemoperfusion) may be considered for critically ill patients.

Many toxic ingestions can be managed solely with good supportive care. Attention to detail with regard to management of the airway and appropriate ventilatory support are keys to a good outcome. Many overdoses involve central nervous system (CNS) depressants in which, once a secure airway is obtained, the rest of the management often revolves around waiting for metabolism and excretion of the drugs in question. Understanding the physiology of a particular ingestion is also important. Rather than advocating rote memorization of pharmacology and mechanism of action of each drug, an understanding of how a particular class of drugs acts allows the clinician to anticipate potential complications and be prepared to respond appropriately.

Discussion on the management of each of the clinical entities presented in this article assumes that some form of basic laboratory evaluation for acute intoxication has been performed. At a minimum this should include serum acetaminophen and electrolyte levels, an ECG, and blood glucose concentration. The history that is obtained from the patient is frequently incorrect; however, these basic screening

Department of Emergency Medicine, Detroit Receiving Hospital, Children's Hospital of Michigan Regional Poison Control Center, Wayne State University, Hutzel Building, 4707 Street Antoine, Suite 302, Detroit, MI 48201, USA
E-mail address: mhedge@dmc.org

Crit Care Clin 28 (2012) 587–600
http://dx.doi.org/10.1016/j.ccc.2012.07.009
0749-0704/12/$ – see front matter © 2012 Elsevier Inc. All rights reserved.

evaluations will address many of the concerns with acute ingestions. More specific laboratory evaluation can be tailored from this starting point. These screening tests will evaluate for possible acid-base disturbances, hypoglycemia, cardiac conduction abnormalities, and acetaminophen intoxication. As screening tests they will provide some basic information but should also provoke further investigation or institution of appropriate therapeutic interventions.

NEWER ANTIDEPRESSANT DRUGS

Collectively, the newer antidepressants interfere with neuronal reuptake of serotonin, norepinephrine, dopamine, or combinations thereof, and include several classes and numerous specific drugs. Examples include the norepinephrine-dopamine reuptake inhibitor bupropion, the selective serotonin reuptake inhibitors (SSRIs) citalopram and escitalopram, and the serotonin-norepinephrine reuptake inhibitors (SNRIs) duloxetine and venlafaxine. These drugs are currently marketed for the treatment of a variety of disorders including anxiety, bipolar disorder, depression, fibromyalgia, migraine, and neuropathic pain syndromes. Therapeutically, these drugs increase concentrations of certain biogenic amines in the synaptic clef by inhibiting their uptake into the presynaptic neuron through inhibition of specific transporters.[1] The drugs have variable affinity to these receptors.[2] The oldest class of these drugs, the SSRIs, are a great step forward over the tricyclic antidepressants with regard to limiting toxicity, although there is still some amount of sedation associated with the resulting increase in serotonin-induced neurotransmission. Thus, the SNRIs were brought to the therapeutic marketplace. Unfortunately the inhibition of norepinephrine reuptake, as opposed to just serotonin, has resulted in increased cardiovascular and neurologic complications related to catecholamine excess, such as seizures, hypertension, and various tachydysrhythmias. Other drugs in this class have varying degrees of affinity for the rapid sodium influx channels and this, in turn, can result in prolongation of the QRS complex[3] and seizures via increased excitatory neurotransmission and disorganized depolarization.[4,5] Two specific examples provide some insight with regard to clinical toxicity and management.

Venlafaxine is absorbed over a somewhat protracted period, reportedly having continued absorption over 8 to 10 hours. There is an active metabolite, O-desmethyl-venlafaxine and, depending on the CYP2D6 phenotype, metabolism can result in accumulation or rapid clearance with poor pharmacologic response to the drug.[2,6,7] Clinically, intoxicated patients present with some degree of CNS depression, ranging from minor alterations in level of consciousness to coma.[8,9] Cardiac symptoms are frequently related to a hyperadrenergic state, with tachycardia and hypertension. Seizures have also been reported in the overdose setting.[10,11] Although venlafaxine has been reported to increase QRS duration, the mechanism is unclear.[12] Animal study findings suggest that sodium channel affinity characteristics are different than typical Vaughan-Williams (V-W) class I antidysrhythmic drugs, but venlafaxine affects sodium channels in a rate-independent fashion.[3] Although therapeutic plasma alkalinization is frequently recommended, it is unclear whether it is benificial.[13] Gastrointestinal (GI) decontamination should consist of single-dose activated charcoal for patients who present within 1 hour postingestion. Whole bowel irrigation (WBI) should be considered for cases involving extended release preparations to limit prolonged or continued absorption of the drug from the GI tract.[14,15] Treatment of intoxication starts with a secure airway and appropriate ventilator support. Seizures should be treated aggressively with benzodiazepines and barbiturates.[14,16–18] Phenytoin is thought to have limited benefit in toxin-induced seizures[19,20]; many of these seizures are related to diffuse problems with neurotransmission as opposed to an irritable focus that serves as an initiation point leading to generalized seizures.

Bupropion is another example of this class of drugs that should have some comment, largely due to the frequency and timing of seizures that are associated with overdoses or at doses that are just outside the therapeutic range.[21–24] An increased incidence of seizures has been noted at the upper limit of therapeutic dosing, 450 mg/d, prompting a change in the package labeling to reduce the maximum daily dose to 300 mg. An extended release preparation is also available, and can substantially delay the onset of symptoms. The time to onset of seizures can be up to 20 hours or more postingestion.[25,26] There is some question whether the parent compound or a metabolite is responsible for the cardiac toxicity. QT interval prolongation has been reported frequently with ingestions of this drug.[27,28]

Lipid emulsions have recently been gaining support for the treatment of several intoxications. The most rigorous data is associated with long-acting local anesthetic intoxication.[29] Although an exact mechanism of action is debated, the lipid sink theory predominates.[30] This theory suggests that lipid emulsion therapy creates an intravascular lipid compartment such that drugs with high lipophilicity will move from the aqueous phase of plasma, where interaction with particular receptors occurs, to the lipid phase, where the drug has relatively limited ability to interact with a particular receptor. This treatment modality is being applied to several intoxications associated with severe cardiac and neurologic symptoms, including venlafaxine, with varying degrees of success.[17,31] Benefit is fairly well established with local anesthetic intoxication, but it remains to be seen if this therapy can be more broadly applied to intoxications with other lipophilic drugs. The therapy itself is relatively safe and, in the setting of severe intoxication, potential benefit will outweigh the risk as a rescue therapy. The guidelines put out by the Association of Anesthetists of Great Britain and Ireland state that for local anesthetic toxicity a bolus of 1.5 mL/kg of a 20% lipid emulsion up to 3 times, followed by an infusion of the 20% lipid emulsion at a rate of 0.25 to 0.5 mL/kg/min for 60 minutes, should be given. This dosing scheme has been adapted to other intoxications.

This class of drugs increases excitatory neurotransmission and, in overdoses, the excessive stimulation can develop into a constellation of symptoms called the serotonin syndrome. This can occur either through a single large drug ingestion or, more commonly, from use of multiple drugs that have a similar mechanism of action or that inhibit drug metabolism and lead to drug accumulation. This is a spectrum disorder with relatively minor cases presenting with slight tremor and diarrhea to lethal cases with severe hyperthermia and rigidity.[32] The classic syndrome is described as a cluster of clinical signs that can include altered mentation, hyperthermia, autonomic instability, and neuromuscular abnormalities.[33] There are currently several different diagnostic criteria for serotonin syndrome, each with varying degrees of sensitivity and specificity. There are several types of 5-hydroxytryptamine (5-HT) or serotonin receptors, each with multiple subtypes, but knowledge of the exact molecular pathology and development of this syndrome is limited. Activation of the 5-HT$_{2A}$ receptor is thought to be primarily responsible for development of the syndrome, whereas the 5-HT$_{1A}$ receptor serves a modulatory function by increasing intrasynaptic concentrations of serotonin. The importance of recognizing mild cases needs to be stressed because failure to appreciate a minor case can lead to inadvertent administration of another pharmaceutical agent that could exacerbate the syndrome, potentially with lethal consequences. Although presence of any of these clinical features should prompt consideration of this syndrome, the presence of hyperthermia is particularly concerning. Loss of neuromuscular control sets off a cascade of events resulting in coagulopathy, rhabdomyolysis, renal injury, and, ultimately, death.[33–35]

Aggressive cooling methods should be instituted to treat hyperthermia, with the goal of decreasing muscular activity that is responsible for the generation of heat. The initial approach should include liberal use of benzodiazepines to control agitation and excess motor activity. If sedation is unsuccessful, neuromuscular blockade should be considered, assuming the patient is intubated and receiving mechanical ventilation. Use of a nondepolarizing paralytic should be strongly considered because the use of a depolarizing paralytic, such as succinylcholine, in a patient that has some amount of rhabdomyolysis could potentially elevate plasma potassium levels to a lethal level. The use of physical restraints should also be discouraged because isotonic work increases thermogenesis. Although neuromuscular blockade will substantially decrease thermogenesis, aggressive use of sedation should still be used to limit excessive excitatory neurotransmission in the CNS. Electroencephalography should be considered because the patient could potentially have status epilepticus that is unrecognized secondary to therapeutic paralysis.

Antagonist therapy with cyproheptadine should be considered.[36] This drug has antagonist properties at 5-HT$_{2A}$ receptors. The initial therapeutic approach should start with a dose of 8 to 12 mg followed by another 2 mg every 2 hours until some degree of control is established. This can be followed by 4 to 8 mg every 6 hours for the first 24 hours, at which point decreasing or withdrawing the drug could be considered. Drawbacks of this therapy include the lack of a parenteral formulation. Alternative therapies include olanzapine and chlorpromethazine. Olanzapine has been successful at treating serotonin syndrome at a dose of 10 mg, although this therapy has not been rigorously studied.[33,37] Chlorpromethazine, which may be administered by the intramuscular route, has been recommended at a dose of 50 to 100 mg.[38,39] Risperidone has also been used successfully in an animal model of serotonin syndrome.[40]

ATYPICAL NEUROLEPTIC DRUGS

The atypical neuroleptic agents aripiprazole, clozapine, olanzapine, quetiapine, risperidone, and others offer an improved side-effect profile compared with earlier generations of neuroleptic drugs by somewhat lessened binding affinity for dopamine receptors. Both the typical and atypical neuroleptic drugs as a class are somewhat nonspecific with regard to binding affinity. These drugs exhibit antagonism at dopamine, muscarinic acetylcholine, alpha-1 adrenergic, histamine, and serotonin receptors, as well as affecting delayed rectifying potassium channels and ligand-gated sodium channels. The scattered and diverse binding affinity makes prediction of the patient's clinical presentation difficult.

The atypical neuroleptic drugs have a lower binding affinity for dopamine receptors, which limits development of drug-induced Parkinson disease, while still controlling the positive symptoms of schizophrenia, such as thought disorders, hallucinations, and paranoia. Additionally, they have agonist properties at 5-HT$_{1A}$ receptors[41] and this feature is thought to improve the negative symptoms of schizophrenia, lessening depression, apathy, and anhedonia.

Acute overdoses present with varying degrees of CNS depression with possible loss of protective airway reflexes and lack of an appropriate ventilatory response. Seizures have been reported and are thought to be related to inhibition of gamma-aminobutyric acid (GABA) A channels, impeding function of the ligand-gated chloride channel.[42–44]

Cardiovascular toxicity is mediated by several different pathways.[45] Antagonism of muscarinic acetylcholine receptors typically produces sinus tachycardia. The tachycardia can also be a compensatory response to the peripheral alpha-adrenergic antagonism in an attempt to maintain blood pressure. Decreased peripheral vascular resistance results in increased cardiac output through either increasing stroke volume or heart rate to maintain a given blood pressure. Neuroleptic drugs also disrupt the cell depolarization cycle, by either blockade of the voltage-gated sodium channel or, more commonly, by blockade of the potassium delayed rectifier.[46,47] Management of each of these complications is very different and treatment of the sodium channel blockade can potentially worsen the performance of the potassium channel.

The voltage-gated sodium channel is best studied in relationship to intoxication with the tricyclic antidepressants and their treatment recommendations have been extrapolated to other ingestions, unfortunately without clear supportive evidence. Blockade of the voltage-gated sodium channel is evaluated by ECG and is considered significant if the QRS duration exceeds 100 milliseconds or if the patient has right axis deviation in the terminal 40 milliseconds of the QRS complex. The latter manifests as a positive deflection of greater than 3 mm in the terminal 40 milliseconds of the QRS complex in lead augmented voltage right arm (aVR) and can be a precursor of degradation to a wide complex ventricular dysrhythmia. This development has been poorly studied in the setting of neuroleptic drug overdose. Although plasma alkalinization is frequently recommended for patients with a widened QRS complex, it is unclear whether this intervention is of any benefit. There is some evidence in the literature suggesting improvement of cardiac conduction with the infusion of 3% sodium chloride solution to induce a minor degree of hypernatremia.[48]

Management of inhibition of the potassium delayed rectifier channel consists primarily of increasing plasma magnesium and potassium concentrations to the upper limit of normal to improve the flow of the particular ion species through the channel when it opens.

A rare complication of atypical neuroleptic drug use, thought to occur less frequently than with the older neuroleptic agents such as haloperidol, is neuroleptic malignant syndrome (NMS).[49] Although the exact pathophysiology is poorly understood, it is an idiopathic reaction likely related to excessive dopamine receptor antagonism or dopamine depletion.[50,51] Antagonism of acetylcholine is also thought to be contributory to its development. The syndrome is characterized by altered mental status, hyperthermia, rhabdomyolysis, and autonomic instability. The diagnosis of NMS is sometimes difficult, partially due to the rather nebulous diagnostic criteria. A recent consensus panel agreed on several diagnostic criteria, including recent dopamine antagonist exposure or dopamine agonist withdrawal, hyperthermia, rigidity, mental status alteration, elevated plasma creatine kinase activity, sympathetic nervous system lability, tachycardia plus tachypnea, and a negative evaluation for alternative causes.[52] NMS frequently presents with an indolent course and many patients are sent to emergency departments as possible meningitis, pneumonia, urosepsis, or worsening dementia. Rhabdomyolysis is the result of sustained muscle contraction (ie, increased resting tone). The byproducts of muscle cell lysis are elevations in plasma potassium, creatine kinase, and myoglobin, resulting in nephrotoxicity and hyperkalemia.[53] This syndrome largely can be managed conservatively by withdrawal of the offending medication, sedation to lessen muscle tone, restoration of intravascular volume status, and active cooling. Other rescue therapies have been used, including electroconvulsive therapy, benzodiazepines, bromocriptine, dantrolene, and neuromuscular blockade (mostly based on case reports).[54–57] Goals of therapy are reduction of thermogenesis, decreased resting muscular tone, and, in return, reduction of hyperthermia. The presentation of this syndrome is indolent and resolution is also delayed; in one case series the mean time to resolution was 27 days.[58]

ANTICONVULSANTS

Many anticonvulsant overdoses will not require care in the intensive care unit (ICU). However, as with all intoxications, "the dose makes the poison." Many patients will present with some degree of neurologic dysfunction, such as ataxia or CNS depression. Phenobarbital is a notable exception and may require active management of the airway and even require vasopressor support, depending on the level of intoxication. Two anticonvulsant drugs, carbamazepine and valproic acid, are the focus of this section.

The therapeutic mechanism of action of carbamazepine is via blockade of the fast sodium influx channel and agonist effect at the adenosine-1 receptor on presynaptic neurons. Stimulation of adenosine-1 receptors results in a G-protein–mediated decrease in calcium release from the endoplasmic reticulum. Stabilization of the sodium channel limits depolarization of the neuron as a whole, whereas limitation of calcium release into the cytosol of the neuron decreases vesicle exocytosis and release of excitatory neurotransmitters into the synaptic cleft. Metabolism of carbamazepine results in conversion to carbamazepine-10, 11-expoxide, which is cardiotoxic and behaves similarly to V-W class Ia or Ic antiarrhythmic drugs, potentially causing conduction disturbances, QRS widening, and ventricular arrhythmias. Accumulation of this active metabolite has been reported secondary to drug–drug interactions with lamotrigine, phenytoin, phenobarbital, and valproic acid.[59,60] Conduction disturbances may be delayed as the parent compound is metabolized to the toxic metabolite.

Clinical presentation of carbamazepine intoxication is similar to other forms of anticholinergic intoxication, with mydriasis, dry mouth, tachycardia, decreased bowel sounds, urinary retention, and agitated delirium. The diagnostic approach should include an ECG and serial carbamazepine levels to guide therapy.[61]

Aggressive supportive care continues to be the mainstay of therapy. Active control of a potentially compromised airway and appropriate sedation to control delirium and prevent hyperthermia are cornerstones of early management. Early GI decontamination with a single dose of activated charcoal to limit absorption of the drug is indicated. Ideally this should be administered in the first hour after ingestion to be effective, although the antimuscarinic effects of carbamazepine theoretically extend this window of opportunity secondary to delayed gastric emptying. In the setting of rising drug levels, WBI with an isotonic polyethylene glycol solution should be considered to limit drug absorption.[62,63] However, this treatment may be contraindicated in patients lacking bowel sounds because of the drug's effects on gastric motility.

Presenting signs of CNS toxicity include agitated delirium, sedation, and seizures.[64,65] The delirium should be treated with benzodiazepines to control agitation. Attempts should be made to limit the use of physical restraints because fixed points for isotonic exertion could result in hyperthermia, a concerning possibility in the setting of anticholinergic symptoms and likely impaired thermoregulation. Seizures should be controlled with GABAergic drugs, namely benzodiazepines, barbiturates, and, possibly, propofol.[66–68] Although these interventions have not been rigorously studied with this ingestion, this is the same pharmacologic approach to many forms of toxin-induced seizures.

Concerning ECG features include QRS duration greater than 100 milliseconds, right axis deviation in the terminal 40 milliseconds of the QRS complex, and a terminal R wave greater than 3 mm in lead aVR. In the appropriate clinical setting these features should prompt consideration for plasma alkalinization using intravenous (IV) sodium bicarbonate. Practically speaking, this is accomplished using a bolus of 50 to 100 mEq of sodium bicarbonate followed by a continuous IV infusion consisting of 150 mEq in a liter of 5% dextrose with 20 mEq of potassium chloride at an initial rate of 1.5 to 2 times the maintenance hydration rate. The goal of therapy should be a narrowing of the QRS complex or a target arterial pH of 7.45 to 7.55. If the QRS complex continues to increase beyond 100 milliseconds despite alkalinization, there is increasing potential for seizures and ventricular dysrhythmia. Lidocaine, a class Ib antiarrhythmic drug, is a rational choice for ventricular dysrhythmias in this setting. The proposed benefit is that lidocaine theoretically competes with carbamazepine at the sodium channel binding site and improves channel conduction and cellular depolarization.

Carbamazepine levels should be assayed every 4 hours until a downward trend is established. For patients taking carbamazepine therapeutically for seizure disorders, treatment to increase elimination will need to be tailored so as not to drive the level into the subtherapeutic range. When levels increase to 20 µg/mL consideration should be given to the use of multidose activated charcoal (MDAC) as an enhanced elimination strategy.[69] MDAC hastens drug elimination in this instance by so-called GI dialysis, with the intestinal mucosa serving as the dialysis membrane. The drug is bound to charcoal in the intestinal lumen and subsequently excreted. MDAC can also be used to interrupt enteroenteric or enterohepatic recirculation. Carbamazepine is one of five drugs that have class 1 evidence to support MDAC use for enhancing elimination.[63] Depending on the patient's mental status and ability to protect the airway, MDAC can be given orally or via orogastric tube. There are no truly standardized dosing regimens, but 0.25 to 0.5 g/kg every 4 to 6 hours is frequently recommended.

When the carbamazepine level exceeds 30 µg/mL, consideration needs to be given for more invasive modes of elimination. Charcoal hemoperfusion is the preferred method of extracorporeal elimination; however, availability is often limited owing to the expense of the cartridges, their short shelf-life, and infrequency of use.[70,71] There are case reports of using high-flux hemodialysis with clinical improvement. The difficulty of extracorporeal removal measures is predicting when conservative management is going to fail, requiring a more invasive measure while the patient is still stable enough to tolerate the procedure.

Valproic acid (VPA) is a short branched-chain fatty acid commonly prescribed as an anticonvulsant for general and focal seizure disorders. This drug is also FDA approved for bipolar disorder and is frequently used off-label for treatment of migraine, trigeminal neuralgia, and other neuropathic pain syndromes.

The mechanism of action is not entirely clear on a molecular level. The anticonvulsant properties seem to be mediated through increased CNS GABA concentrations.[72,73] There seem to be inhibition of GABA transaminase and succinate semialdehyde dehydrogenase, enzymes responsible for the metabolism of GABA. There is also data suggesting that VPA is inhibitory to the function of N-methyl-d-aspartate (NMDA) glutamate receptor. The combination of increasing inhibitory neurotransmission and decreasing excitatory neurotransmission slows repetitive neuronal firing, resulting in decreased epileptiform activity.

Metabolism of VPA is mainly by β-oxidation in the mitochondria but also occurs by ω-oxidation on the endoplasmic reticulum. At least nine separate metabolites have been identified. The metabolites formed on the endoplasmic reticulum have been implicated in much of the toxicity in acute overdoses and toxicity associated with chronic therapeutic dosing.

Clinical presentation in the acute overdose setting is that of a sedative-hypnotic toxidrome, with CNS depression, ataxia, confusion, loss of protective airway reflexes, and hypotension reported.[74–76] Loss of other homeostatic reflexes also has been reported, including loss of thermoregulation.[77] Laboratory evaluation for these ingestions should include serial serum VPA levels, transaminase activities, and ammonia levels.[78–80]

Carnitine depletion is another method by which VPA causes toxicity. This depletion potentiates VPA toxicity by shunting metabolism from β-oxidation to ω-oxidation with generation of toxic metabolites.[81] Carnitine is required to shuttle fatty acids into the mitochondria and is also necessary for proper functioning of the urea cycle.[82,83] Carnitine depletion thus results in hyperammonemia, which can occur during therapeutic dosing as well as a complication of acute overdose.[84] This complication is more common in patients with nutritional deficiency or high-demand metabolic states such as burn injury, sepsis, and the neonatal period.

Management of VPA intoxication early on is primarily one of airway management. Sometimes patients will present with an opioid toxidrome appearance provoking the use of naloxone as antidotal therapy.[85–87] Although this has not been particularly successful, a few cases have been reported. Circulatory support frequently can be achieved by intravascular volume expansion with crystalloid solutions. Patients sometimes require vasopressor support. Typical recommendations are for direct-acting pressors, instead of indirect-acting drugs such as dopamine. There is little evidence to support this recommendation, although the rationale is that an indirect-acting pressor will need to be converted to epinephrine or norepinephrine and, subsequently, secreted before there is any effect on blood pressure. Frequently, the cause of hypotension in sedative intoxications is related to loss vasomotor regulation with the sympathetic system not secreting appropriate amounts of catecholamines to support normal vascular tone and cardiac output.

After ventilation and circulatory issues are addressed, the next priority should be gastric decontamination. Early single-dose activated charcoal is indicated. VPA is frequently marketed as an extended release preparation, which introduces the potential for delayed rise in VPA levels and prolonging or worsening the intoxication.[88,89] For patients with VPA levels that continue to rise, consideration should be given for WBI to prevent further absorption of the drug.

The pharmacologic properties of VPA, including its low volume of distribution, make this drug amenable to methods of enhancing elimination. High protein binding makes the drug less amenable to standard dialysis therapies, although the protein binding saturates in the overdose setting, thereby increasing the free fraction of the drug available for dialytic removal.[90] These same properties also make VPA amendable to MDAC as a method of enhancing elimination. Although there is a lack of strong evidence that MDAC enhances elimination, there are suggestions that it may be helpful.[79,91] Several dialysis methods have been tried and, although charcoal hemoperfusion is probably the most rational choice for enhancing elimination, lack of availability has made this prohibitive.[88,92,93] High flux hemodialysis has also demonstrated substantial declines in plasma half-life of VPA and should be considered.[94,95] MDAC should be given when VPA levels are in the range of 175 to 200 μg/mL. WBI should be considered when drug levels suggest continued absorption, as evidenced by levels that continue to rise or plateau. Forms of extracorporeal elimination, namely hemodialysis, high-flux hemodialysis, or charcoal hemoperfusion, should be considered when drug levels are in excess of 700 μg/mL, more conservative measures fail, and clinical instability or multiorgan failure occur.[76,79,96–98] There have been case reports describing the use of a molecular absorbent recycling system for treating acute intoxications, but limitations of access to this system render it impractical currently.[99]

Carnitine supplementation, while not truly antidotal, may provide some benefit in the setting of VPA intoxication by theoretically shunting metabolism away from the more toxic ω-oxidation and shuttling the drug into the mitochondria where β-oxidation occurs.[100] Supplementation of carnitine in patients who are carnitine depleted could improve urea cycle function, decreasing plasma ammonia levels by conversion to urea.[101] Dosing is extrapolated from recommendations by the Pediatric Neurology Advisory Committee for carnitine supplementation in children with signs of chronic intoxication and include recommendations for use of IV levocarnitine. The dosing recommendations are 150 to 200 mg/kg per day, either orally or IV, to a maximum of 3 g/day, given in 3 divided doses.[79,102] There are a few studies examining the safety of L-carnitine, but no adverse effects have been reported in this somewhat limited data set.

Clinical presentation should guide therapy, although the use of an early aggressive approach to the critically intoxicated patient can result in an improved outcome.[103]

SUMMARY

Although these intoxicants and syndromes are diverse in their presentation and physiology, there are some constants throughout these exposures. Early and aggressive supportive care, particularly airway protection and appropriate ventilatory support, will limit the potential complications and facilitate control in the unstable patient. Hyperthermia must be controlled; anticholinergic intoxication, neuroleptic malignant syndrome, serotonin syndrome, sympathomimetic intoxication, and temperature are the markers for morbidity and mortality. Much of the hyperthermia is derived from excessive muscular activity that needs to be suppressed either though rapid dose-escalation of a benzodiazepine or by neuromuscular blockade. There are some instances in which specific pharmacologic therapies may be beneficial, such as cyproheptadine in the case of serotonin syndrome or bromocriptine in the case of neuroleptic malignant syndrome. Toxin-induced seizures should be controlled with GABAergic, drugs such as benzodiazepines, barbiturates, or propofol. Circulatory support may be required and should be initiated with volume support followed by direct-acting pressors in the case of hypotension. Hyperadrenergic states will sometimes require suppression to control a hypertensive emergency or demand ischemia in an overworked myocardium, but short-acting drugs, such as nitroprusside or esmolol, would be preferred. Cardiac conduction abnormalities should be addressed with plasma alkalinization, in the case of QRS prolongation, or optimization of plasma potassium and magnesium concentrations, in the case of QT interval prolongation. GI decontamination with single-dose charcoal or WBI should be undertaken when appropriate. Methods of enhancing elimination—multidose activated charcoal, hemodialysis, or charcoal hemoperfusion—may be considered for critically ill patients. Levocarnitine is likely beneficial in the setting of severe VPA intoxication or hyperammonemia related to this anticonvulsant. There is some case-based literature suggesting temporal improvement of cardiovascular and CNS toxicity with the use of lipid emulsions. Although the evidence is limited for so-called lipid rescue therapy, it is relatively safe, may be beneficial, and, in a moribund patient, the benefit will greatly outweigh the risk.

REFERENCES

1. Foley KF, DeSanty KP, Kast RE. Bupropion: pharmacology and therapeutic applications. Expert Rev Neurother 2006;6(9):1249–65.

2. Montgomery SA. Tolerability of serotonin norepinephrine reuptake inhibitor anti-depressants. CNS Spectr 2008;13(7 Suppl 11):27–33.
3. Khalifa M, Daleau P, Turgeon J. Mechanism of sodium channel block by venla-faxine in guinea pig ventricular myocytes. J Pharmacol Exp Ther 1999;291(1):280–4.
4. Ayers S, Tobias JD. Bupropion overdose in an adolescent. Pediatr Emerg Care 2001;17(2):104–6.
5. Waring WS, Gray JA, Graham A. Predictive factors for generalized seizures after deliberate citalopram overdose. Br J Clin Pharmacol 2008;66(6):861–5.
6. Lobello KW, Preskorn SH, Guico-Pabia J, et al. Cytochrome P450 2D6 pheno-type predicts antidepressant efficacy of venlafaxine: a secondary analysis of 4 studies in major depressive disorder. J Clin Psychiatry 2010;71(11):1482–7.
7. Stahl SM, Grady MM, Moret C, et al. SNRIs: their pharmacology, clinical efficacy, and tolerability in comparison with other classes of antidepressants. CNS Spectr 2005;10(9):732–47.
8. Fantaskey A, Burkhart KK. A case report of venlafaxine toxicity. J Toxicol Clin Toxicol 1995;33(4):359–61.
9. Chan AN, Gunja N, Ryan CJ. A comparison of venlafaxine and SSRIs in delib-erate self-poisoning. J Med Toxicol 2010;6(2):116–21.
10. White CM, Gailey RA, Levin GM, et al. Seizure resulting from a venlafaxine over-dose. Ann Pharmacother 1997;31(2):178–80.
11. Thundiyil JG, Kearney TE, Olson KR. Evolving epidemiology of drug-induced seizures reported to a Poison Control Center System. J Med Toxicol 2007;3(1):15–9.
12. Isbister GK. Electrocardiogram changes and arrhythmias in venlafaxine over-dose. Br J Clin Pharmacol 2009;67(5):572–6.
13. Glassman AH, Preud'homme XA. Review of the cardiovascular effects of hetero-cyclic antidepressants. J Clin Psychiatry 1993;54(Suppl):16–22.
14. Kumar VV, Isbister GK, Duffull SB. The effect of decontamination procedures on the pharmacodynamics of venlafaxine in overdose. Br J Clin Pharmacol 2011;72(1):125–32.
15. Djogovic D, Hudson D, Jacka M. Gastric bezoar following venlafaxine overdose. Clin Toxicol (Phila) 2007;45(6):735.
16. Bosse GM, Spiller HA, Collins AM. A fatal case of venlafaxine overdose. J Med Toxicol 2008;4(1):18–20.
17. Hillyard SG, Barrera-Groba C, Tighe R. Intralipid reverses coma associated with zopiclone and venlafaxine overdose. Eur J Anaesthesiol 2010;27(6):582–3.
18. Howell C, Wilson AD, Waring WS. Cardiovascular toxicity due to venlafaxine poisoning in adults: a review of 235 consecutive cases. Br J Clin Pharmacol 2007;64(2):192–7.
19. Sharma AN, Hoffman RJ. Toxin-related seizures. Emerg Med Clin North Am 2011;29(1):125–39.
20. Wills B, Erickson T. Chemically induced seizures. Clin Lab Med 2006;26(1):185–209, ix.
21. Belson MG, Kelley TR. Bupropion exposures: clinical manifestations and medical outcome. J Emerg Med 2002;23(3):223–30.
22. Balit CR, Lynch CN, Isbister GK. Bupropion poisoning: a case series. Med J Aust 2003;178(2):61–3.
23. Boora K, Cummings MR, Marshall DR. Generalized seizure in three adolescents with bupropion overdose. J Child Adolesc Psychopharmacol 2010;20(2):159–60.

24. Harris CR, Gualtieri J, Stark G. Fatal bupropion overdose. J Toxicol Clin Toxicol 1997;35(3):321–4.
25. Donnelly K, Walkowiak HB, Donnelly C, et al. Bupropion toxicokinetic: a case report. Clin Toxicol (Phila) 2010;48(4):385–7.
26. Jepsen F, Matthews J, Andrews FJ. Sustained release bupropion overdose: an important cause of prolonged symptoms after an overdose. Emerg Med J 2003; 20(6):560–1.
27. Isbister GK, Balit CR. Bupropion overdose: QTc prolongation and its clinical significance. Ann Pharmacother 2003;37(7–8):999–1002.
28. Jackson WK, Roose SP, Glassman AH. Cardiovascular toxicity of antidepressant medications. Psychopathology 1987;20(Suppl 1):64–74.
29. Weinberg GL, VadeBoncouer T, Ramaraju GA, et al. Pretreatment or resuscitation with a lipid infusion shifts the dose-response to bupivacaine-induced asystole in rats. Anesthesiology 1998;88(4):1071–5.
30. Mirtallo JM, Dasta JF, Kleinschmidt KC, et al. State of the art review: intravenous fat emulsions: current applications, safety profile, and clinical implications. Ann Pharmacother 2010;44(4):688–700.
31. Cave G, Harvey M. Intravenous lipid emulsion as antidote beyond local anesthetic toxicity: a systematic review. Acad Emerg Med 2009;16(9):815–24.
32. Kolecki P. Isolated venlafaxine-induced serotonin syndrome. J Emerg Med 1997;15(4):491–3.
33. Boyer EW, Shannon M. The serotonin syndrome. N Engl J Med 2005;352(11): 1112–20.
34. Flanagan RJ. Fatal toxicity of drugs used in psychiatry. Hum Psychopharmacol 2008;23(Suppl 1):43–51.
35. Rajapakse S, Abeynaike L, Wickramarathne T. Venlafaxine-associated serotonin syndrome causing severe rhabdomyolysis and acute renal failure in a patient with idiopathic Parkinson disease. J Clin Psychopharmacol 2010;30(5):620–2.
36. Graudins A, Stearman A, Chan B. Treatment of the serotonin syndrome with cyproheptadine. J Emerg Med 1998;16(4):615–9.
37. Bever KA, Perry PJ. Olanzapine: a serotonin-dopamine-receptor antagonist for antipsychotic therapy. Am J Health Syst Pharm 1998;55(10):1003–16.
38. Steinberg M, Morin AK. Mild serotonin syndrome associated with concurrent linezolid and fluoxetine. Am J Health Syst Pharm 2007;64(1):59–62.
39. Gillman PK. Serotonin syndrome treated with chlorpromazine. J Clin Psychopharmacol 1997;17(2):128–9.
40. Nisijima K, Yoshino T, Ishiguro T. Risperidone counteracts lethality in an animal model of the serotonin syndrome. Psychopharmacology (Berl) 2000;150(1):9–14.
41. Meltzer HY, Massey BW. The role of serotonin receptors in the action of atypical antipsychotic drugs. Curr Opin Pharmacol 2011;11(1):59–67.
42. Centorrino F, Price BH, Tuttle M, et al. EEG abnormalities during treatment with typical and atypical antipsychotics. Am J Psychiatry 2002;159(1):109–15.
43. Yokota K, Tatebayashi H, Matsuo T, et al. The effects of neuroleptics on the GABA-induced Cl- current in rat dorsal root ganglion neurons: differences between some neuroleptics. Br J Pharmacol 2002;135(6):1547–55.
44. Amann BL, Pogarell O, Mergl R, et al. EEG abnormalities associated with antipsychotics: a comparison of quetiapine, olanzapine, haloperidol and healthy subjects. Hum Psychopharmacol 2003;18(8):641–6.
45. Tan HH, Hoppe J, Heard K. A systematic review of cardiovascular effects after atypical antipsychotic medication overdose. Am J Emerg Med 2009;27(5): 607–16.

46. Oulis P, Florakis A, Markatou M, et al. Corrected QT interval changes during electroconvulsive therapy-antidepressants-atypical antipsychotics coadministration: safety issues. J ECT 2011;27(1):e4–6.

47. Eyer F, Pfab R, Felgenhauer N, et al. Clinical and analytical features of severe suicidal quetiapine overdoses—a retrospective cohort study. Clin Toxicol (Phila) 2011;49(9):846–53.

48. McCabe JL, Menegazzi JJ, Cobaugh DJ, et al. Recovery from severe cyclic antidepressant overdose with hypertonic saline/dextran in a swine model. Acad Emerg Med 1994;1(2):111–5.

49. Caroff SN, Mann SC. Neuroleptic malignant syndrome and malignant hyperthermia. Anaesth Intensive Care 1993;21(4):477–8.

50. Gillman PK. Neuroleptic malignant syndrome: mechanisms, interactions, and causality. Mov Disord 2010;25(12):1780–90.

51. Baguley IJ. The excitatory: inhibitory ratio model (EIR model): an integrative explanation of acute autonomic overactivity syndromes. Med Hypotheses 2008;70(1):26–35.

52. Gurrera RJ, Caroff SN, Cohen A, et al. An international consensus study of neuroleptic malignant syndrome diagnostic criteria using the Delphi method. J Clin Psychiatry 2011;72(9):1222–8.

53. Boutaud O, Roberts LJ II. Mechanism-based therapeutic approaches to rhabdomyolysis-induced renal failure. Free Radic Biol Med 2011;51(5):1062–7.

54. Stoner SC, Berry A. Suspected neuroleptic malignant syndrome during quetiapine-clozapine cross-titration. J Pharm Pract 2010;23(1):69–73.

55. Tsai MC, Huang TL. Severe neuroleptic malignant syndrome: successful treatment with high-dose lorazepam and diazepam: a case report. Chang Gung Med J 2010;33(5):576–80.

56. Gortney JS, Fagan A, Kissack JC. Neuroleptic malignant syndrome secondary to quetiapine. Ann Pharmacother 2009;43(4):785–91.

57. van Maldegem BT, Smit LM, Touw DJ, et al. Neuroleptic malignant syndrome in a 4-year-old girl associated with alimemazine. Eur J Pediatr 2002;161(5):259–61.

58. Tural U, Onder E. Clinical and pharmacologic risk factors for neuroleptic malignant syndrome and their association with death. Psychiatry Clin Neurosci 2010;64(1):79–87.

59. Potter JM, Donnelly A. Carbamazepine-10,11-epoxide in therapeutic drug monitoring. Ther Drug Monit 1998;20(6):652–7.

60. Tutor-Crespo MJ, Hermida J, Tutor JC. Relative proportions of serum carbamazepine and its pharmacologically active 10,11-epoxy derivative: effect of polytherapy and renal insufficiency. Ups J Med Sci 2008;113(2):171–80.

61. Ciszowski K, Szpak D, Jenner B. The influence of carbamazepine plasma level on blood pressure and some ECG parameters in patients with acute intoxication. Przegl Lek 2007;64(4–5):248–51.

62. Sano R, Takahashi K, Kominato Y, et al. A case of fatal drug intoxication showing a high-density duodenal content by postmortem computed tomography. Leg Med (Tokyo) 2011;13(1):39–40.

63. Tenenbein M. Position statement: whole bowel irrigation. American Academy of Clinical Toxicology; European Association of Poisons Centres and Clinical Toxicologists. J Toxicol Clin Toxicol 1997;35(7):753–62.

64. Graudins A, Peden G, Dowsett RP. Massive overdose with controlled-release carbamazepine resulting in delayed peak serum concentrations and life-threatening toxicity. Emerg Med (Fremantle) 2002;14(1):89–94.

65. Sullivan JB Jr, Rumack BH, Peterson RG. Acute carbamazepine toxicity resulting from overdose. Neurology 1981;31(5):621–4.
66. Baptiste SL, Tang HM, Kuzniecky RI, et al. Comparison of the antiepileptic properties of transmeningeally delivered muscimol, lidocaine, midazolam, pentobarbital and GABA, in rats. Neurosci Lett 2010;469(3):421–4.
67. Myhrer T, Enger S, Aas P. Pharmacological therapies against soman-induced seizures in rats 30 min following onset and anticonvulsant impact. Eur J Pharmacol 2006;548(1–3):83–9.
68. Myhrer T, Nguyen NH, Enger S, et al. Anticonvulsant effects of $GABA_A$ modulators microinfused into area tempestas or substantia nigra in rats exposed to soman. Arch Toxicol 2006;80(8):502–7.
69. Vale JA, Krenzelok EP, Barceloux GD. Position statement and practice guidelines on the use of multi-dose activated charcoal in the treatment of acute poisoning. American Academy of Clinical Toxicology; European Association of Poisons Centres and Clinical Toxicologists. J Toxicol Clin Toxicol 1999;37(6):731–51.
70. Pilapil M, Petersen J. Efficacy of hemodialysis and charcoal hemoperfusion in carbamazepine overdose. Clin Toxicol (Phila) 2008;46(4):342–3.
71. Bek K, Doçak Ş, Özkaya, et al. Carbamazepine poisoning managed with haemodialysis and haemoperfusion in three adolescents. Nephrology (Carlton) 2007;12(1):33–5.
72. Hariton C, Ciesielski L, Simler S, et al. Distribution of sodium valproate and GABA metabolism in CNS of the rat. Biopharm Drug Dispos 1984;5(4):409–14.
73. Johannessen CU. Mechanisms of action of valproate: a commentatory. Neurochem Int 2000;37(2–3):103–10.
74. Katiyar A, Aaron C. Case files of the Children's Hospital of Michigan Regional Poison Control Center: the use of carnitine for the management of acute valproic acid toxicity. J Med Toxicol 2007;3(3):129–38.
75. Lee WL, Yang CC, Deng JF, et al. A case of severe hyperammonemia and unconsciousness following sodium valproate intoxication. Vet Hum Toxicol 1998;40(6):346–8.
76. Thanacoody RH. Extracorporeal elimination in acute valproic acid poisoning. Clin Toxicol (Phila) 2009;47(7):609–16.
77. Robinson P, Abbott C. Severe hypothermia in association with sodium valproate overdose. N Z Med J 2005;118(1223):U1681.
78. Houghton BL, Bowers JB. Valproic acid overdose: a case report and review of therapy. MedGenMed 2003;5(1):1. Available at: http://www.medscape.com/viewarticle/445062. Accessed January 23, 2012.
79. Jung J, Eo E, Ahn KO. A case of hemoperfusion and L-carnitine management in valproic acid overdose. Am J Emerg Med 2008;26(3):388.e3–4.
80. Khoo SH, Leyland MJ. Cerebral edema following acute sodium valproate overdose. J Toxicol Clin Toxicol 1992;30(2):209–14.
81. Ishikura H, Matsuo N, Matsubara M, et al. Valproic acid overdose and L-carnitine therapy. J Anal Toxicol 1996;20(1):55–8.
82. Tein I. Carnitine transport: pathophysiology and metabolism of known molecular defects. J Inherit Metab Dis 2003;26(2–3):147–69.
83. Oechsner M, Steen C, Stürenburg HJ, et al. Hyperammonaemic encephalopathy after initiation of valproate therapy in unrecognised ornithine transcarbamylase deficiency. J Neurol Neurosurg Psychiatr 1998;64(5):680–2.
84. Eyer F, Felgenhauer N, Gempel K, et al. Acute valproate poisoning: pharmacokinetics, alteration in fatty acid metabolism, and changes during therapy. J Clin Psychopharmacol 2005;25(4):376–80.

85. Espinoza O, Maradei I, Ramírez M, et al. An unusual presentation of opioid-like syndrome in pediatric valproic acid poisoning. Vet Hum Toxicol 2001;43(3): 178–9.
86. Montero FJ. Naloxone in the reversal of coma induced by sodium valproate. Ann Emerg Med 1999;33(3):357–8.
87. Roberge RJ, Francis EH III. Use of naloxone in valproic acid overdose: case report and review. J Emerg Med 2002;22(1):67–70.
88. Graudins A, Aaron CK. Delayed peak serum valproic acid in massive divalproex overdose—treatment with charcoal hemoperfusion. J Toxicol Clin Toxicol 1996; 34(3):335–41.
89. Ingels M, Beauchamp J, Clark RF, et al. Delayed valproic acid toxicity: a retrospective case series. Ann Emerg Med 2002;39(6):616–21.
90. van den Broek MP, Sikma MA, Ververs TF, et al. Severe valproic acid intoxication: case study on the unbound fraction and the applicability of extracorporeal elimination. Eur J Emerg Med 2009;16(6):330–2.
91. Vannaprasaht S, Tiamkao S, Sirivongs D, et al. Acute valproic acid overdose: enhance elimination with multiple-doses activated charcoal. J Med Assoc Thai 2009;92(8):1113–5.
92. Franssen EJ, van Essen GG, Portman AT, et al. Valproic acid toxicokinetics: serial hemodialysis and hemoperfusion. Ther Drug Monit 1999;21(3):289–92.
93. Matsumoto J, Ogawa H, Ameyama R, et al. Successful treatment by direct hemoperfusion of coma possibly resulting from mitochondrial dysfunction in acute valproate intoxication. Epilepsia 1997;38(8):950–3.
94. Engbersen R, Kramers C. Enhanced extracorporeal elimination of valproic acid in overdose. Neth J Med 2004;62(9):307–8.
95. Kane SL, Constantiner M, Staubus AE, et al. High-flux hemodialysis without hemoperfusion is effective in acute valproic acid overdose. Ann Pharmacother 2000;34(10):1146–51.
96. Johnson LZ, Martinez I, Fernández MC, et al. Successful treatment of valproic acid overdose with hemodialysis. Am J Kidney Dis 1999;33(4):786–9.
97. Meek MF, Broekroelofs J, Yska JP, et al. Valproic acid intoxication: sense and non-sense of haemodialysis. Neth J Med 2004;62(9):333–6.
98. Singh SM, McMormick BB, Mustata S, et al. Extracorporeal management of valproic acid overdose: a large regional experience. J Nephrol 2004;17(1):43–9.
99. Dichtwald S, Dahan E, Adi N, et al. Molecular adsorbent recycling system therapy in the treatment of acute valproic acid intoxication. Isr Med Assoc J 2010;12(5):307–8.
100. Lheureux PE, Penaloza A, Zahir S, et al. Science review: carnitine in the treatment of valproic acid-induced toxicity—what is the evidence? Crit Care 2005; 9(5):431–40.
101. Lheureux PE, Hantson P. Carnitine in the treatment of valproic acid-induced toxicity. Clin Toxicol (Phila) 2009;47(2):101–11.
102. Perrott J, Murphy NG, Zed PJ. L-carnitine for acute valproic acid overdose: a systematic review of published cases. Ann Pharmacother 2010;44(7–8): 1287–93.
103. Licari E, Calzavacca P, Warrillow SJ, et al. Life-threatening sodium valproate overdose: a comparison of two approaches to treatment. Crit Care Med 2009; 37(12):3161–4.

Toxigenic and Metabolic Causes of Ketosis and Ketoacidotic Syndromes

Martina M. Cartwright, PhD, RD[a],*, Waddah Hajja, MD[b],
Sofian Al-Khatib, MD[b], Maryam Hazeghazam, MD, PhD[c],
Dharmashree Sreedhar, MD[d], Rebecca Na Li, MD[e],
Edna Wong-McKinstry, MD[f], Richard W. Carlson, MD, PhD[b,g,h]

KEYWORDS

- Ketosis • Ketoacidosis • Diabetic ketoacidosis • Alcoholic ketoacidosis
- Acidosis management • Toxic ingestions • Alcohol ingestion
- Ketoacidotic syndromes

KEY POINTS

- The phenomenon of diabetic ketoacidosis (DKA) has been well described and is a frequent cause of severe metabolic acidosis with a high anion gap (HAG), ketosis, and hyperglycemia.
- The mnemonic MUDPILES aids in the differential diagnosis of HAG and includes assessment of methanol poisoning, uremia, DKA and alcoholic ketoacidosis, paraldehyde intoxication, iron or isoniazid overdose, lactic acidosis, ethylene glycol, and salicylate intoxication.
- Early identification of the causes of HAG metabolic acidosis is paramount to timely treatment and patient outcomes because severe acidotic syndromes may result in coma, encephalopathy, renal failure, and death.

Disclosures: None.
[a] Department of Nutritional Sciences, University of Arizona, Shantz Building, Room 309, Tucson, AZ 85721, USA; [b] Department of Medicine, Maricopa Medical Center, 2601 East Roosevelt, Phoenix, AZ 85008, USA; [c] Department of Psychiatry and Medicine, Maricopa Medical Center, 2601 East Roosevelt, Phoenix, AZ 85008, USA; [d] Department of Internal Medicine, Maricopa Medical Center, 4849 East Roosevelt, Phoenix, AZ 85008, USA; [e] Department of Internal Medicine, Sutter Pacific Medical Foundation, 1375 Sutter Street, San Rafael, CA 94904, USA; [f] Department of Internal Medicine, University of Arizona College of Medicine, 1501 North Campbell Avenue, Tucson, AZ 85724, USA; [g] University of Arizona College of Medicine, 550 E. Van Buren Street, Phoenix, AZ 85004, USA; [h] Mayo Clinic College of Medicine, 13400 E. Shea Blvd, Scottsdale, AZ 85259, USA
* Corresponding author.
E-mail address: drmartinac@mac.com

Crit Care Clin 28 (2012) 601–631
http://dx.doi.org/10.1016/j.ccc.2012.07.001
0749-0704/12/$ – see front matter © 2012 Elsevier Inc. All rights reserved.
criticalcare.theclinics.com

Diabetic ketoacidosis (DKA) has been well described and is a frequent cause of severe metabolic acidosis with a high anion gap (HAG), ketosis, and hyperglycemia. However, HAG with ketosis has numerous other causes and many of these conditions may be encountered in the critical care setting. The mnemonic MUDPILES aids in the differential diagnosis of HAG and includes assessment of methanol poisoning, uremia, DKA and alcoholic ketoacidosis (AKA), paraldehyde intoxication, iron or isoniazid overdose, lactic acidosis, ethylene glycol, and salicylate intoxication. However, MUDPILES does not address less common, but important, causes of HAG metabolic acidosis that are also accompanied by ketoacidosis. Early identification of the causes of HAG metabolic acidosis is paramount to timely treatment and patient outcomes because severe acidotic syndromes may result in coma, encephalopathy, renal failure, and death.[1,2]

This article reviews multiple causes and characteristics of HAG ketoacidotic syndromes encountered in the critical care setting and discusses clinical features that may assist in differential diagnosis.

KETONES AND KETONE METABOLISM

Ketoacidosis is defined as an increase in ketone body concentration, together with a decrease of serum bicarbonate and pH. Ketogenesis, the production of ketone bodies, takes place in the liver, within the mitochondria of perivenous hepatocytes. When carbohydrate availability is significantly reduced, the body resorts to use of ketones as a primary energy source. This process is tightly regulated by a series of biochemical reactions and regulatory hormones (**Fig. 1**). Ketone metabolism is affected by age, the fasting versus fed state, basal metabolic rate, macronutrient intake and balance, liver glycogen stores, and amino acid mobilization from muscle.

The 3 ketone bodies are acetoacetate (AcAc), 3-hydroxybutyrate (3HB), and acetone (Ac), which are produced by hepatic β oxidation of fatty acids to form acetyl

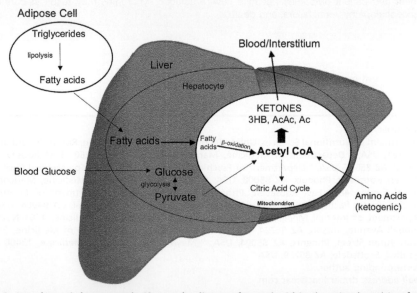

Fig. 1. Intrahepatic ketogenesis. Ketone bodies are formed within the mitochondria of perivenous hepatocytes. Ketones are produced in response to low glucose levels and absence of glycogen. AcAc, acetoacetate; Ac, acetone; CoA, coenzyme A; 3HB, β-hydroxybutyrate.

coenzyme A (CoA) (**Fig. 2**). Fatty acid β oxidation involves cleavage of the fatty acyl group liberating a 2-carbon acetyl CoA unit. The β carbon is oxidized to a keto group; hence the term β oxidation. AcAc may be reduced by β-hydroxybutyrate dehydrogenase to 3HB in a reversible reaction defined by the equilibrium of the ratio of oxidized/reduced nicotinamide adenine dinucleotide ($NAD^+/NADH$) within the mitochondria (**Fig. 3**).[3]

Ac is formed by spontaneous decarboxylation of AcAc. Ketone production is increased to spare glucose use and reduce proteolysis when glucose supply is limited, with ketones serving as an energy source for tissues, such as the brain, during fasting and starvation.[4] The liver can produce up to 185 g of ketones per day.[4] The ketoacids AcAc and 3HB alter metabolic pH, whereas Ac is the ketone body responsible for the sweet breath odor in patients with ketosis. Unlike AcAc and 3HB, Ac does not contribute to acidosis.

Total ketone levels during normal states are less than 0.5 mmol/L.[4,5] Even brief periods of fasting or exercise result in an increase in plasma ketones. Ketosis is the general term that reflects increased plasma ketones. Hyperketonemia is a ketone level greater than 1.0 mmol/L and ketoacidosis is defined as a level greater than 3.0 mmol/L.[4] The ketone body ratio reflects the amount of 3HB relative to AcAc. The ratio is almost always greater than 1.0 and increases markedly with prolonged fasting and with certain pathologic conditions, especially when the intrahepatic redox potential is altered.[6]

Ketolysis refers to the breakdown of ketone bodies in extrahepatic tissues to produce energy (**Fig. 4**). Two important enzymes are involved in ketolysis with regeneration of acetyl CoA from AcAc: succinyl CoA:3-ketoacid transferase (SCOT), which converts AcAc to acetoacetyl CoA, and methylacetoacetyl CoA thiolase (MAT), which cleaves acetoacetyl CoA to form 2 acetyl CoA molecules.[4,7] Multiple toxicities and pathologic conditions result in ketoacidosis, including diabetes, starvation coupled with physiologic stress, ethanol toxicity, other alcohol ingestions, drug toxicities, and inborn errors of ketone metabolism.

Assessment of Ketonemia

The presence of acetone is easily detected by the characteristic sweet odor of breath because Ac is readily excreted by the lungs. However, the relative contributions of AcAc, 3HB, and Ac cannot be quantified from bedside assays or the usual laboratory analysis of ketones.[8,9] The gold standard for detection of ketones, the urine ketone

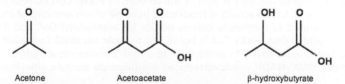

Acetone   Acetoacetate   β-hydroxybutyrate

Fig. 2. Structures of the 3 main ketone bodies. There are 3 ketone bodies: AcAc, 3HB, and Ac. 3HB is not a ketone, but is considered a ketone body for historical reasons. Ketosis occurs when ketone body concentration is pathologically increased. The hallmarks of ketosis are fruity breath and detectable urinary ketones caused by high acetone levels. Acetone, formed from spontaneous decarboxylation of AcAc, cannot be converted to acetyl CoA, but is excreted in the urine and on the breath. Unlike AcAc and 3HB, which are anions of carboxylic acids, acetone is a neutral molecule with no ionic charge. Ketoacidosis or the chronic increase of AcAc and 3HB concentration lowers blood pH and often results in numerous metabolic and clinical complications. 3HB levels are significantly increased in patients experiencing DKA and alcoholic ketoacidosis.

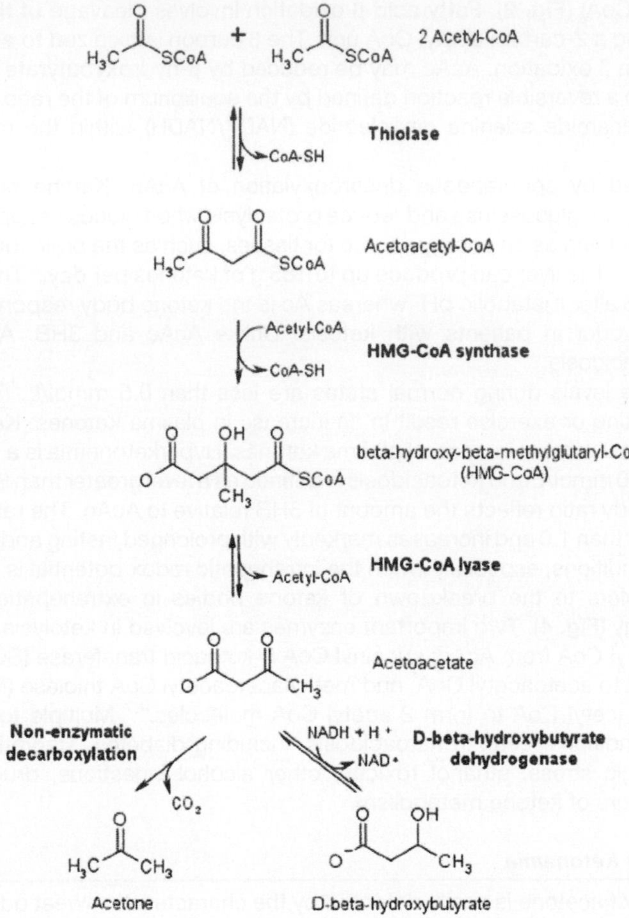

Fig. 3. Ketogenesis in the liver. Ketogenesis is the process that results in ketone body production as a result of fatty acid breakdown. Fatty acids are enzymatically dissembled by β oxidation to form acetyl CoA. Acetyl CoA is oxidized and energy is transferred to the citric acid cycle (TCA) via electrons transferred from NADH, guanosine triphosphate (GTP), and flavin adenine dinucleotide (FADH2). If the amount of acetyl CoA exceeds the capacity of the TCA or if the TCA cycle activity is suppressed because of low amounts of oxaloacetate, the acetyl CoA is used to synthesize ketone bodies via acetoacetyl CoA and β-hydroxy-β-methylglutaryl (HMG) CoA. HMG CoA is converted to AcAc via HMG CoA lyase with AcAc being converted spontaneously to acetone or to β-hydroxybutyrate via β-hydroxybutyrate dehydrogenase. NAD+/NADH, oxidized/reduced nicotinamide adenine dinucleotide.

dip-stick test (Ketostix; Bayer, Pittsburgh, PA; Ames, Elkhart, IN), has several limitations because this technique uses the Legal nitroprusside reaction, which only detects AcAc and Ac, but not 3HB.[10] Moreover, the Legal assay is affected by air and substances such as captopril (Capoten), N-acetylcysteine (Mucomyst), dimercaprol (British antilewisite), as well as penicillamine (Cuprimine), which may interfere with the results.[11] Furthermore, urinary ketones do not accurately reflect blood levels, and are affected by renal function.[10,12] Quantitation of 3HB and AcAc would optimally allow the clinician to follow changes in these compounds during the course of therapy. Until recently, methods to quantify 3HB have not been widely available. However, both

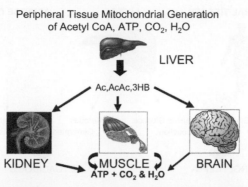

Peripheral Tissue Mitochondrial Generation
of Acetyl CoA, ATP, CO_2, H_2O

LIVER

Ac,AcAc,3HB

KIDNEY — MUSCLE — BRAIN
ATP + CO_2 & H_2O

Fig. 4. Ketolysis and peripheral tissue mitochondrial generation of acetyl CoA, ATP, CO_2, and H_2O. Ketolysis refers to the breakdown of ketone bodies in extrahepatic tissues to produce energy. Two important enzymes are involved in ketolysis with regeneration of acetyl CoA from AcAc: succinyl CoA:3-ketoacid transferase (SCOT), which converts AcAc to acetoacetyl CoA; and methylacetoacetyl CoA thiolase (MAT), which cleaves AcAc CoA into 2 acetyl CoA molecules. ATP, adenosine triphosphate; CO_2, carbon dioxide; H_2O, water.

bedside and laboratory devices for direct measurement of 3HB are now available and provide reliable determination of 3HB from microsamples of blood or other fluids.[13–16] The advent of 3HB technology should be a valuable tool in the management of ketosis, including titration of insulin therapy. In addition, the ratio of 3HB to AcAc may be useful in the differential diagnosis of ketoacidotic syndromes.[6,16,17]

DKA

DKA, a potentially life-threatening condition of severe metabolic acidosis coupled with a HAG, is clinically the most frequently encountered form of metabolic acidosis, accounting for a substantial number of admissions to critical care units. Although typically seen in type I diabetes mellitus (DM), DKA is seen with increasing frequency among type II diabetic patients of certain ethnic groups[18] or those suffering from stressful metabolic events.[19,20] Mortality is low if patients seek medical attention promptly, although mortalities of up to 13% have been reported.[21] Clinical hallmarks of DKA are fruity breath caused by acetone, Kussmaul breathing, signs and symptoms of volume depletion, and altered mentation. Laboratory criteria for DKA include hyperglycemia, ketonemia and ketonuria, and metabolic acidosis.[22,23] An absolute or relative lack of insulin is required for the development of DKA, but concomitant increases of counterregulatory hormones, including glucagon, catecholamines, growth hormone, and cortisol play important pathogenic roles. Lipolysis and hepatic ketogenesis are also key factors in development of DKA.[24–27] Mechanisms that account for metabolic and fluid derangements in DKA are shown in **Fig. 5**.

Precipitating factors for DKA include infections; errors or poor compliance in the implementation of diabetic regimen; myocardial infarction; trauma; pancreatitis or other acute medical or psychological crises; and drugs, such as corticosteroids, sympathomimetic agents, as well as certain other medications, illicit drugs, and alcohol.[25–28]

DKA and Atypical Antipsychotic Medications

Metabolically fragile diabetic patients with a history of poor glycemic control are the most frequently encountered patients with DKA. However, increases in DKA have been noted in patients using atypical antipsychotic medications.[19,28,29] Atypical

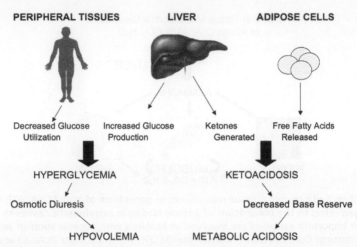

PERIPHERAL TISSUES   **LIVER**   **ADIPOSE CELLS**

Decreased Glucose   Increased Glucose   Ketones   Free Fatty Acids
Utilization   Production   Generated   Released

HYPERGLYCEMIA   KETOACIDOSIS

Osmotic Diuresis   Decreased Base Reserve

HYPOVOLEMIA   METABOLIC ACIDOSIS

Fig. 5. DKA. An absolute or relative lack of insulin is required for the development of DKA, but concomitant increases of counterregulatory hormones, including glucagon, catecholamines, growth hormone, and cortisol, play an important pathogenic role. Lipolysis and hepatic ketogenesis are also key factors in development of DKA. Hyperglycemia results from increased liver production of glucose and a concurrent decrease in peripheral use of glucose. Ketoacidosis results from increased free fatty acid release from adipose (fat) tissue and liver generation of ketones. Hyperglycemia triggers osmotic diuresis and hypovolemia. A decrease in base reserve from ketoacidosis results in metabolic acidosis. DKA is a potentially life-threatening condition that requires immediate medical attention and is a frequent cause of hospital admissions. (*Data from* Umpierrez GE, Khajavi M, Kitabchi AE. Review: diabetic ketoacidosis and hyperglycemic hyperosmolar nonketotic syndrome. Am J Med Sci 1996;311(5):225–33.)

antipsychotic drugs (AAPs) including clozapine (Clozaril, Fazacio), risperidone (Risperdal), olanzapine (Zyprexa, Relprevv), quetiapine (Seroquel), ziprasidone (Geodon), and aripiprazole (Abilify) have been widely prescribed to treat a spectrum of psychiatric disorders. As a drug class, AAPs have shown clinical efficacy compared with traditional antipsychotics for treatment of schizophrenia, with a lower incidence of extrapyramidal symptoms and tardive dyskinesia compared with conventional medications.[29] Improved drug tolerance and clinical psychiatric outcomes have prompted a surge in AAP prescriptions for bipolar disorder, posttraumatic stress disorder, and dementia with psychosis. The increasing use of AAPs has coincided with an increase in DKA in patients not previously diagnosed with diabetes.[29,30]

AAPs are associated with significant and sudden metabolic side effects, including excessive weight gain, obesity, glucose intolerance, and new-onset type II DM.[30] DKA and hypertriglyceridemia have been reported with initiation of AAP therapies.[31,32] Jin and colleagues[32] analyzed 45 published cases of new-onset DM following AAP initiation and found that 42% developed DKA. The mean duration of AAP exposure before the DKA episode was 19 (range 2–24) weeks, with 14% developing DM or DKA within 1 month after starting AAP therapy.[32] Koller and colleagues[33–35] performed a retrospective analysis of 805 cases of new-onset DM or exacerbation of existing DM in patients who were nascent to AAPs. DKA was reported in 100 of 289 patients who were receiving olanzapine, 80 of 384 taking clozapine, and 36 of 132 who were prescribed risperidone. DKA has also been reported with aripiprazole use.[36] The incidence of DKA in patients newly prescribed AAPs occurred in the absence of any notable preexisting illness or metabolic stress. Patients who present with signs of

DKA without a history of DM should therefore be evaluated for the use of AAPs. Although DKA can develop at any time during AAP therapy, clinicians should be cognizant of the often-observed short duration between institution of AAP therapy and development of DM. DKA may therefore be the first symptom of new-onset DM in patients receiving AAPs.

DKA and Illicit Drug Use

Common precipitating causes of DKA include infection, concurrent illness, and failure to comply with a diabetic management regimen.[23–25] Patients may be financially or otherwise unable to obtain diabetic medications and equipment. Others discontinue therapy because of psychological or social factors. In the past few years there has been an increase in reports of patients who developed DKA in association with concomitant alcohol or illicit drug use. In some instances, these patients have presented with more severe acidosis or hyperglycemia than those with other precipitating issues.[37–39] In a review of 60 consecutive patients with DKA at our institution, 63% presented with noncompliance as a major precipitating factor.[40,41] Acute alcohol abuse accounted for one-fourth of these cases; and one-third were related to cocaine or amphetamine abuse. Alcohol abuse is also associated with development of DKA, and patients who present with abdominal pain and DKA are more likely to have severe acidosis and a recent history of alcohol or cocaine abuse.[38]

Cocaine leads to marked increases in catecholamines with effects on counterregulatory hormones such as adrenocorticotropic hormone, cortisol, and glucagon.[42–45] These counterregulatory factors, plus the effect of drug abuse on diabetic regimen compliance, likely account for the strong association of cocaine abuse and DKA episodes. Cocaine abusers who develop DKA have few concurrent precipitating factors such as infection but high admission serum glucose levels. Such patients usually respond rapidly to DKA management.[39]

Other illicit agents have also been implicated in the development of DKA.[46–48] Fatal episodes that included DKA were associated with sertraline and methadone overdose.[46] The sudden development of DKA has similarly been observed in patients taking the street drug ecstasy (3,4-methylenedioxymethamphetamine [MDMA]). This drug can cause hyponatremia, severe hyperthermia, and a variety of metabolic changes that may precipitate DKA.[47] MDMA stimulates release of serotonin, dopamine, and norepinephrine, as well as antidiuretic hormone.[49] Toxicologic studies together with historical information and clinical features may therefore pinpoint illicit drug use as a factor in the development of DKA.

In addition to AAPs and illicit drugs, rare cases of DKA have been reported with other prescription drugs and some over-the-counter herbal dietary aids. Use of the bronchodilator terbutaline (Brethine, Bricanyl) may lead to insulin resistance and the development of DKA that is likely caused by the counterregulatory effects of the drug.[50] The immunosuppressant mizoribine, of the imidazole class of drugs, has been associated with development of DKA in an otherwise stable diabetic patient.[51]

Two diabetic patients developed DKA following use of the original formulation of Metabolife 356, an over-the-counter herbal appetite suppressant that contained ephedra and guarana, a herbal source of caffeine.[52] Side effects of ephedra and caffeine include tachycardia, hypertension, hyperglycemia, and increased catecholamine levels.[53,54] Although not considered to be the sole cause of DKA in these patients, the combination of ephedra and caffeine was a likely contributor. In 2001, Metabolife 356 was reformulated after several reports of adverse effects associated with ephedra.[55] Other appetite suppressant products that contain a combination of caffeine and ephedra are currently available.

NUTRITIONAL CAUSES OF KETOACIDOSIS

The simplest form of ketosis occurs in starvation and involves carbohydrate depletion with free fatty acid mobilization. Starvation-induced ketosis is generally mild and not life threatening. During starvation, glycogenolysis and gluconeogenesis offset potential hypoglycemia, and are accompanied by lipolysis and ketogenesis.[56] When glucose is scarce, ketones provide an alternative energy source to the brain and other tissues. Short-term fasting is usually associated with mild acidosis. After an overnight fast, the body enters the basal or postabsorptive state with release and oxidation of fatty acids, glycogenolysis, and liberation of amino acids from muscle. After 12 to 24 hours of fasting, additional free fatty acids are released from adipose tissue and ketone production increases. Fasting beyond 2 days is associated with low insulin levels, depletion of liver glycogen, and protein catabolism. Glucose production shifts to glycerol and glucogenic amino acids. Glucagon and other counterregulatory hormones increase. Severe, life-threatening ketoacidosis is possible when starvation is complicated by a stressful event, such as pregnancy, extreme exercise, prolonged emesis, or undiagnosed hyperthyroidism.[57-64]

Eating disorders and deranged eating patterns classified as eating disorders not otherwise specified are associated with extreme starvation and may result in profound metabolic complications that require immediate treatment and hospitalization.[65] In recent years, a disordered eating pattern termed orthorexia nervosa has been recognized and is characterized by the obsessive desire to eat only foods deemed healthy or pure. The orthorexic is driven to eat a rigid selection of certain foods. Variations of orthorexia include rawism and fruitarianism. Individuals who follow such rigid diets may suffer from nutritional deficiencies and metabolic complications. Severe ketoacidosis, ketonuria, and metabolic acidosis have been reported in a fruitarian patient.[66]

Therapeutic Ketogenic Diets

Nonpathogenic ketosis with normoglycemia frequently occurs with consumption of therapeutic ketogenic diets. These high-fat, high-protein, low-carbohydrate diets promote ketosis by depleting carbohydrate stores, allowing the body to convert fat and protein into energy.[67] The resulting ketosis is usually mild and temporary and is associated with side effects such as bad breath, constipation, and dehydration.[68-70] Electrolyte imbalances and kidney stones have been reported.[71-73]

The use of therapeutic ketogenic diets for the treatment of epileptic seizures dates to biblical times.[74] Numerous studies have confirmed the efficacy of the ketogenic diet as an adjunct to pharmacologic control of seizures, even in those who are not responsive to medications.[74-76] Ketogenic diets may be beneficial to adults with Alzheimer disease, Parkinson disease, and amyotrophic lateral sclerosis,[77,78] although more study is required to recommend widespread use in these conditions.

Alcoholic Ketoacidosis

Alcoholic ketoacidosis (AKA) was first recognized as a clinical syndrome in 1940 by Dillon and colleagues.[79] AKA is characterized by HAG metabolic acidosis and ketosis. Some experts prefer to designate this syndrome as alcoholic acidosis, because complex mixed acid-base disturbances are usually present.[80-82] In AKA, unless 3HB is measured, the severity of ketosis may be underestimated, because the ratio of 3HB to AcAc is higher in AKA than DKA.[83] Serum glucose is normal to low in AKA; only 11% of patients with AKA in the series by Wrenn and colleagues[84] presented with hyperglycemia. Since the syndrome was initially documented, subsequent reports have confirmed clinical features.[81,85,86]

Patients with AKA have a history of alcohol abuse and present with severe acidemia following a binge drinking episode that is often coupled with malnutrition, nausea, severe vomiting, dehydration, gastritis, or pancreatitis.[17,87,88] Gastrointestinal signs and symptoms predominate, together with features of volume depletion. Mentation is abnormal in approximately 15% of patients.[84,87] In addition to acidosis that may include lactic acidosis, multiple electrolyte disturbances are commonly observed. Acid-base derangements are complex and may include double and triple acid-base defects.

Although starvation plays a role in the genesis of AKA, the pathophysiology is complex (**Fig. 6**). Three inciting events are (1) suppression of insulin and excess glucagon precipitated by poor nutritional intake; (2) a high NADH/NAD$^+$ ratio related to alcohol metabolism; and (3) hypovolemia caused by poor food intake and vomiting.[89–93]

Ethanol is metabolized by alcohol dehydrogenase and aldehyde dehydrogenase to acetate. Acetate is then converted to acetyl CoA, a substrate that can be oxidized to carbon dioxide, condensed into ketones, or converted to fat.[80] Gluconeogenesis is suppressed and the ketoacids AcAc and 3HB are produced in response. Hypovolemia

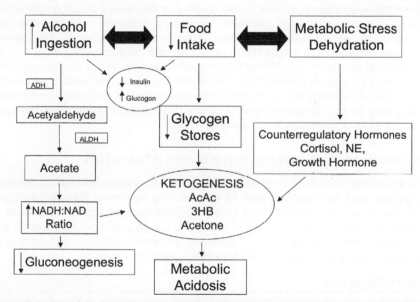

Fig. 6. The interrelationship between high ethanol intake, reduced food consumption and metabolic stress in ketogenesis. Alcoholism and binge drinking are often associated with ketosis. Many alcoholics and chronic binge drinkers are malnourished because of decreased caloric intake.[91,92] In addition, alcoholics and the malnourished are often immunocompromised and suffer from metabolic stress.[88] All 3 conditions can lead to enhanced ketogenesis through 3 distinct pathways. First, in the case of excessive alcohol consumption, ethanol is metabolized to acetaldehyde and acetate, resulting in increased NADH/NAD$^+$ ratio[80,90] and reduced gluconeogenesis. High levels of NADH and low glucose availability enhances ketogenesis, with profound increases in serum 3HB levels that can contribute to ketoacidosis. Poor food intake causes a decrease in insulin and glycogen stores. As glucose becomes limited In starvation, ketogenesis ensues to provide energy to body tissues. Metabolic stress, such as infection, fever, and hypermetabolic conditions (trauma, burns, sepsis), trigger counterregulatory hormone release and ketogenesis.[88] All 3 conditions may cause metabolicacidosis. ADH, alcohol dehydrogenase; ALDH, aldehyde dehydrogenase; NE, norepinephrine.

stimulates the sympathetic nervous system through increases in counterregulatory factors such as catecholamines, cortisol, glucagon, and growth hormone. The result is ketogenesis and ketosis, enhanced lipolysis, increase of free fatty acids, and increases in lactate. Umpierrez and colleagues[83] observed that the hormonal profiles of AKA and DKA are characterized by similar decreases in insulin and increases of counterregulatory hormones, but differ in plasma glucose and levels of 3HB. The hallmark of AKA is HAG and ketoacidosis in the absence of hyperglycemia.[83] Overall, AKA is characterized by decreased blood pH, plasma bicarbonate, and insulin. Free fatty acids, cortisol, and the ratio of 3HB to AcAc are increased. The patient with AKA usually presents with tachycardia, orthostatic hypotension, and a sweet breath odor. Electrolyte imbalances and comorbidities are common.

In uncomplicated AKA the prognosis is good, but up to 10% experience sudden cardiac arrest.[81,94] Very high levels of 3HB as well as hypokalemia, hypomagnesemia, and increased lactate have been found at autopsy.[81,95–99]

Treatment of AKA is straightforward and includes rapid fluid loading with isotonic saline to repair extracellular fluid deficits, glucose administration to replete glycogen stores, as well as thiamine supplementation and correction of electrolyte defects. Dextrose administration increases insulin levels and decreases glucagon secretion. Insulin or bicarbonate therapy are rarely necessary. Thiamine prevents Wernicke encephalopathy and Korsakoff syndrome. Glucose helps to interrupt ketogenesis and reverse the abnormal NADH/NAD$^+$ ratio. Although hyperphosphatemia may be documented in approximately 25% of patients admitted with AKA, a similar proportion present with hypophosphatemia.[84] For those with hypophosphatemia on presentation, as acidemia is corrected, severe hypophosphatemia is a potential complication, and may lead to life-threatening complications.[99] Phosphate repletion is therefore indicated if initial phosphorus levels are low.

ISOPROPANOL, ACETONE, AND PROPYLENE GLYCOL INTOXICATION

AKA is a condition specific to long-term consumption of ethanol; however, other alcohols, glycols, and ketones can lead to serious, and sometime fatal, ketoacidotic events. The American Association of Poison Control Centers reports thousands of accidental and intentional ingestions of methanol, ethylene glycol, isopropanol, and other related compounds each year.[100] Methanol and ethylene glycol can lead to toxic ketoacidosis and are discussed elsewhere in this issue by Kruse.

Isopropanol Ingestion

Isopropanol (isopropyl alcohol, 2-propanol), or rubbing alcohol, is found in multiple household and automotive products and is frequently taken as a substitute for ethanol (Box 1). Rubbing alcohol contains up to 70% isopropanol and is the most commonly ingested isopropanol-containing product. More than 7000 rubbing alcohol ingestions were reported in 2010 to United States poison control centers with no fatalities, although 3 deaths were reported caused by cleaning agents and other products containing isopropanol.[100] Topical application with inhalation of isopropyl vapor may also lead to toxicity in children after sponge baths.[101]

Isopropyl alcohol is rapidly absorbed from the stomach and mucous membranes and converted to acetone by the action of alcohol dehydrogenase (ADH). Acetone is excreted through the lungs and kidneys. Ingestion of isopropanol results in gastric irritation, central nervous system (CNS) depression, hypotension, and, with high doses, hemodynamic instability with shock (Box 2).[89,102–104] Although hyperosmolality and high levels of acetone are observed, ketoacidosis is uncommon; if metabolic

---

Box 1
Common products containing isopropanol

Rubbing alcohol

Hair tonics

Permanent wave solution

Liquid detergents

Paint removers

Cosmetics

Rug cleaners

Windshield deicers

Dog repellents

Radiator stop leak

Stain and rust removers

Hand sanitizers

---

acidosis occurs, it is related to accumulation of lactate because of hypoperfusion, or the development of renal failure. Fatalities have been reported in patients with coma and hypotension.[1]

As little as 20 mL (50% solution) may induce symptoms in adults.[105] Serum levels greater than 150 mg/dL lead to coma and hypotension, although 1 study reported

---

Box 2
Isopropanol intoxication

1. Rapid absorption from stomach, mucous membranes
2. Onset of toxicity: less than 1 hour after ingestion
3. Signs and symptoms
    a. Gastrointestinal irritation, abdominal pain, nausea, vomiting, diarrhea, bleeding
    b. CNS depression
    c. Hypotension, shock
    d. Renal failure
4. Laboratory findings
    a. Ketonemia and ketonuria
    b. Hyperosmolality
    c. Increased blood lactate level
    d. Renal failure (or spurious creatinine increase)
    e. Rhabdomyolysis
5. Therapy
    a. Supportive care
    b. Hemodialysis: for hemodynamic instability, severe CNS depression, isopropanol levels greater than 200 mg/dL

---

that levels greater than 400 mg/dL were associated with these findings.[103] Abdominal pain, nausea, vomiting, and diarrhea may develop within 30 minutes of ingestion, together with altered mentation.

Of increasing concern is the intentional or accidental consumption of alcohol-based hand sanitizers. Hand disinfectants have become a commonplace alternative to hand washing. Most hand sanitizers contain short-chain alcohols such as 1-propanol or 2-propanol and ethanol. In 2006, United States poison control centers reported more than 11,000 exposures to hand sanitizers, including 9600 related to children.[106] Cases of hospitalized or imprisoned alcoholics consuming large volumes of 60% ethanol or isopropanol-containing hand disinfectants have been reported.[107–109] Some sanitizers contain a mixture of alcohols, which can result in mixed acidosis. Metabolism of 1-propanol by ADH leads to propionic acid production with a HAG metabolic acidosis, whereas 2-propanol metabolism leads to acetone formation but no acidosis. A hospitalized patient who ingested a lethal dose of hand disinfectant containing 1-propanol and 2-propanol required intubation within 30 minutes of ingestion, and developed a mixed acidosis with HAG and ketonuria.[110] Clinicians should be aware of potential intoxications from hand sanitizers, particularly in clinical settings where these products are ubiquitous. In sudden cases of mixed acidosis that may include ketosis, patients should be evaluated promptly for toxic ingestion of hand sanitizers.

For isopropanol ingestion, because of rapid absorption and significant gastritis, emesis, gastric lavage, and activated charcoal are unlikely to be effective within 1 hour of ingestion, and are contraindicated in the presence of CNS depression. Hemodialysis should be implemented for severe intoxications that produce hypotension or coma, or with levels greater than 200 mg/dL.[89,111] Hypotension is related in part to peripheral vasodilation and may require aggressive fluid infusion as well as vasoactive agents.[112,113] Dialysis is effective in removing isopropanol.[89] Inhibition of ADH by fomepizole or ethanol is not indicated.

Acetone

Acetone (2-propanone) is an uncommon intoxication that can occur after ingestion or dermal absorption of acetone, or from ingestion or inhalation of fumes from various solvents that contain acetone. Acetone is found in some fingernail polish removers, solvents for glues, varnishes, and rubber cements, and in some solvents for fiberglass resin.[114,115] The agent is rapidly absorbed through the lungs and gastrointestinal systems and is excreted unchanged through the lung or kidney. Toxicity includes altered mental status that may progress to coma, respiratory depression, and hyperglycemia.[115,116] Vomiting commonly occurs after ingestion. The half-life of acetone is 19 to 31 hours. Prolonged observation is indicated after intoxication. There is no antidote.

Propylene Glycol

Propylene glycol (1,2-propanediol [PG]) is used as a solvent for intravenous (IV), oral, and topical pharmaceutical agents including diazepam (Valium), phenytoin (Dilantin), lorazepam (Ativan), phenobarbital, pentobarbital, etomidate, nitroglycerin, and digoxin. PG is also found in some dermal preparations, including sulfadiazine cream. Metabolic acidosis from toxic levels of PG is associated with increased lactate levels.[117] PG is oxidized by ADH to lactic acid. Ketosis is not typically a component of PG toxicity, but hemodynamic instability with hypotension and bradycardia, as well as CNS depression, seizures, and hypoglycemia, can occur. Hemodialysis may be required for unstable patients.

DRUG TOXICITIES
Salicylate Poisoning

Salicylates have been used for treatment of pain for more than 2500 years. Hippocrates, Dioscorides, and Galen used willow leaves to treat a variety of conditions, and warned of overdosing.[118–120] Salicylates are found in several prescription and over-the-counter pain relievers, antipyretics, and antiinflammatory medication as well as natural herbal remedies that contain willow, poplar bark, or oil of wintergreen. Because of the wide availability of salicylate in the form of aspirin (acetylsalicylic acid), salicylate overdose remains a common intoxication, despite other nonsteroidal antiinflammatory agents such as ibuprofen and acetaminophen having largely replaced aspirin as principal pain medications consumed by the public. However, rates of poisoning remain high among elderly, chronic aspirin users.[121–123]

When ingested, aspirin is rapidly converted to its active metabolite, salicylic acid (orthohydroxybenzoic acid), which is absorbed through the stomach and small intestine. Salicylate is distributed throughout most body tissues and transcellular fluids; in pregnant women, salicylate enters the choroid plexus and crosses the placental barrier. The volume of distribution is approximately 170 mL/kg, which increases markedly with high therapeutic doses because of protein binding.[124] Aspirin is hydrolyzed by the gastrointestinal mucosa, as well as the liver, plasma, and red blood cells. Approximately 80% of salicylate in plasma is bound to albumin and other proteins. Therapeutic doses of salicylic acid are metabolized in the liver and cleared within 2 to 3 hours, although chronic ingestion can increase the half-life to more than 20 hours.[121,125] Additional metabolism occurs with formation of glucuronides. Metabolites are collected in the urine, although urinary excretion is depends on urine pH. Enhanced excretion can be achieved by alkalinization.

Low doses of aspirin (75–81 mg/d) irreversibly acetylate a serine residue within the active site of cyclooxygenase (COX). This action irreversibly blocks formation of thromboxane A2, which inhibits platelet aggregation and produces an antithrombotic effect. Larger doses of up to 4 g/d inhibit both COX-1 and COX-2, which reduce production of certain prostaglandins and account for analgesic and antipyretic effects. Very high doses (4–8 g/d) are antiinflammatory and are used for rheumatic disorders.[126] Therapeutic plasma levels of aspirin may therefore reach 30 mg/dL in patients taking high doses. Plasma concentrations greater than 40 mg/dL are associated with tinnitus, fever, vertigo, a variety of gastrointestinal complaints, and altered mentation.

Symptoms of intoxication occur when levels exceed 40 mg/dL and the lethal adult dose is 10 to 30 g, or approximately thirty-five 325-mg tablets.[1,125] Salicylate toxicity interferes with aerobic metabolism and thus affects virtually all organs. **Table 1** depicts the systemic effects of salicylate poisoning. In aspirin intoxication, cellular glucose metabolism proceeds, resulting in production of carbon dioxide and water. However, because aspirin uncouples mitochondrial oxidative phosphorylation adenosine triphosphate (ATP) formation is aborted, leading to increased anaerobic metabolism and accumulation of lactate. In addition, ketone production is upregulated.[127] Ketones, which increase as a result of free fatty acid liberation from adipose tissue lipolysis, are shunted to tissues and used as an energy source. The metabolic acidosis of salicylate intoxication is related to a combination of salicylic acid, lactic acidosis, and ketoacidosis.[128,129]

In addition, hyperglycemia may develop with salicylate poisoning, although hypoglycemia is more common, in part because of glycogen depletion. Hypoglycemia leads to corresponding decreases of CNS glucose (neuroglycopenia), and dangerously low CNS glucose levels may develop despite normal serum levels. Mental status

Table 1 Organ system toxicity of salicylates	
Organ	**Toxicity Symptoms**
Ear	Tinnitus, deafness
Lung	Permeability pulmonary edema, acute lung injury, acute respiratory distress syndrome, hypoxemia, respiratory alkalosis (early), respiratory acidosis (late)
Gastrointestinal	Nausea, vomiting, gastritis, upper gastrointestinal bleeding, pylorospasm, bezoars (may inhibit activated charcoal therapy)
Renal	Proteinuria, acute renal failure (especially with agents containing phenacetin or hemodynamic instability), tubular injury
Blood	Decreased platelet function, hypoprothrombinemia
Musculoskeletal	Heat production, rhabdomyolysis
Liver	Glycogen depletion, lactic acidosis, uncoupling of oxidative phosphorylation, ketogenesis, Reye syndrome (children), hepatic failure
CNS	Confusion, delirium, seizures, coma, cerebral edema, neuroglycopenia
Metabolic	Hypoglycemia, anion gap metabolic acidosis, fever, diaphoresis, hypokalemia

changes are common in severe salicylate intoxications and cerebral edema may be a fatal event. Children experience a more rapid progression to metabolic acidosis.[121] Patients typically manifest metabolic acidosis along with primary respiratory alkalosis early in the course of the poisoning; respiratory acidosis is a late finding, unless severe pulmonary edema has affected carbon dioxide elimination.

Toxic levels of salicylate lead to adverse effects on both cyclooxygenase and lipoxygenase pathways with production of a variety of prostaglandins including thromboxane A2, as well as leukotrienes.[130–135] Increases of these prostaglandins have been linked to increases in vascular permeability with development of acute respiratory distress syndrome and other organ dysfunction. An early correlate of potentially serious salicylate intoxication is proteinuria, which may herald subsequent development of respiratory permeability and pulmonary edema.[136]

Identifying Salicylate Poisoning

In 1960, pediatrician AK Done developed the salicylate intoxication nomogram,[137] which became a standard for evaluating toxicity of salicylate ingestions. However, the Done nomogram was developed for the pediatric population and may not be appropriate for adults, especially those who use aspirin over a prolonged period, those who use time-released preparations, and those with renal insufficiency. Moreover, because salicylates are not eliminated by first-order toxicokinetics, the nomogram may be of limited usefulness.[138] Serial salicylate levels, rather than use of the Done nomogram, may be more helpful in the management of toxic ingestions. Recent studies suggest a greater correlation with clinical findings when using serial measurements of salicylate rather than the nomogram and, therefore, routine use of the nomogram is discouraged.[139–141]

Chronic intoxication may be associated with lower serum salicylate values, therefore levels should be monitored frequently because bezoar formation by clumps of pills, enteric-coated tablets, and other factors may affect absorption and symptoms of intoxication.[142] Although serum salicylate levels should be measured routinely, early diagnosis may be facilitated by use of the point-of-care ferric chloride test of urine.[143] However, there are limitations to using this test because a single aspirin can render a positive result.[121]

Treatment of Salicylate Toxicity

Lavage of gastric contents and activated charcoal can significantly reduce the salicylate poison burden. Some experts recommend multiple-dose activated charcoal, although it is not considered standard therapy. Whole bowel irrigation with polyethylene glycol may reduce absorption in cases of enteric-coated aspirin ingestion.[144]

Priorities of management include stabilization of cardiorespiratory status as well as rehydration and correction of metabolic and electrolyte disturbances, particularly hypoglycemia and hypokalemia. Serum and urine alkalinization with sodium bicarbonate reduces CNS toxicity and enhances urinary excretion. Carbonic anhydrase inhibitors should be avoided because they enhance plasma acidity.

Patients who are massively poisoned may have hemodynamic instability and require aggressive fluid loading, including colloids as well as use of vasoactive drugs. Patients who manifest such toxicity should be considered for hemodialysis, because progressive pulmonary edema and acute respiratory distress syndrome may result. Considerations for hemodialysis in severe salicylate intoxication are shown in **Box 3**.[1,144] Fatalities have resulted from failure to institute hemodialysis in patients with severe intoxications who were not responding to supportive measures. Alkalemia should be achieved using bicarbonate therapy and, if the patient is intubated, increased minute volume with respiratory alkalosis assured by mechanical ventilation.

Isoniazid Poisoning

Isoniazid (isonicotinic acid hydrazide [INH]) is an antimicrobial used in tuberculosis therapy and prophylaxis. Because of the widespread use of INH, accidental and intentional intoxication is seen throughout the world. Patients may also take additional doses of INH for missed doses, resulting in toxicity. The structure of INH includes a pyridine nucleus and is similar to pyridoxine (vitamin B_6) and niacin (vitamin B_3 or nictotinic acid). The drug is effectively absorbed from the small intestine with high plasma levels attained within 2 hours.[145] There is little protein binding, but INH binds to the active form of vitamin B_6, pyridoxal 5'-phosphate, to form INH-pyridoxal hydrazones, which inhibit glutamate decarboxylase. This enzyme is involved in the synthesis of the inhibitory neurotransmitter γ-aminobutyric acid (GABA). INH also inhibits pyridoxal 5'-phosphate synthesis, thereby further interfering with GABA synthesis.

The primary metabolism of INH is via hepatic acetylation. The rate of acetylation varies with ethnic groups. Metabolites of INH are potent hepatotoxins and liver

---

Box 3
Considerations for hemodialysis in salicylate intoxication

Hemodynamic instability

Progressive CNS dysfunction

Uncontrolled acid-base, metabolic, or electrolyte defects

Renal failure

Very high or increasing serum salicylate levels (>90 mg/dL), respiratory failure, pulmonary edema, acute respiratory distress syndrome

damage has been documented with chronic therapeutic doses. Mild toxicity may be seen with ingestion of less than 1.5 g. Fatalities secondary to isoniazid therapy, although rare, can occur with acute ingestion of 6 to 10 g.[146] Toxicity is related to deficiencies of vitamin B_6 and GABA, and to hepatic injury. Signs and symptoms of intoxication can appear within 45 minutes of ingestion of 80 to 150 mg/kg, but may be delayed for up to 2 or more hours when peak absorption occurs.[147] Severe neurotoxicity is the major manifestation and is seen with doses greater than 200 mg/kg.[147,148] Findings include nausea, vomiting, visual changes, fever, metabolic acidosis, hypocalcemia, ketonemia and ketonuria, seizures, coma, and death.[149–151]

The clinical triad of INH toxicity includes coma, seizures, and severe metabolic acidosis. In addition, the presence of hyperglycemia and ketosis may lead to a misdiagnosis of DKA.[147,148,152] The presence of neurologic findings, especially seizures, is an important clue to INH poisoning. Because INH reacts with pyridoxine and results in pyridoxine deficiency as well as GABA deficiency, a major clinical problem is intractable seizures that are resistant to conventional anticonvulsant therapies.

HAG metabolic acidosis is characteristic of severe INH poisonings, although the cause of the metabolic acidosis is multifactorial. High lactate levels are observed as well as ketonemia.[153,154] Rhabdomyolysis and renal failure may occur as a result of refractory seizures. Ketogenesis leads to production of 3HB and accompanying ketoacidosis.[155]

Management of INH Poisoning

Asymptomatic patients should receive activated charcoal within 1 to 2 hours after ingestion; symptomatic patients should receive IV pyridoxine at a dose equivalent to the amount of isoniazid ingested in milligrams.[152] This dose may be repeated every 10 minutes to help control seizures. If the dose of ingested INH is unknown, 5 g IV may be given and repeated for refractory seizures. Aggressive supportive treatment should be instituted for unresponsive patients or those with recurrent seizures. Urinary alkalinization promotes INH clearance, but hemodialysis may be needed for severe poisonings. Treatment of seizures should be directed to repletion of GABA by IV administration of pyridoxine and a potent GABA agent such as the benzodiazepine lorazepam. Phenobarbital may also be used for refractory seizures, but phenytoin is not indicated for INH-induced seizures.

ORPHAN DISEASES: INBORN ERRORS OF KETONE METABOLISM

Several inborn errors of metabolism are associated with severe ketoacidosis: succinyl CoA:3-ketoacid CoA transferase (SCOT) deficiency, mitochondrial 2-methyacetoacetyl CoA thiolase (MAT or T2) deficiency, and methylmalonyl coenzyme A mutase deficiency.[156] SCOT and T2 deficiencies are characterized by abnormally high levels of ketones with periodic ketoacidotic episodes and no clinical symptoms in between episodes. Methylmalonyl CoA mutase deficiency produces infantile ketoacidotic coma.

SCOT is an enzyme that facilitates transfer of the CoA portion of succinyl CoA to AcAc to form acetoacetyl CoA. In the absence of glucose, extrahepatic tissues require SCOT to use ketones as an energy source. SCOT deficiency, a rare disease, is characterized by intermittent ketoacidotic events that typically manifest in early infancy.[157] Symptoms include persistent ketosis with frequent episodes of ketoacidosis.[157,158] The latter often develops following fasting, fever, infection, or other metabolically stressful events. SCOT deficiency is often initially diagnosed following a severe, if not fatal, ketoacidotic episode. These children frequently present with tachycardia, secondary to severe metabolic acidosis, and a history of failure to thrive, feeding difficulties, vomiting, and lethargy.[159] Lactate, pyruvate, and glucose are usually normal during a ketoacidotic event, whereas urinary ketones are increased. The differential diagnosis includes other possible causes of ketoacidosis including diabetes and ingestion of salicylate or other poisons.[157] If a young child repeatedly presents with ketoacidosis, an assay for SCOT should be performed to exclude deficiency. Permanent ketosis or ketonuria is considered a pathogenic characteristic of complete SCOT deficiency. However, mild mutations result in incomplete SCOT deficiency; these individuals with partial enzyme activity present with intermittent ketosis.[160,161]

The goal of SCOT deficiency treatment is to limit and treat stressful physiologic events that may promote ketoacidosis. Fasting should be avoided by providing a diet rich in carbohydrate with limited protein. In times of acute illness, adequate calories, fluids, and electrolytes should be provided. Normal growth and development is expected.[160]

Mitochondrial 2-methyacetoacetyl CoA thiolase (T2) deficiency is a rare autosomal recessive disorder of isoleucine and ketone metabolism that causes acute episodes of ketoacidosis and hypoglycemia or hyperglycemia. Unlike SCOT deficiency, and despite state-mandated newborn screening programs, early neonatal diagnosis is rare, with most infants diagnosed between 6 and 20 months of age.[162,163] Characterized by intermittent ketoacidotic events, vomiting and lethargy, it is a highly variable disorder observed in many different ethnic groups. The disorder can result in normal development or lead to severe cognitive impairment or death.

In contrast with SCOT deficiency, persistent ketosis does not occur in T2 deficiency. Instead, an increase in urinary excretion of several organic acids, such as 2-methyl-3-hydroxybutyric acid, tiglylglycine and occasionally 2-methylacetoacetic acid, is observed. After ruling out other possible causes of repeated ketoacidotic events in children, an organic acid profile and T2 enzyme test should be used to distinguish T2 deficiency from SCOT deficiency.[164] It is suggested that T2 deficiency may be underdiagnosed and should be considered in young children who present with sporadic ketoacidotic events and no history of diabetes or toxic ingestions.[165] Prognosis is good if the condition is identified early and measures are taken to avoid and treat metabolically stressful events that promote ketosis.

Methylmalonyl CoA mutase deficiency is an autosomal recessive disorder characterized by ketoacidotic coma, dehydration, increased ammonia, and thrombocytopenia. Children with the subacute form, observed in early childhood, present with vomiting and hypotonia, plus growth and psychomotor retardation.[166] The diagnosis is indicated by increased urinary organic acids, acylcarnitine chromatography that shows high levels of methyl malonic acid and propionylcarnitine, along with measurement of methylmalonyl CoA mutase activity. Treatment includes antibiotics to limit growth of propionic acid–producing intestinal bacteria and dietary protein restriction.[166]

Table 2 provides a summary of the laboratory and clinical features observed in the most common causes of HAG metabolic acidosis and ketoacidosis. Although each metabolic syndrome is characterized by increases in ketones, the degree of electrolyte imbalances, hydration status, and other laboratory findings vary based on the duration of the disorder or degree of toxic exposure. Therefore, the clinical signs and symptoms are unique to the cause and, as such, require specific medical management. **Table 3** summarizes the most common ketoacidotic syndromes and their corresponding past medical history characteristics, clinical features, and treatment recommendations. Response to therapy is often determined by improvement in symptoms and reductions in ketone levels.

Table 2
Summary of common laboratory findings and clinical features of selected ketotic and ketoacidotic syndromes[a]

Laboratory and Condition Clinical Features	DKA	Starvation or High-Protein Diets	Alcoholic Ketoacidosis	Salicylate Poisoning	Isopropyl Alcohol Toxicity	Isoniazid Toxicity	Errors of Metabolism (Orphan Diseases)
Blood glucose	↑↑↑	—	N or ↓	↓	—	↑↑	—
Urinary ketones	↑↑	↑	↑	↑	↑↑	↑	↑
Blood Ketones							
Acetoacetate	↑↑	↑	↑↑	↑↑	↑	↑	↑
Acetone	↑	↑	↑	↑↑	↑↑	↑	↑
3HB	↑↑	↑	↑↑↑	↑↑	↑	↑	↑
Counterregulatory Hormones							
Cortisol	↑↑	↑	↑↑	—	—	—	—
Epinephrine	↑↑	↑	↑↑	—	—	—	—
Glucagon	↑↑↑	—	↑↑↑	—	—	—	—
Growth Hormone	↑	—	↑	—	↑	—	↑
Anion gap	↑↑↑	—	↑	↑	—	—	—
Plasma Electrolytes							
Potassium	↑↓	—	↓	—	—	↑↑↑	—
Sodium	—	—	↓	↓	—	—	—
Magnesium	—	—	↓	↓	—	—	—
Phosphate	—	—	↓	↓	—	—	—

Vitamin Depletion							
Pyridoxine	—	—	↓↓	—	—	↓↓	—
B₁₂	—	—	↓↓↓	—	—	—	—
Thiamin	—	—	↓↓↓	—	—	—	—
Riboflavin	—	—	↓↓↓	—	—	—	—
Niacin	—	—	↓↓↓	—	—	—	—
Dehydration/fluid loss	↑↑↑	↑	↑↑	↑	—	—	—
Proteinuria	—	—	—	↑↑	—	—	—
Metabolic Acidosis	↑↑↑	↑	↑	↑↑	—	—	—
Fruity breath	+++	+	+++	—	—	—	—
Constipation	—	++	—	—	—	—	—
Nausea and vomiting	+++	—	+++	+++	+++	—	+++
Increased plasma lactate	+	+	+	—	—	+++	—
Mental status changes	+++	—	++	—	—	++	—
Hypotension	+	—	—	—	+	—	—
Coma	+	—	++	++	+	—	—
Positive DIC profile	—	—	—	—	—	+++	+++
Refs	18–42,46	68–75	81,84–93,167	1,121,142–144	1,102–105	145–152	156–166

ᵃ Laboratory and clinical features observed in the most common metabolic and ketoacidotic syndromes. Arrows represent the degree of increase or decrease from normal values of a particular laboratory value: ↑, mildly increased; ↑↑, moderately increased; ↑↑↑, severely increased; ↓, mildly decreased; ↓↓, moderately decreased; ↓↓↓, severely decreased; ↑↓, prominent initial increase followed by prominent decrease during insulin treatment. Plus signs represent the frequency of observing a particular clinical feature: +, rarely observed; ++, occasionally observed; +++, frequently observed; −, means that the particular clinical feature has not been observed or has not been reported; DIC, disseminated intravascular coagulation; N, normal value.

Table 3
Past medical history, clinical features and selected treatments for common causes of ketotic and ketoacidotic syndromes

Condition	Past Medical History	Clinical Features	Treatment	References
Starvation ketoacidosis	Limited food intake (<500 kcal/d) Weight loss diets Alcoholism Anorexia nervosa	Bad breath Constipation Dehydration Electrolyte imbalance	Increase caloric intake Increase carbohydrate intake	68–75
Ketogenic diets	Low-carbohydrate weight loss diet Eg, 20–60 g carbohydrate/d, Atkins diet Pediatric epilepsy ketogenic diet for seizure disorders	Kidney stones Delayed growth Menstrual irregularities	Monitor growth in pediatric epileptics on ketogenic diets	
Diabetic ketoacidosis	Type I DM Poor insulin compliance Impaired insulin pump Recent fever, infection, stress, surgery Type II diabetes mellitus Diet/medication compliance Recent use of steroids or clozapine Precipitating factors: Drug abuse (eg, cocaine) Atypical antipsychotics Other prescription drugs Poor glycemic control	Thirst Nausea, vomiting Weakness Fatigue Altered consciousness Palpitations Dehydration Altered electrolytes Increased glucose Fruity odor to breath Ketoacidosis, ketonuria, ketosis	Fluid repletion (0.9% saline) 500–1000 mL/h for first 1–2 h 300–500 mL/h for 8–12 h Insulin therapy Electrolyte replacement Treat infection (if present) and other acute illnesses Other interventions to prevent relapse	18–42,46
Alcoholic ketoacidosis	Chronic alcoholism Binge drinking episode Malnutrition, poor food intake	Nausea, vomiting, dehydration Gastritis Pancreatitis Tachycardia	Fluids Glucose Electrolyte repletion B vitamin therapy	81,84–93,167

Condition	Predisposing conditions	Clinical features	Treatment	References
Isopropyl alcohol poisoning	Suicide attempt Alcoholism Accidental ingestion	Orthostatic hypotension Sweet breath odor Electrolyte imbalances B vitamin deficiencies Ketoacidosis, ketonuria, ketosis Gastric irritation CNS depression Hypotension Cardiovascular collapse (high dose) Ketonemia, ketonuria	Fluids Inotropes for hypotension Hemodialysis if high doses Consider gastric lavage if <1 h after ingestion Anticipate other complications Infection Aspiration pneumonia Pancreatitis Gastrointestinal bleeding	1,102–105
Salicylate poisoning	Suicide attempt Accidental ingestion	Gastric irritation Nausea/vomiting Tinnitus Metabolic/respiratory disturbances Seizures, coma Liver failure Pulmonary edema Proteinuria Hypoglycemia Ketoacidosis, ketonuria, ketosis	Stabilize respiratory and cardiovascular systems Activated charcoal Bowel irrigation Rehydration Electrolyte replacement Alkalization treatment as required	1,121,142–144
Isoniazid poisoning	Tuberculosis Accidental ingestion Suicide attempt	Metabolic acidosis Seizures Coma Pyridoxine deficiency Ketosis, ketonuria Lactic acidosis Hyperglycemia Hypokalemia Positive disseminated intravascular coagulation profile	If asymptomatic and within 1–2 h after ingestion, use activated charcoal and IV pyridoxine Aggressive support for nonresponders: Urinary alkalinization Hemodialysis	145–152

(continued on next page)

Table 3
(continued)

Condition	Past Medical History	Clinical Features	Treatment	References
Orphan diseases				156,157,160
SCOT deficiency	Intermittent ketoacidotic events in early infancy coupled with: Failure to thrive Feeding difficulties Ketoacidotic events common after fever, infection, fasting	Persistent ketosis with frequent ketoacidosis Tachycardia Severe metabolic acidosis Vomiting, lethargy Lactate, pyruvate, and glucose usually normal Increased urinary ketones	Limit/treat stressful physiologic events that promote ketoacidosis Avoid fasting Limit dietary protein Provide adequate fluids, calories, and electrolytes during acute illness	162,166
T2 deficiency	Intermittent ketoacidotic events between 6–20 mo of age	Ketosis is not persistent Increased urinary excretion of several organic acids Vomiting, lethargy		
Methylmalonyl coenzyme A mutase deficiency	Ketoacidotic events in early childhood	Ketoacidotic coma Dehydration Increased ammonia Thrombocytopenia Vomiting Hypotonia Growth and psychomotor retardation Increased urinary organic acids Increased methyl malonic acid and propionyl carnitine	As listed earlier, along with antibiotics to limit growth of propionic acid-producing gastrointestinal bacteria	

SUMMARY

In addition to DKA there are numerous causes of HAG metabolic acidosis with ketoacidosis. These processes include common syndromes such as starvation, AKA, and certain intoxications, as well as rare disorders. DKA may be precipitated by a variety of toxicologic causes. Careful consideration of the patient's medical, social, and medication history is paramount to appropriate diagnosis and subsequent therapy. As ketone detection methodologies advance, the identification of the various ketoacidotic syndromes will be facilitated.

ACKNOWLEDGMENTS

The authors are indebted to the Maricopa Medical Center library staff for their assistance with the preparation of this article.

REFERENCES

1. Mokhlesi B, Leikin J, Murray P, et al. Adult toxicology in critical care: part II: specific poisonings. Chest 2003;123(3):897–922.
2. Goldberg PA, Inzucchi SE. Critical issues in endocrinology. Clin Chest Med 2003;24(4):583–606.
3. Lieberman M, Marks AD, Smith CM. Oxidation of fatty acids and ketone bodies. In: Lieberman M, Marks AD, editors. Marks' basic medical biochemistry. 3rd edition. Philadelphia: Wolters Kluwer/Lippincott Williams & Wilkins; 2009. p. 421–42.
4. Laffel L. Ketone bodies: a review of physiology, pathophysiology and application of monitoring to diabetes. Diabetes Metab Res Rev 1999;15(6):412–26.
5. Mitchell GA, Kassovska-Bratinova S, Boukaftane Y, et al. Medical aspects of ketone body metabolism. Clin Invest Med 1995;18(3):193–216.
6. Bohan JS. Chemical measurements in ketoacidosis. Arch Intern Med 1999; 27(17):2089.
7. Fukao T, Lopaschuk GD, Mitchell GA. Pathways and control of ketone body metabolism: on the fringe of lipid biochemistry. Prostaglandins Leukot Essent Fatty Acids 2004;70(3):245–51.
8. Carmant L. Assessing ketosis: approaches and pitfalls. Epilepsia 2008; 49(Suppl 8):20–2.
9. Khan AS, Talbot JA, Tieszen KL, et al. Evaluation of a bedside blood ketone sensor: the effects of acidosis, hyperglycaemia and acetoacetate on sensor performance. Diabet Med 2004;21(7):782–5.
10. Hendy GW, Schwab T, Soliz T. Urine ketone dip test as a screen for ketonemia in diabetic ketoacidosis and ketosis in the emergency department. Ann Emerg Med 1997;29(6):735–8.
11. Csako G, Elin RJ. Unrecognized false positive ketones from drugs containing free sulfhydryl groups [letter]. JAMA 1990;269(13):1634.
12. Taboulet P, Haas L, Porcher R, et al. Urinary acetoacetate or capillary beta-hydroxybutyrate for the diagnosis of ketoacidosis in the emergency department setting. Eur J Emerg Med 2004;11(5):251–8.
13. Porter WH, Yao HH, Karounos DG. Laboratory and clinical evaluation of assays for beta hydroxybutyrate. Am J Clin Pathol 1997;107(13):353–8.
14. Fulop M, Murthy V, Michilli A, et al. Serum beta-hydroxybutyrate measurement in patients with uncontrolled diabetes mellitus. Arch Intern Med 1999;159(4):381–4.
15. Timmons JA, Meyer P, Maturen A, et al. Use of beta-hydroxybutyric acid levels in the emergency department. Am J Ther 1998;5(3):159–63.

16. Zur M, Moccio RJ, Nichols JH. Evaluation of the [beta]-hydroxybutyrate ketone test on the STAT-Site M analyzer. Point of Care 2008;7(2):60–3.

17. Palmer JP. Alcoholic ketoacidosis: clinical and laboratory presentation, pathophysiology and treatment. Clin Endocrinol Metab 1983;12(2):381–9.

18. Banerji MA, Chaiken RL, Huey H, et al. GAD antibody negative NIDDM in adult black subjects with diabetic ketoacidosis and increased frequency of human leukocyte antigen DR3 and DR4. Flatbush diabetes. Diabetes 1994;43(6): 741–5.

19. Expert panel on the diagnosis, classification of diabetes mellitus. Diagnosis and classification of diabetes mellitus. Diabetes Care 2004;27(Suppl 1):S5–10.

20. Westphal SA. The occurrence of diabetic ketoacidosis in non-insulin-dependent diabetes and newly diagnosed diabetic adults. Am J Med 1996;101(1):19–24.

21. Efstathiou SP, Tsiakou AG, Tsioulos DI, et al. A mortality prediction model in diabetic ketoacidosis. Clin Endocrinol 2002;57(5):595–601.

22. Kitabchi AE, Umpierrez GE, Murphy MB, et al. Management of hyperglycemic crises in patient with diabetes. Diabetes Care 2001;24(1):131–53.

23. Kitabchi AE, Umpierrez GE, Murphy MB. Diabetic ketoacidosis and hyperglycemic hyperosmolar site. In: DeFronzo RA, Ferrannini E, Keen H, et al, editors. International textbook of diabetes mellitus. 3rd edition. Chichester (United Kingdom): John Wiley & Sons; 2004. p. 1101–20.

24. Kitabchi AE, Rose BD. Clinical features and diagnosis of diabetic ketoacidosis and hyperosmolar hyperglycemic state in adults. Waltham (MA): UptoDate; 2007. Available at: http://www.uptodate.com/contents/treatment-of-diabetic-ketoacidosis-and-hyperosmolar-hyperglycemic-state-in-adults. Accessed January 20, 2012.

25. Fleckman AM. Diabetic ketoacidosis. Endocrinol Metab Clin North Am 1993; 22(2):181–207.

26. Umpierrez GE, Khajavi M, Kitabchi AE. Review: diabetic ketoacidosis and hyperglycemic hyperosmolar nonketotic syndrome. Am J Med Sci 1996; 311(5):225–33.

27. Umpierrez GE, Murphy MB, Kitabchi AE. Diabetic ketoacidosis and hyperglycemic hyperosmolar syndrome. Diabetes Spectrum 2002;15(1):28–36.

28. American Diabetes Association, American Psychiatric Association, American Association of Clinical Endocrinologists, North American Association for the Study of Obesity. Consensus development conference on antipsychotic drugs and obesity and diabetes. J Clin Psychiatry 2004;65(2):267–72.

29. Jin H, Meyer JM, Jeste DV. Atypical antipsychotics and glucose dysregulation: a systematic review. Schizophr Res 2004;71(2–3):195–212.

30. Ucok A, Gaebel W. Side effects of atypical antipsychotics: a brief overview. World Psychiatry 2008;7(1):58–62.

31. Henderson DC, Cagliero E, Gray C, et al. Clozapine, diabetes mellitus, weight gain and lipid abnormalities: a five year naturalistic study. Am J Psychiatry 2000;157(6):975–81.

32. Jin H, Meyer M, Jeste DV. Phenomenology of and risk factors for new onset diabetes mellitus and diabetic ketoacidosis associated with atypical antipsychotics: an analysis of 45 published cases. Ann Clin Psychiatry 2002;14(1):59–64.

33. Koller EA, Doraiswamy PM. Olanzapine associated diabetes mellitus. Pharmacotherapy 2002;22(7):841–52.

34. Koller E, Schneider B, Bennett K, et al. Clozapine associated diabetes. Am J Med 2001;111(9):716–23.

35. Koller E, Cross JT, Doraiswamy PM, et al. Risperidone associated diabetes mellitus: a pharmacovigilance study. Pharmacotherapy 2003;23(6):735–44.

36. Kibby KJ, Roberts AM, Nicholson GC. Diabetic ketoacidosis and elevated serum lipase in the setting of aripiprazole therapy. Diabetes Care 2010;33(7):e96.
37. Lee P, Greenfield JR, Campbell LV. "Mind the gap" when managing ketoacidosis in type I diabetes. Diabetes Care 2008;31(7):e58.
38. Umpierrez G, Freire AX. Abdominal pain in patients with hyperglycemic crises. J Crit Care 2002;17(1):63–7.
39. Warner EA, Greene GS, Buchsbaum MS, et al. Diabetic ketoacidosis associated with cocaine abuse. Arch Intern Med 1998;158(16):1799–802.
40. Sreedhar D, Hazeghazam MH, Li RN, et al. Serum bicarbonate vs closure of anion gap (AG) in diabetic ketoacidosis (DKA). Crit Care Med 2008;36 (2 Suppl 12):A69.
41. Hazeghazam MH, Sreedhar D, Li NR, et al. The importance of correcting anion gap for albumin and evaluation of hyperchloremia in the management of diabetic ketoacidosis [abstract A21]. J Diabetes Sci Technol 2010;4(2):456/A21. Abstracts of International Hospital Diabetes Meeting, October 8–9, 2010. Available at:. http://www.journalofdst.org/March2011/PDF/Abstract/VOL-5-2-MTG2-IHDM2010-ABSTRACTS.pdf. Accessed April 5, 2012.
42. Mendelsen JH, Teoh SK, Mello NK, et al. Acute effects of cocaine on plasma adrenocorticotropic hormone, luteinizing hormone and prolactin levels in cocaine-dependent men. J Pharmacol Exp Ther 1992;263(2):505–9.
43. Beesch CM, Negus BH, Keffer JH, et al. Effects of cocaine on cortisol secretions in humans. Am J Med Sci 1995;310(2):61–4.
44. Gerich JE, Karam JH, Fosham PH. Stimulation of glucagon secretion by epinephrine in man. J Clin Endocrinol Metab 1973;37(3):479–81.
45. Keller U, Gerber PP, Stauffacher W. Stimulatory effect of norepinephrine on ketogenesis in normal and insulin-deficient humans. Am J Physiol 1984;247(6 Pt 1): E732–9.
46. Byard RW, Riches KJ, Kostakis C, et al. Diabetic ketoacidosis–a possible complicating factor in deaths associated with drug overdose: two case reports. Med Sci Law 2006;46(1):81–4.
47. Gama MP, de Souza BV, Ossowski AC, et al. Diabetic ketoacidosis complicated by the use of ecstasy: a case report. J Med Case Rep 2010;4(1):240–3.
48. Seymor HR, Gilmand D, Quin JD. Severe ketoacidosis complicated by ecstasy and prolonged exercise. Diabet Med 1996;13(10):908–9.
49. Hartung TK, Schofield E, Short AI, et al. Hyponatremic states following 3,4-methylenedioxymethamphetamine (MDMA, "ecstasy") ingestion. QJM 2002;95(7): 431–7.
50. Tibaldi JM, Lorber DL, Nerenberg A. Diabetic ketoacidosis and insulin resistance with subcutaneous terbutaline infusion: a case report. Am J Obstet Gynecol 1990;163(2):509–10.
51. Mori S, Ebihara K. A sudden onset of diabetic ketoacidosis and acute pancreatitis after introduction of mizoribine therapy in a patient with rheumatoid arthritis. Mod Rheumatol 2008;18(6):634–8.
52. Case CC, Maldonado M. Diabetic ketoacidosis associated with Metabolife: a report of two cases. Diabetes Obes Metab 2002;4(6):402–6.
53. Astrup A, Toubro S, Cannon S, et al. Thermogenic, metabolic, and cardiovascular effects of a sympathomimetic agent, ephedrine: a double-blind placebo-controlled study. Curr Ther Res 1990;48(6):1087–100.
54. Haller CA, Benowitz NL. Adverse cardiovascular and central nervous system effects associated with dietary supplements containing ephedra alkaloids. N Engl J Med 2000;343(25):1833–8.

55. United States General Accounting Office. Dietary supplements containing ephedra. health risks and FDA's oversight. Washington, DC: US General Accountability Office; 2003. Available at: http://www.gao.gov/assets/120/110228.pdf. Accessed April 4, 2012.
56. Gwen OE, Caprio S, Reichard GA Jr, et al. Ketosis of starvation: a revisit and new perspectives. Clin Endocrinol Metab 1983;12(2):359–79.
57. Hoffer LJ. Metabolic consequences of starvation. In: Shils ME, Olson JA, Shike M, et al, editors. Modern nutrition in health and disease. 9th edition. Baltimore (MD): Lippincott Williams & Wilkins; 1999. p. 645–55.
58. Mahoney CA. Extreme gestational starvation ketoacidosis: case report and review of pathophysiology. Am J Kidney Dis 1992;20(3):276–80.
59. Toth H, Greenbaum L. Severe acidosis caused by starvation and stress. Am J Kidney Dis 2003;42(5):16–9.
60. Burbos N, Shiner AM, Morris E. Severe metabolic acidosis as a consequence of acute starvation in pregnancy. Arch Gynecol Obstet 2009;279(3):399–400.
61. Miaskiewicz S, Levey GS, Owen O. Severe metabolic ketoacidosis induced by starvation and exercise. Am J Med Sci 1989;297(3):178–80.
62. Owen D, Little S, Leach R, et al. A patient with an unusual aetiology of a severe ketoacidosis. Intensive Care Med 2008;34(5):971–2.
63. Bartels PD, Kristensen LO, Heding LG, et al. Development of ketonemia in fasting patients with hyperthyroidism. Acta Med Scand 1979;205(Suppl 624):43–7.
64. Wood ET, Kinlaw WB. Nondiabetic ketoacidosis caused by severe hyperthyroidism. Medscape. 2004. Available at: www.medscape.com/viewarticle/488880. Accessed September 20, 2011.
65. Cartwright MM. Eating disorder emergencies: understanding the complexities of the hospitalized eating disordered patient. Crit Care Nurs Clin North Am 2004;16(4):515–30.
66. Causso C, Arrieta F, Hernández J, et al. Severe ketoacidosis secondary to starvation in a frutarian patient. Nutr Hosp 2010;25(6):1049–52.
67. Freeman JM, Kossoff EH. Ketosis and the ketogenic diet, 2010: advances in treating epilepsy and other disorders. Adv Pediatr 2010;57(1):315–29.
68. Sondike SB, Copperman N, Jacobson MS. Effects of a low carbohydrate diet on weight loss and cardiovascular risk factors in overweight adolescents. J Pediatr 2003;142(3):253–8.
69. Westman EC, Yancy WS, Edman JS, et al. Effect of 6-month adherence to a very low carbohydrate program. Am J Med 2002;113(1):30–6.
70. Yancy WS, Olsen MK, Guyton JR, et al. A low carbohydrate ketogenic diet versus a low fat diet to treat obesity and hyperlipidemia. Ann Intern Med 2004;140(10):769–77.
71. Agnew B. Rethinking Atkins. New research suggests that the famous low-carb diet may be safe–at least in the short term. Diabetes Forecast 2004;57(4): 64–6, 68–70.
72. Rollo I. Understanding the implications of adopting the Atkins' diet. Nurs Times 2003;99(43):20–1.
73. Furth SL, Casey JC, Pyzik PL, et al. Risk factors for urolithiasis in children on the ketogenic diet. Pediatr Nephrol 2000;15(1–2):125–8.
74. Wheless J. The history of the ketogenic diet. Epilepsia 2008;49(8):3S–5S.
75. Kossoff EH. More fat and fewer seizures: dietary therapies for epilepsy. Lancet Neurol 2004;3(7):415–20.
76. Mady MA, Kossoff EH, McGregor AL, et al. The ketogenic diet: adolescents can do it too. Epilepsia 2003;44(6):847–51.

77. Gasior M, Rogawski MA, Hartman AL. Neuroprotective and disease modifying effects of the ketogenic diet. Behav Pharmacol 2006;17(5–6):431–9.
78. Henderson ST. Ketone bodies as a therapeutic for Alzheimer's disease. Neurotherapeutics 2008;5(3):470–80.
79. Dillon ES, Dyer WW, Smelo LS. Ketone acidosis in non-diabetic adults. Med Clin North Am 1940;24:1813–22.
80. Halperin ML, Hammeke M, Josse RG, et al. Metabolic acidosis in the alcoholic: a pathophysiologic approach. Metabolism 1983;32(3):308–15.
81. McGuire LC, Cruickshank AM, Munro PT. Alcoholic ketoacidosis. Emerg Med J 2006;23(6):417–20.
82. Shull PD, Rapoport J. Life-threatening reversible acidosis caused by alcohol abuse. Nat Rev Nephrol 2010;6(9):555–9.
83. Umpierrez GE, DiGirolamo M, Tulvin JA, et al. Differences in metabolic and hormonal milieu in diabetic and alcohol induced ketoacidosis. J Crit Care 2000;15(2):52–9.
84. Wrenn KD, Slovis CM, Minion GE, et al. The syndrome of alcoholic ketoacidosis. Am J Med 1991;91(2):119–28.
85. Cooperman MT, Davidoff F, Spark R, et al. Clinical studies of alcoholic ketoacidosis. Diabetes 1974;23(5):433–9.
86. Levy LJ, Duga J, Girgis M, et al. Ketoacidosis in association with alcoholism in nondiabetic subjects. Ann Intern Med 1973;78(2):213–9.
87. Cuevas-Korensky CE, Kruse JA, Carlson RW. Characteristic findings in patients with alcoholic ketoacidosis. Chest 1991;100(Suppl 2):81S.
88. Weissman C. The metabolic response to stress: an overview and update. Anesthesiology 1990;73(2):308–27.
89. Kraut JA, Kurtz I. Toxic alcohol ingestions: clinical features, diagnosis and management. Clin J Am Soc Nephrol 2008;3(1):208–25.
90. Reuler JB, Poorman J. Anion and osmolal gaps in a patient with alcoholism. West J Med 1993;158(2):191–4.
91. Elisaf M, Merkouropoulos M, Tsianos EV, et al. Acid-base and electrolyte abnormalities in alcoholic patients. Miner Electrolyte Metab 1994;20(5):274–81.
92. Kamel KS, Gowrishankar M, Gougoux A, et al. Metabolic acidosis in the alcoholic: an emphasis on intracellular events. Endocrinologist 1995;5(4):278–85.
93. Thomasen JL, Simonsen KW, Felby S, et al. A prospective toxicology analysis in alcoholics. Forensic Sci Int 1997;90(1–2):33–40.
94. Yanagawa Y, Sakamoto T, Okada Y. Six cases of sudden cardiac arrest in alcoholic ketoacidosis. Intern Med 2008;47(2):113–7.
95. Brinkman B, Fechner B, Karger B, et al. Ketoacidosis and lactic acidosis–frequent causes of death in alcoholics. Int J Legal Med 1998;111(3):115–9.
96. Kadiš P, Balažic J, Ferlan-Marolt V. Alcoholic ketoacidosis: a cause of sudden death in chronic alcoholics. Forensic Sci Int 1999;103:S53–9.
97. Pounder DJ, Stevenson RJ, Taylor KK. Alcoholic ketoacidosis at autopsy. J Forensic Sci 1998;43(4):812–6.
98. Thomsen J, Felby S, Theilade P, et al. Alcoholic ketoacidosis as a cause of death in forensic cases. Forensic Sci Int 1995;75(2–3):163–70.
99. Yalamanchili S, Rempe S, Puri N, et al. Profound, reversible myopathy with severe hypophosphatemia in a patient with diabetic ketoacidosis. Resid Staff Physician 2005;51(6):35–8.
100. Bronstein AC, Spyker DA, Cantilena LR Jr, et al. 2010 annual report of the American Association of Poison Control Centers' National Poison Data System (NPDS): 28th annual report. Clin Toxicol 2011;49(10):910–41.

101. Lewin GA, Oppenheimer PR, Wingert WA. Coma from alcohol sponging. J Am Coll Emerg Physicians 1977;6(4):165–7.
102. Lehman AJ, Chase HF. The acute and chronic toxicity of isopropyl alcohol. J Lab Clin Med 1944;29:561–7.
103. Lacouture PG, Wason S, Abrams A, et al. Acute isopropyl alcohol intoxication: diagnosis and management. Am J Med 1983;75(4):680–6.
104. Kulig K, Duffy JP, Linden CH, et al. Toxic effects of methanol, ethylene glycol and isopropyl alcohol. Top Emerg Med 1984;6(2):14–28.
105. Fuller HC, Hunter OB. Isopropyl alcohol. J Lab Clin Med 1927;12:326–49.
106. Bronstein AC, Spyker DA, Cantilina LR Jr, et al. American Association of Poison Control Centers. NPDS annual reports. Clin Toxicol 2007;45(8):815–917.
107. Doyon S, Welsh C. Intoxication of a prison inmate with an ethyl alcohol-based hand sanitizer. N Engl J Med 2007;356(5):529–30.
108. Thanarajasingam G, Diedrich DA, Mueller PS. Intentional ingestion of ethanol-based hand sanitizer by a hospitalized patient with alcoholism. Mayo Clin Proc 2007;82(10):1288–9.
109. Emadi A, Coberly L. Intoxication of a hospitalized patient with isopropanol based hand sanitizer. N Engl J Med 2007;356(5):530–1.
110. Vujasinovic M, Kocar M, Kramer K, et al. Poisoning with 1-propanol and 2-propanol. Hum Exp Toxicol 2007;26(12):975–8.
111. Jammalamadaka D, Faissi R. Ethylene glycol, methanol and isopropyl alcohol intoxication. Am J Med Sci 2010;339(3):276–81.
112. Zaman F, Pervez A, Abreo K. Isopropyl alcohol intoxication: a diagnostic challenge. Am J Kidney Dis 2002;40(3):E12.
113. Chan KM, Wong ET, Matthews WS. Severe isopropanolemia without acetonemia or clinical manifestations of isopropanol intoxication. Clin Chem 1993;39(9): 1922–5.
114. Hayden SR, Kallus L, McCuskey CF. Aldehydes, ketones, ethers and esters. In: Viccellio P, editor. Emergency toxicology. 2nd edition. Philadelphia: Lippincott-Raven; 1998. p. 292.
115. Gamis AS, Wasserman GS. Acute acetone intoxication in a pediatric patient. Pediatr Emerg Care 1988;4(1):24–6.
116. Gitelson S, Werozberger A, Herman JB. Coma and hyperglycemia following drinking of acetone. Diabetes 1966;15(11):810–1.
117. Sivlott ML. Methanol, ethylene glycol and other toxic alcohols. Other toxic alcohols. In: Shannon MW, Borron SW, Burns MJ, editors. Haddad & Winchester's clinical management of poisoning and drug overdose. 4th edition. Philadelphia: WB Saunders; 2007. p. 625.
118. Rainsford KD. History and the development of the salicylates. In: Rainsford KD, editor. Aspirin and related drugs. London: Taylor & Francis; 2004. p. 1–5.
119. Rodnan GP, Benedek TG. Early history of antirheumatic drugs. Arthritis Rheum 1970;13(2):145–65.
120. Haas H. History of antipyretic analgesic therapy. Am J Med 1983;75(5A):1–3.
121. Waseem M, Aslam M, Gernsheimer J. Salicylate toxicity. In: Medscape 2011. Available at: http://emedicine.medscape.com/article/1009987-overview. Accessed November 16, 2011.
122. Durnas C, Cusack BJ. Salicylate intoxication in the elderly. Recognition and recommendations on how to prevent it. Drugs Aging 1992;2(1):20–34.
123. Litovitz TL, Smikstein L, Felberg L, et al. 1996 annual report of the American Association of Poison Control Centers Toxic Exposure Surveillance System. Am J Emerg Med 1997;15(5):447–500.

124. Burke A, Smyth E, FitzGerald GA. Analgesic-antipyretic agents; pharmaco-therapy of gout. In: Brunton LL, Chabner BA, Knollmann BC, editors. Goodman and Gillman's pharmacologic basis of therapeutics. 12th edition. New York: McGraw-Hill; 2006. p. 689.
125. Krenzelok EP, Kerr F, Proudfoot A. Salicylate toxicity. In: Haddad LM, Shannon MW, Winchester JF, editors. Clinical management of poisoning and drug overdose. 3rd edition. Philadelphia: WB Sanders; 1998. p. 675–87.
126. Abramson SB, Howard R. Aspirin: mechanism of action, major toxicities and use in rheumatic diseases. Waltham (MA): UptoDate; 2012. Available at: http://www.uptodate.com/contents/aspirin-mechanism-of-action-major-toxicities-and-use-in-rheumatic-diseases. Accessed January 30, 2012.
127. Miyahara JT, Karler R. Effect of salicylate on oxidative phosphorylation and respiration of mitochondrial fragments. Biochem J 1965;97(1):194–8.
128. Bartels PD, Lund-Jacobsen H. Blood lactate and ketone body concentrations in salicylate intoxication. Hum Toxicol 1986;5(6):363–6.
129. Gabow PA, Anderson RJ, Potts DE, et al. Acid-base disturbances in the salicylate poisoning in adults. Arch Intern Med 1978;138(10):1481–4.
130. Togo K, Suzuki Y, Yoshimaru T, et al. Aspirin and salicylates modulate IgE-mediated leukotriene secretion in mast cells through a dihydropyridine receptor-mediated Ca2+ influx. Clin Immunol 2009;131(1):146–56.
131. Lapenna D, Ciofani G, Pierdomenico SD, et al. Inhibitory activity of salicylic acid on lipoxygenase-dependent lipid peroxidation. Biochim Biophys Acta 2009; 1790(1):25–30.
132. Buchanan MR, Butt RW, Hirsh J, et al. Role of lipoxygenase metabolism in platelet function: effect of aspirin and salicylate. Prostaglandins Leukot Med 1986;21(2):157–68.
133. Tremoli E, Maderna P, Eynard A, et al. In vitro effects of aspirin and non steroidal anti-inflammatory drugs on the formation of 12-hydroxyeicosatetraenoic acid by platelets. Prostaglandins Leukot Med 1986;23(2–3):117–22.
134. Cerletti C. Interaction of non-steroidal anti-inflammatory drugs on platelet cyclo-oxygenase and lipoxygenase activity. Int J Tissue React 1985;7(4):309–12.
135. Jung TT, Hwang AL, Miller SK, et al. Effect of leukotriene inhibitor on cochlear blood flow in salicylate ototoxicity. Acta Otolaryngol 1995;115(2):251–4.
136. Hormaechea E, Carlson RW, Rogove H, et al. Hypovolemia, pulmonary edema and protein changes in severe salicylate poisoning. Am J Med 1979;66(6): 1046–50.
137. Done AK. Salicylate intoxication: significance of measurements of salicylate in blood in cases of acute ingestion. Pediatrics 1960;26(5):800–7.
138. Krenzelok EP, Kerr F, Proudfoot AT. Salicylate toxicity. In: Haddad LM, Shannon MW, Winchester JF, editors. Clinical management of poisoning and drug overdose. 3rd edition. Philadelphia: WB Saunders; 1998. p. 682.
139. Dugandzic RM, Tierney MG, Dickinson GE, et al. Evaluation of the validity of the Done nomogram in the management of acute salicylate intoxication. Ann Emerg Med 1989;18(11):1186–90.
140. Flomenbaum NE. Salicylates. In: Flomenbaum NE, Goldfrank LR, Hoffman RS, et al, editors. Goldfrank's toxicologic emergencies. 8th edition. New York: McGraw-Hill; 2006. p. 550–64.
141. Boyer EW. Aspirin poisoning in adults. Waltham (MA): UptoDate; 2011. Available at: http://www.uptodate.com/contents/aspirin-poisoning-in-adults?source=search_result&search=boyer+aspirin+poisoning+in+adults&selectedTitle=1%7E52. Accessed January 13, 2012.

142. O'Malley GF. Emergency department management of the salicylate-poisoned patient. Emerg Med Clin North Am 2007;25(2):333–46.
143. Hoffman RJ, Nelson LS, Hoffman RS. Use of ferric chloride to detect salicylate-containing poisons. J Toxicol Clin Toxicol 2002;40(5):547–9.
144. Dargan PI, Wallace CI, Jones AL. An evidence based flowchart to guide the management of acute salicylate (aspirin) overdose. Emerg Med J 2002;19(3):206–9.
145. Shannon MW. Isoniazid. In: Shannon MW, Winchester JF, editors. Clinical management of poisoning and drug overdose. 3rd edition. Philadelphia: WB Saunders; 1998. p. 721.
146. Alvarez FG, Guntupalli KK. Isoniazid overdose: four case reports and a review of the literature. Intensive Care Med 1995;21(8):641–4.
147. Romero JA, Kuczler FJ Jr. Isoniazid overdose: recognition and management. Am Fam Physician 1998;57(4):749–52.
148. Temmerman W, Dhondt A, Vandewoude K. Acute isoniazid intoxication: seizures, acidosis and coma. Acta Clin Belg 1999;54(4):211–6.
149. Cameron WM. Isoniazid overdose. Can Med Assoc J 1978;2(6145):127–8.
150. Kingston RL, Saxena K. Management of acute isoniazid overdosages. Clinical Toxicology Consultant 1980;2(2):37–44.
151. Sullivan EA, Geoffroy P, Weisman R, et al. Isoniazid poisonings in New York City. J Emerg Med 1998;16(1):57–9.
152. Orlowski JP, Paganini EP, Pippenger CE. Treatment of a potentially lethal dose of isoniazid ingestion. Ann Emerg Med 1988;17(1):73–6.
153. Kelso T, Toll HW, Pinkerton DC, et al. Death due to intentional overdose of isoniazid. A case report. J Forensic Sci 1965;10(3):313–8.
154. Bear ES, Hoffman PF, Siegel SR, et al. Suicidal ingestion of isoniazid. An uncommon cause of metabolic acidosis and seizures. Southampt Med J 1976;69(1):31–2.
155. Pahl MV, Vaziri ND, Ness R, et al. Association of beta-hydroxybutyric acidosis with isoniazid intoxication. Clin Toxicol 1984;22(2):167–76.
156. Sass JO. Inborn errors of ketogenesis and ketone body utilization. J Inherit Metab Dis 2012;35(1):23–8.
157. Fukao T. Succinyl-CoA: 3-keotacid CoA transferase (SCOT) deficiency. In: Orphanet encyclopedia. Orphanet; 2006. Available at: www.orpha.net/data/patho/GB/uk-scot.pdf. Accessed December 20, 2011.
158. Middleton B, Day R, Lombes A, et al. Infantile ketoacidosis associated with decreased activity of succinyl-CoA: 3-ketoacid CoA-transferase. J Inherit Metab Dis 1987;10(Suppl 2):273s–5s.
159. Niezen-Koning KE, Wanders RJA, Ruiter JPN, et al. Succinyl-CoA: acetoacetate transferase deficiency: identification of a new patient with a neonatal onset and review of the literature. Eur J Pediatr 1997;156(11):870–3.
160. Fukao T, Song XQ, Mitchell GA, et al. Enzymes of ketone body utilization in human tissues: protein and mRNA levels of succinyl-coenzyme A (CoA): 3-ketoacid CoA transferase and mitochondrial and cytosolic acetoacetyl-CoA thiolases. Pediatr Res 1997;42(4):498–502.
161. Fukao T, Sass JO, Kursula P, et al. Clinical and molecular characterization of five patients with succinyl-Co A: 3-ketoacid CoA transferase (SCOT) deficiency. Biochim Biophys Acta 2011;1812(5):619–24.
162. Mitchell GA, Fukao T. Inborn errors of ketone body catabolism. In: Scriver CR, Beaudet AL, Sly WS, et al, editors. Metabolic and molecular bases of inherited disease. 8th edition. New York: McGraw-Hill; 2001. p. 2327–56.

163. Sarafoglou K, Matern D, Redlinger-Grosse K, et al. Siblings with mitochondrial acetoacetyl-CoA thiolase deficiency not identified by newborn screening. Pediatrics 2011;128(1):e246–50.
164. Sovik O. Mitochondrial 2-methylacetoacetyl-CoA thiolase deficiency: an inborn error of isoleucine and ketone body metabolism. J Inherit Metab Dis 1993; 16(1):46–54.
165. Thummler S, Dupont D, Acquaviva C, et al. Different clinical presentation in siblings with mitochondrial acetoacetyl-Co A thiolase deficiency and identification of two novel mutations. Tohoku J Exp Med 2010;220(1):27–31.
166. Saudubray JM, Specola N, Middleton B, et al. Hyperketotic states due to inherited defects of ketolysis. Enzyme 1987;38(1):80–90.
167. Ansstas G, Robinson I, Rubinchick S, et al. Alcoholic ketoacidosis. Medscape. 2011. Available at: http://emedicine.medscape.com/article/116820-overview. Accessed July 25, 2011.

North American Poisonous Bites and Stings

Dan Quan, DO[a,b],*

KEYWORDS

- Envenomations • Poisonous bites • Poisonous stings • North America

KEY POINTS

- North American scorpion, arachnid, Hymenoptera, and snake envenomations cause clinically significant problems.
- Critical care management of envenomed patients can be challenging for clinicians.
- Although the animals are located in specific geographic areas, patients envenomed may travel to endemic areas and present to health care facilities remote from the exposure.

This article focuses on the management of the most common North American scorpion, arachnid, Hymenoptera, and snake envenomations that cause clinically significant problems. Water creatures and less common animal envenomations are not covered in this article. Critical care management of envenomed patients can be challenging for clinicians. Although the animals are located in specific geographic areas, patients envenomed on passenger airliners and those who travel to endemic areas may present to health care facilities distant from the exposure.

HYMENOPTERA

This taxonomic order, Hymenoptera, consists of bees, ants, and wasps. These insects have stingers that can cause local reactions and anaphylaxis in susceptible patients. Confusion often exists regarding the differences between bees and wasps. **Table 1** illustrates some of the key differences between relevant Hymenoptera.[1–4]

Wasps are neither bees nor ants and they have hairless, smooth bodies. They can sting multiple times because their stingers are smooth and retractable. Wasps feed on all types of sugary substances whereas bees feed on flower nectar. Bee stingers are barbed so a bee is likely to eviscerate itself after a single sting.

[a] Department of Emergency Medicine, Maricopa Medical Center, 2601 East Roosevelt Road, Phoenix, AZ 85008, USA; [b] Department of Emergency Medicine, University of Arizona College of Medicine - Phoenix, Phoenix, AZ, USA
* Department of Emergency Medicine, Maricopa Medical Center, 2601 East Roosevelt Road, Phoenix, AZ 85008, USA.
E-mail address: Dan_Quan@dmgaz.org

Crit Care Clin 28 (2012) 633–659
http://dx.doi.org/10.1016/j.ccc.2012.07.010
0749-0704/12/$ – see front matter © 2012 Elsevier Inc. All rights reserved.
criticalcare.theclinics.com

Table 1		
Hymenoptera characteristics		
Insect	Envenomation Mechanism	Nest
Bees	Barbed stinger (stings once)	Hives, above or below ground; vertical flat wax honeycomb
Wasps (including hornets and yellow jackets)	Smooth stinger (may sting repeatedly)	Hollowed-out trees or in-ground burrows; paper-like combs, often horizontal
Ants (fire ants)	Modified ovipositor (female)	Ground mounds

Data from Refs.[1–4]

Hybridized bees are often called Africanized bees or killer bees in the lay press. In 1957, European honeybees crossbred with African species in Brazil, South America. Unfortunately the crossbreeding did not improve the aggressive nature of the African species. Gradually the hybridized bees made their way from South America in the mid-1950s through Central America, landing in the Southwestern United States in the 1990s. Their migration continues to spread northward each year. Hybridized bees are more aggressive than their European counterparts and they defend their nests farther.[5]

Ants are social insects that form nests in the ground. The ants with the most significance in North America are the black imported fire ant (*Solenopsis richteri*), the red imported fire ant (*Solenopsis invicta*), and the harvester ant (*Pogonomyrmex* species). Fire ants were introduced into the Southeastern United States port of Mobile, Alabama, in 1939 from Brazil.[6,7] They have spread rapidly throughout the United States. Harvester ants are located primarily in the Southwestern United States. These insects can cause reactions similarly to stings from other hymenoptera species. The mechanism of envenomation is through a stinger much like a bee or wasp. The ant grasps its pray with mandibles and injects them with a stinger located at the tip of the gaster (ie, the caudal end of the abdomen).[8]

Hymenopteran venom can cause varying effects depending on the amount injected, the number of stings, and the host's immune system reaction. These can range from local reactions to significant reactions, such as life-threatening anaphylaxis. Components of the venom include peptides, vasoactive substances, and enzymes causing catecholamine release, mast cell degranulation, and pain (**Table 2**).[4,9–13]

The severity of envenomation reactions cannot be predicted.[14] Allergic reactions from Hymenoptera occur through immunoglobulin E (IgE)-mediated reactions or type I hypersensitivity. These reactions are a consequence of previous exposure to Hymenopteran venom causing antibodies to be produced. On subsequent exposure, a reaction occurs

Table 2	
Major hymenopteran venom components and actions	
Venom Component	Action
Melittin	Increases cell membrane permeability
Phospholipase A2	Major antigen and allergen; coagulopathy
Hyaluronidase	Increases tissue permeability
Serotonin	Pain
Acetylcholine	Pain

when mast cell degranulation occurs, releasing several substances, including histamine. The reaction may be quick and severe.[15] The most severe reactions can cause tissue edema, erythema, cardiovascular collapse, respiratory distress from bronchospasm, severe urticaria, and death. Treatment of severe reactions includes antihistamines, corticosteroids, inhaled β-adrenergic agonists, and epinephrine.

Cross-reactions between Hymenoptera species may occur. Those with reactions to fire ant stings are likely to have a reaction to bee and wasp stings. The reverse may also be true. Those with bee venom reactions are unlikely to have a significant reaction to wasp stings.[7,16]

Patients with significant envenomation may require ICU admission for frequent monitoring and development of severe systemic symptoms. Otherwise mild to moderately symptomatic patients can be admitted for observation to a monitored bed.

Evaluation of these patients should be tailored as patient specific (**Table 3**). Those with comorbid conditions, such as coronary artery disease, should be scrutinized more closely than healthy individuals without medical problems.

Minor local reactions consist of mild edema, erythema, pain, and pruritus and may be symptomatically treated and carefully monitored. Moderate to severe reactions may occur from large envenomations. These are not mediated through IgE.

Depending on the Hymenoptera species, a significant number of hybridized bee stings is considered approximately 50.[17] Patients with 50 or more stings should be observed for systemic symptoms for up to 24 hours. Delayed systemic problems (renal, hematologic, and neurologic) can occur 8 to 24 hours postenvenomation.[5] The median lethal dose from honeybee envenomation is estimated through animal models to be 19 stings per kilogram body weight.[18]

Removal of stingers should be performed to avoid foreign body reactions from the retained stingers. The technique of scraping or squeezing the stingers was once debated. Theoretically, squeezing the stinger may inject further venom into the wound. The venom apparatus continues to contract, however, propagating venom into the wound even after the bee is disemboweled. Removing stingers quickly by any method results in less venom injected into the wound.[19] In patients with multiple stings, the amount of venom left in the venom sac is minimal so any method would be satisfactory for removal.

Systemic signs and symptoms consist of nausea, vomiting, abdominal pain, rhabdomyolysis, renal injury, coagulopathy, serum transaminase elevations, seizures,

Table 3
Laboratory testing in severe envenomations by Hymenoptera

Test	Potential Findings
Complete blood cell count	Anemia, thrombocytopenia, leukocytosis
Serum urea nitrogen, creatinine, electrolytes	Acute kidney injury
Serum transaminases	Liver involvement
Prothrombin time	Coagulopathy (DIC)
Serum creatine kinase	Rhabdomyolysis
Plasma fibrinogen	DIC
Urinalysis	Hematuria
Cardiac biomarkers	Myocardial infarction
Chest radiograph	Pulmonary edema
Electrocardiogram	Myocardial infarction

headache, disseminated intravascular coagulation (DIC), myocardial infarction, stroke, and edema. Specific treatments should be tailored for each of these issues. It is imperative that patients with allergic and anaphylactic reactions be discharged with a prescription for a subcutaneous epinephrine autoinjector (EpiPen).

Type III hypersensitivity may occur in those patients with significant envenomation. These reactions manifest as joint pain, fever, swelling, and rash approximately 5 to 10 days after envenomation. Often called serum sickness, the treatment includes corticosteroids and supportive care but rarely requires hospitalization.

SPIDERS (ARACHNIDA)

Arachnids have a worldwide distribution but cause a few clinically significant envenomations despite public belief that implicates them as a common cause of cutaneous abscess formation. In North America, there are only a few species of arachnids that can cause significant clinical problems.

Loxosceles reclusa (Brown Recluse)

The brown spider has a characteristic violin-shaped area on its back. The genus, *Loxosceles*, is distributed worldwide. Some species cause significant clinical findings whereas others do not. The spider lives in woodpiles and feeds at night. The female spiders are more likely to envenomate than the male spiders and to bite when provoked. The species that causes clinically significant findings in the United States is *L reclusa*. Distribution of this particular spider is limited to the Southeastern United States (**Fig. 1**).[20]

The venom of *L reclusa* consists of several enzymes that affect human tissue. Important enzymes include sphingomyelinase D and hyaluronidase.[21,22] These enzymes cause a series of reactions, leading to tissue damage by way of inflammatory mediators. Eventually tissue necrosis occurs, with some severe wounds requiring skin grafting. Other spiders can cause necrotic wounds that may be similar in appearance to bites from *L reclusa* but less severe.

Diagnosis of an envenomation caused by *L reclusa* is through identification of the spider, if available. There are no routine laboratory tests to confirm envenomation. Laboratory tests in severe envenomations should include those that detect hemolysis,

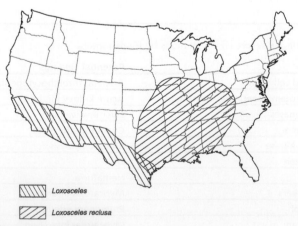

Loxosceles

Loxosceles reclusa

Fig. 1. *Loxosceles* species distribution.

hematuria, and coagulopathy. **Table 4** serves as a guide for testing in severe envenomations by *Loxosceles*.

Clinical symptoms of envenomation may not be immediate because the spider bite may not be initially noticed but often it presents as a stinging pain. As the wound blisters and bleeds over the next 24 to 48 hours, it eventually forms a necrotic lesion during the next 5 to 7 days.[23–25] The wound eschar ulcerates over the next 1 to 2 weeks and may require skin grafting and débridement at a later date.

Typically, bites by *L reclusa* do not require ICU admission except in cases of systemic loxoscelism, which occurs 24 to 72 hours after the bite. This syndrome presents with fever, chills, nausea, vomiting, arthralgias, DIC, rhabdomyolysis, and hemolysis.[24,26–29] Severe cases involve respiratory failure, soft tissue edema, renal failure, and rarely death. Management of systemic symptoms is mainly supportive with standard treatments, such as mechanical ventilation, blood product transfusions, and hemodialysis as necessary.[23]

Antivenom treatment of *Loxosceles* species is not available in the United States but is available in Brazil, Argentina, Peru, and Mexico.[30] Treatment with steroids, antihistamines, and prophylactic antibiotics is not recommended. Antibiotics should be started in patients with signs and symptoms of infection. Dapsone was believed to help with decreasing leukocyte aggregation at the bite site reducing tissue damage.[31–33] Results with dapsone use are mixed. Without a well-designed clinical trial to support its use, it should not be used routinely.[24] Early excision of the bite site is not recommended because scarring is likely to occur.[34] Hyperbaric oxygen therapy has been used with mixed results; its use is not recommended.[33,35–37] On discharge from a hospital, patients should be referred to a specialist who can manage the wound for healing and possible débridement.

Latrodectus Species (Black Widow Spiders)

Black widow spiders (*Latrodectus mactans*) belong to the general category of *Latrodectus* species, which are similar around the world. There are many subspecies, but their venoms and characteristics are similar. The spiders live in woodpiles and garages, particularly in dark places. They feed primarily at night with their meals consisting of insects. Black widow female spiders are much larger than their male counterparts. Because of their size, female spiders are responsible for all significant human bites because their fangs are long enough to penetrate through skin. Often after mating, the female spider eats the male spider, giving this arachnid the name, black widow.

Table 4
Laboratory testing in severe envenomations caused by *L reclusa*

Test	Potential Findings
Complete blood cell count	Anemia, thrombocytopenia, leukocytosis
Serum urea nitrogen, creatinine, electrolytes	Acute kidney injury
Serum transaminase activity	Liver involvement
Prothrombin time	Coagulopathy (DIC)
Serum creatine kinase activity	Rhabdomyolysis
DIC panel	DIC: fibrinogen ($\downarrow$), fibrin(ogen) split products ($\uparrow$), D-dimer ($\uparrow$)
Urinalysis	Hematuria
Coombs test	Hemolysis

The bite of the black widow generally results in the onset of intense pain, with or without evidence of fang marks or the classic target sign. There may be local sweating due to local norepinephrine release at the bite site. The onset of symptoms is generally within 30 to 60 minutes and lasts 24 to 48 hours. The venom contains α-latrotoxin, which causes catecholamine release through neurotransmitter stimulation of norepinephrine and acetylcholine into synaptic terminals.[38,39] The result is severe muscle spasm, tachycardia, high blood pressure, agitation, pain, diaphoresis, and anxiety. The envenomation may cause abdominal muscle spasms and symptoms mimicking acute appendicitis.

Treatment of black widow bites includes pain control with opioids and anxiolytic medications, such as benzodiazepines. Intravenous (IV) fluids may correct dehydration from hyperadrenergic stimulation. Most patients require only pain control without needing admission. Only the most severely symptomatic patients require further care in the hospital. Severely envenomed patients may require high doses of analgesia to control pain. Those with comorbid conditions, such as underlying cardiac or respiratory disease, may require more aggressive supportive care with other agents. Calcium infusions were believed to help the symptoms of black widow bites; however, this intervention has not been proven effective.[40]

Severe black widow envenomation that causes systemic symptoms is known as latrodectism. These symptoms may include facial swelling (latrodectus facies), parvor mortis (feeling of impending doom), tachycardia, chest pain, diaphoresis, conjunctivitis, muscle spasms, nausea, vomiting, abdominal pain, and priapism.[41–45] Rarely, severe hypertension, respiratory depression, compartment syndrome, and gangrene at the bite site have been reported. Death from *Latrodectus* envenomation is rare and has not been reported in decades.

If antivenom is available, the indications are summarized in **Box 1**. Pregnant patients and those with comorbid conditions, such as coronary artery disease or chronic obstructive pulmonary disease, are at high risk and should receive antivenom.[46–49] Merck has manufactured black widow spider antivenin since the 1950s. As of late 2011 this antivenom was still available on a limited basis from the manufacturer. Use of this equine-derived antivenom has been used sparingly in the United States. This may be because of a case report of a death after a patient received this antivenom.[40] The package insert states that either a skin test or conjunctival test should be performed for the possibility of an allergic reaction to antivenom.[50] Skin testing does not exclude the possibility of anaphylaxis to antivenom, and routine skin testing is not recommended.[51] Careful consideration should be performed in those with allergies to horses and horse products as well as patients with asthma because deaths have been reported after antivenom administration.[40,52] The usual dose is one vial, with subsequent administration of additional vials if the symptoms have not resolved. Each vial should be infused over 20 to 30 minutes to avoid anaphylactoid reactions. Time to relief of symptoms after antivenom treatment averages 31 minutes.[41,53] Serum sickness, which manifests as fever, joint pain, and rash, has often occurred with this antivenom.

Box 1 **Indications for *Latrodectus mactans* antivenin**
Uncontrolled hypertension
Respiratory difficulties
Pregnancy
Intractable pain

SCORPION

Scorpions are located throughout the Southwestern United States. There are many species of scorpions in North America but only one causes clinically relevant symptoms. The *Centruroides sculpturatus*, also known as *Centruroides exilicauda*, is colloquially referred to as the bark scorpion. These scorpions are located in the Southwestern United States, especially in Arizona, California, New Mexico, Texas, and Nevada. Scorpions have been transported to other non-native areas as stowaways, causing surprise and pain.[54,55]

Scorpions have several distinctive anatomic features. These parts are the pinchers, or pedipalps, and grabbers, or chelicerae, which assist moving food to its mouth; the tail or metasomal segments; and the telson, or stinger (venom apparatus). The exoskeleton is made of chitin. The chemical, β-carboline, contained in the exoskeleton causes the scorpion to fluoresce under ultraviolet light.[56]

Scorpion venom is injected into its victim to cause immobilization through neurotoxic effects. The venom contains many components but the effect on humans is centered on the sodium channels. Sodium channels are dual-gated channels that are affected by the inhibited closure of one of these gates, thereby depleting the channel for sodium. This results in repeated action potentials generated stimulating the neuron. Clinically these effects manifest as muscle jerking, opsoclonus (rapid, irregular, and nonrhythmic eye movements), tongue fasciculations, and loss of muscle control. Opsoclonus is often referred to as nystagmus; however, these 2 entities are separate. Nystagmus is a rhythmic oscillation of the eyeballs, with alternating fast-phase and slow-phase movements within a particular plane, whereas opsoclonus is unpredictable in both movement and direction.

Venom effects are especially worrisome in infants, children, and elderly patients. The most severe symptoms occur when there is loss of the airway muscles coupled with increased salivation causing the inability to control secretions, leading to respiratory failure. Pancreatitis is not a common finding in envenomations by *Centruroides* but is associated with those stung by Buthidae, a scorpion indigenous to Trinidad.[57]

Symptom onset may occur immediately to 15 minutes after envenomation.[58] The severity of symptoms may depend on the amount of antivenom injected into the victim. Half-life of the venom ranges from 313 minutes to 515 minutes.[59] Generally, minimal to no local wound effects are seen. There may be erythema and pruritus. Local symptoms include pain and paresthesia at the bite site and may progress proximally in the affected limb. A grading scale has been developed for scorpion envenomations, and a summary of these signs and symptoms is given in **Table 5**.[60]

Table 5	
Centruroides scorpion severity grade	
Grade I	Pain or paresthesia at the sting site
Grade II	Pain or paresthesia at the sting site and remote areas
Grade III	Cranial nerve and autonomic dysfunction[a] or somatic skeletal neuromuscular dysfunction[b]
Grade IV	Both cranial nerve and somatic skeletal neuromuscular dysfunction

[a] Cranial nerve dysfunction: blurred vision, opsoclonus, hypersalivation, tongue fasciculation, dysphagia, dysphonia, upper airway abnormalities.
[b] Somatic skeletal neuromuscular dysfunction: restlessness, severe involuntary extremity movements (limb jerking).

Poison control center data reveal there were no deaths in 2010 from scorpion enve-nomations.[61] This may be due to the availability of an F(ab′)2 antivenom that has been used on an investigational basis in areas endemic to scorpions.

The management of most scorpion stings includes pain control with nonsteroidal anti-inflammatory agents, opioid medications, and anxiolytic drugs. Antivenom is reserved for those individuals who have severe systemic symptoms, such as grade III or grade IV findings. As of 2011, *Centruroides* (scorpion) immune F(ab′)2 (equine) injection (Anascorp) was Food and Drug Administration approved for use in severely envenomed patients.[62] **Fig. 2** and **Box 2** outline treatment algorithms for using the antivenom. In a randomized, double-blind study, the severity of symptoms were significantly decreased 2 hours after infusion of the antivenom.[63] The most common adverse reactions occurred in approximately 2% of patients. These were mainly vomiting, pyrexia, rash, nausea, and pruritus.[62] Antivenom treatment may not halt all symptoms of envenomation. This is due to the inability of antivenom to reach venom at the level of affected neurons or certain other tissues. In addition, the amount of venom may exceed the antivenom's neutralizing power (ie, insufficient antivenom). Patients treated with antivenom generally are discharged home. Rarely, patients

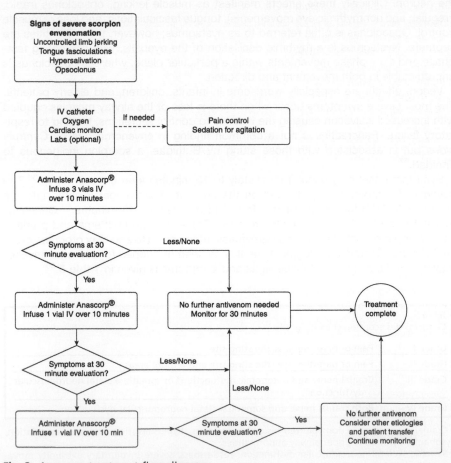

Fig. 2. Anascorp treatment flow diagram.

Box 2
Anascorp dosing

- Give initial dose of 3 vials
  - Reconstitute each vial with 5 mL normal saline
  - Add the contents of the 3 vials to a 50 mL bag of sterile normal saline
  - Infuse IV over 10 minutes minimum
- Monitor patient up to 60 minutes for improvement of signs and symptoms
- Give additional doses, one vial each (up to 2 doses) if symptoms do not improve
  - Reconstitute each vial with 5 mL normal saline
  - Add the contents of the vial to a 50-mL bag of sterile normal saline
  - Infuse IV over 10 minutes minimum
- Monitor patient up to 60 minutes for improvement of signs and symptoms

Data from Anascorp package insert.

---

who continue to have severe symptoms despite antivenom treatment may be observed for 24 hours and be discharged home after symptoms improve.

Severe envenomations (grade III or IV) may be managed without the use of antivenom. Patients are treated with symptomatic relief and may require airway support with mechanical ventilation along with sedation for severe agitation. Ventilated patients require approximately 24 to 48 hours of mechanical ventilation.[64] Complications associated with severe scorpion envenomation include aspiration pneumonitis, rhabdomyolysis, dehydration, and convulsions. The use of corticosteroids, antihistamines, and antibiotics is not routinely recommended. Antibiotics should be reserved for those patients who have signs and symptoms of bacterial infections. Those envenomed by scorpions may continue to complain of numbness, tingling, paresthesia, and pain that may persist for weeks without permanent sequelae.

SNAKES

Snakes play an important role in nature's ecology by controlling the population of rodents and other small animals. Snakes are often feared by hikers, backpackers, campers, and swimmers, including men, women, and children. Treating snakebite patients can be challenging. The most common poisonous snakes encountered in North America belong to the subfamily Crotalinae (family Viperidae) and the subfamily Elapinae (family Elapidae). The subfamily Crotalinae includes the genera *Crotalus*, *Agkistrodon*, and *Sistrurus*. The subfamily Elapinae includes the genus *Micrurus*. These snakes can cause substantial morbidity and mortality in those who have been bitten and envenomed.

Coral Snakes (Elapidae)

Coral snakes belong to the family Elapidae, which includes species that are distributed around the world. In North America, *Micrurus* species are located primarily on the Gulf Coast states of the United States. The 2 clinically relevant species are *Micrurus fulvius fulvius* (Eastern coral snake) and *Micrurus fulvius tenere* (Texas coral snake). The species *Micruroides euryxanthus euryxanthus* (Sonoran or Arizona coral snake) is not considered significantly venomous because the amount of venom delivered is much less than the bites of other coral snakes (**Fig. 3**). Several nonvenomous snakes have a similar appearance to the coral snake, including the king snake and milk snake. The mnemonic, "red on yellow, kill a fellow; red on black, venom lack," holds true only for coral snakes north of Mexico City.[65]

Envenomation by the coral snake occurs through grooved fixed fangs where venom flows down into the wound created by the reptile biting through the victim's skin. Effective envenomation occurs when the snake chews and attaches itself as venom enters the wound.

Coral snake venom contains several components that cause systemic neurotoxic effects and local wounds. Neurologic venom effects are caused by α-neurotoxin.[66] Wound effects are caused primarily by phospholipase A2.[67]

The diagnosis of a coral snake bite may not be readily apparent. The bite site may not be seen and local swelling may not occur. Symptoms of coral snake envenomation include nausea, vomiting, headache, abdominal pain, diaphoresis, paresthesias or numbness, dysphonia, dysphagia, or respiratory insufficiency leading to respiratory failure.[68] Symptoms may be delayed up to 12 h or longer.[69] Careful monitoring of a patient's respiratory status should be performed in the ICU setting and mechanical ventilatory respiratory support should not be delayed when signs and symptoms occur. The use of end-tidal capnometry or capnography, pulse oximetry, and arterial blood gases may be helpful in monitoring a patient's respiratory status. Complete resolution of the neurologic effects takes weeks. Envenomed patients suffer neurologic effects causing paralysis for 3 to 5 days if they are untreated with antivenom.[70]

Severe manifestations (described previously) are associated with the Eastern coral snake (*Micrurus fulvius fulvius*). Envenomation with the Texas coral snake (*Micrurus fulvius tenere*) may not require treatment with antivenom and only require pain control. Bites with this coral snake cause local effects (pain, swelling, erythema, or paresthesia) without neurologic impairment. Patients envenomed by a coral snake west of the Mississippi river may be monitored for 8 hours and treatment with antivenom is considered for those with progressively worsening bites and systemic effects.[71]

The decision to treat with coral snake antivenom must be weighed against the availability of antivenom and geographic consideration of the type of coral snake species that caused the bite. Dosing for the Wyeth coral snake antivenom consists of an initial dose of 5 vials with a repeat dose of 5 vials if symptoms do not improve.[72] In significant envenomations, more than 10 vials may be required. Antivenom is likely not effective once neurologic signs and symptoms occur.[69]

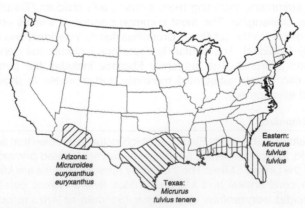

Fig. 3. Coral snake distribution in North America.

Treatment of coral snake envenomations in the United States will be challenging in the coming years because production of the Wyeth North American coral snake antivenom (equine origin) was discontinued in October 2010. The availability of antivenom is limited to stock on hand. Antivenom administration is recommended with significant envenomations, especially east of the Mississippi River, because of the prolonged neurologic effects.

Pit Viper (Crotalinae)

Of all the venomous creatures encountered in North America, bites from Crotalinae, or pit vipers, may be the most deadly. The total number of crotaline exposures reported to US poison control centers in 2010 was 3465 with 1 death reported.[61] **Fig. 4** show the areas where the genera *Crotalus*, *Agkistrodon*, and *Sistrurus* are found. *Crotalus* and *Sistrurus* possess rattles and are called rattlesnakes. *Agkistrodon*, which includes the cottonmouth (*Agkistrodon piscivorus*) and the copperhead (*Agkistrodon contortrix*), lacks rattles.

Pit vipers have poor eyesight, are deaf, and rely on their heat sensing pits as well as their sense of smell to detect prey. Their venom is delivered through sharp, hollow, mobile fangs from venom sacs. The speed and striking distances of the snake can be as fast as 8 feet per second and up to one-half of the snake's body length, respectively.[73]

Venom

Venom composition is complex and unpredictable. Factors that influence the composition vary from species to species, and by geographic location, diet, and time between feedings for the snake.[72] Venom components affect certain body processes.

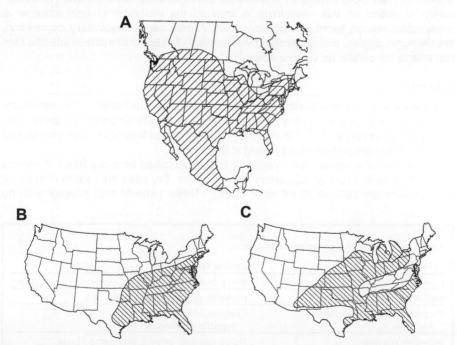

Fig. 4. Distribution of Crotalinae in North America. (A) *Crotalus*, (B) *Agkistrodon*, and (C) *Sistrurus*.

Each of these is essential to immobilize prey and to initiate the digestive process. Venom contains numerous proteins. **Table 6** summarizes some key components of pit viper venom.[65,72]

Pit viper venom causes tissue damage by increasing cell permeability. Blood and fluid from cell damage contribute to wound swelling. Fluid accumulates under the skin causing blebs filled with a mixture of substances resulting from reactions catalyzed by enzymes in the venom. The blebs are often bluish black in color and may swell impressively. Hemorrhage into the surrounding tissue occurs through the venom's effects on hematologic processes.

Hematologic effects of pit viper venom generally affect prothrombin time, fibrinogen, and platelets through consumptive coagulopathy. These reactions occur through a process that resembles DIC. True DIC is generally caused by sepsis, cancer, and endothelial insults activating the coagulation cascade to cause hemolytic anemia and intravascular clotting. DIC can occur in pit viper envenomations but it is rare. The syndrome caused by this venom's thrombin-like protein and other proteolytic enzymes results in fibrinolysis with decreased fibrinogen and thrombocytopenia from platelet aggregation and consumption at the bite site. A disorganized, uncrosslinked fibrin clot forms and is rapidly degraded into fibrin degradation products. Patients do not have problems with clotting because thrombin and factor XIII are not affected by pit viper venom and cross-linked fibrin clots continue to form. D-dimer assay results generally be in the normal range. **Fig. 5** depicts this process.

Neurologic effects are associated with crotalid envenomation, particularly that of the Mohave rattlesnake (*Crotalus scutulatus scutulatus*) and the Southern Pacific rattlesnake (*Crotalus oreganus helleri*). Geographically these rattlesnakes are located in California and Arizona. Mohave toxin A is a neurotoxin in the venom of these rattlesnakes that immobilizes its prey and causes the described tissue effects. The mechanism of action of this neurotoxin is through the inhibition of acetylcholine at presynaptic neuron terminals. Mohave toxin A may cause respiratory depression, cranial nerve palsies, and generalized weakness.[74] **Table 7** summarizes specific clinical effects for certain pit viper species.[75–77]

Diagnosis

The presentation of patients with pit viper bites depends on the severity. The most common clinical findings are fang marks, edema, weakness, pain, diaphoresis, paresthesia, and abnormal pulse rate.[72,78] Patients may not even realize they have been envenomed and have only pain and minimal swelling at the bite site.

The degree of envenomation varies. A bite is classified as a dry bite if it causes little or no swelling and no laboratory abnormalities. Dry bites are reported to occur in approximately 20% of all pit viper bites.[72] Those patients that present with no

Table 6 Summary of key pit viper venom components	
Venom Components	**Clinical Effects**
Low molecular weight polypeptides	Shock from capillary leakage causing third spacing
Metalloproteinases	Hemorrhage into tissues and shock
Thrombin-like glycoproteins, fibrinolysins	Coagulopathy, thrombocytopenia, and hypofibrinogenemia
Digestive enzymes	Tissue damage, edema, and hemorrhage
Myotoxins	Muscle necrosis

significant evidence of pit viper envenomation can be observed for a minimum of 6 hours. Initial blood work should be obtained (**Table 8**) on arrival and repeat complete blood cell count, prothrombin time, and fibrinogen levels obtained in 6 hours to determine if any hematologic venom effects are occurring. Vigilant observation for swelling, bleeding, systemic symptoms (eg, nausea or vomiting), and increasing pain must be performed during this period. Taking measurements of the extremity every 30 minutes monitors for swelling progression (**Fig. 6**). Asymptomatic patients with no laboratory abnormalities during this observation period may be discharged without further treatment. Exceptions to this recommendation are children and lower extremity wounds. Significant swelling may not be evident and may go unnoticed. Conservative observation in the hospital may be warranted in select patients.[80,81]

A summary of pit viper envenomation severity is contained in **Table 9**. Mild bites cause slight local swelling and pain but without laboratory abnormalities. Moderate to severe envenomations are associated with laboratory abnormalities in platelet count, fibrinogen level, and prothrombin time along with significant swelling and pain. Severe envenomations manifest these plus severe respiratory and cardiovascular problems. Systemic signs and symptoms of envenomation include a metallic taste, nausea, vomiting, hypotension, and bradycardia.

Moderate pit viper bites may develop fluid-filled blebs, or blood blisters. If the skin covering the bleb is removed, the tissue beneath may appear dusky and necrotic. Sensation to this exposed area is a good sign that the tissue may not require significant débridement. Insensate areas indicate the wound is necrotic and amputation or significant débridement may be required at a later time. During the acute phase of pit viper treatment, the wounds do not require immediate débridement, but surgical intervention can be considered once control of venom effects are stabilized with antivenom. Severe swelling and lymphangitis generally occur, which may give the impression that the bite is infected. Bacterial infection is rare, however, and antibiotics are only indicated if there is evidence of infection. Hemorrhage and swelling may occur remote from the bite site. There is no specific treatment other than antivenom.

The spread of pit viper venom is propagated by the lymphatic system except in those rare cases of intravascular envenomation. With each movement of the limbs the lymph system transports venom to the central circulation. Eventually, the venom circulates throughout the body via the bloodstream. There may be lymphatic swelling. Tender inguinal and axillary lymph nodes may indicate advancement of venom.

Management

Consultation with a clinician experienced with pit viper bites is recommended, especially for moderate to severe envenomations. Admission to the hospital is based on the severity of the bite. Mild pit viper bites on the upper extremity may be observed for a period of time in the emergency department with frequent limb measurements to monitor for progression of swelling. Laboratory examination of platelet count, fibrinogen level, and prothrombin time should be made on arrival and at 8 hours postbite to assess whether antivenom treatment is required. Lower extremity bites should be observed for a minimum of 24 hours because those compartments are much larger than the upper extremities and significant swelling may go unnoticed. Moderate and severe envenomations require admission to the ICU because antivenom treatment, wound care, cardiopulmonary, and neurologic monitoring are necessary.

Measure the affected extremity at 3 sites of the extremity (see **Fig. 6**) every 30 minutes initially to assess for worsening swelling and to determine the necessity for antivenom treatment. Once antivenom has started to infuse, hourly measurements

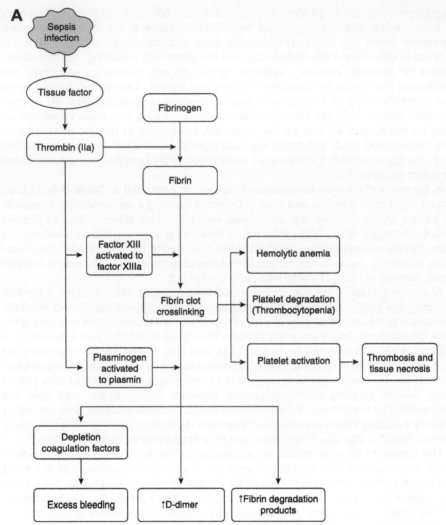

Fig. 5. Hematologic effects of crotaline venom and comparison to DIC. (*A*) DIC and (*B*) pit viper.

should be taken until the swelling has stabilized. Measurements can then be taken every 4 to 6 hours during maintenance antivenom infusions. Recording the measurements on a nursing flow sheet or progress note is essential to monitor for worsening swelling. Uncontrolled pain may be an indication to measure compartment pressures.

Patients should be placed on a cardiac monitor and receive supplemental oxygen. Two large-bore IV catheters should be inserted. Depending on the degree of envenomation, IV fluid boluses of isotonic crystalloid solutions should be instituted, especially in moderate to severe bites. Third spacing of fluids can cause significant swelling in the extremity and deplete intravascular volume leading to hypotension. Decreased urine output may occur in those victims that develop hypotension or rhabdomyolysis, either of which can result in acute kidney injury.

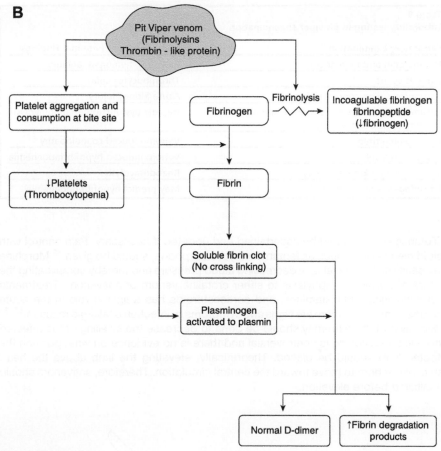

Fig. 5. (continued)

Table 7	
Summary of clinical effects of certain pit viper species	
Species	**Effects**
Mohave rattlesnake (*Crotalus scutulatus scutulatus*)	Neurologic complications from Mohave toxin A
Southern Pacific rattlesnake (*Crotalus oreganus helleri*)	Severe thrombocytopenia, no significant hypofibrinogenemia; neurologic complications (from Mohave toxin A)
Canebrake rattlesnake (*Crotalus horridus atricaudatus*)	Rhabdomyolysis
Copperhead (*Agkistrodon contortrix contortrix*)	Local swelling and pain, but rarely causing severe hematologic effects (antivenom is rarely indicated)
Water moccasin or cottonmouth (*Agkistrodon piscivorus*)	Causes less severe swelling and hematologic effects
Timber rattlesnake (*Crotalus horridus horridus*)	Severe thrombocytopenia, with or without prothrombin time increase; myokymia

Table 8
Laboratory testing in pit viper envenomation

Laboratory Examination	Indications and Potential Findings
Hemoglobin and hematocrit	Bleeding, hemolysis, anemia
Platelet count	Thrombocytopenia
Serum creatinine concentration	Acute kidney injury
Serum aspartate aminotransferase and alanine aminotransferase activity	Hepatic dysfunction, rhabdomyolysis
Prothrombin time	Venom-induced coagulopathy
Fibrinogen level	Venom-induced hypofibrinogenemia
Serum creatine kinase activity	Rhabdomyolysis
Fibrin(ogen) split products[79]	May predict hypofibrinogenemia

Tetanus status should be ascertained and updated if necessary. Pain control with opioid medications, such as fentanyl or hydromorphone, should be given.[82] Morphine may cause histamine release decreasing blood pressure and thereby complicating the picture of possible anaphylaxis to either crotaline venom or antivenom. Treatments with antibiotics, antihistamines, and corticosteroids has a limited role in the acute management unless there are signs and symptoms of infection or allergic reaction.[83–86]

Elevation of the extremity should be done to decrease the swelling of the affected limb. Limb positioning is controversial and there is no evidence on what position the affected limb should be placed. Theoretically, elevating the limb above the heart can cause venom to move toward the central circulation. Therefore, antivenom should be initiated before elevation.

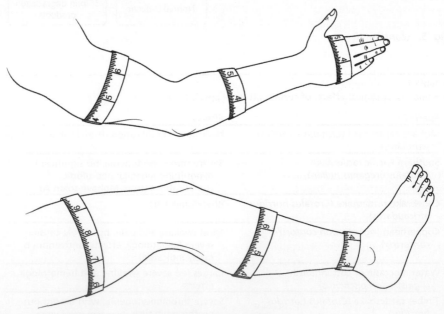

Fig. 6. Measuring the extremity to monitor for swelling.

Table 9		
Pit viper envenomation severity		
Mild	**Moderate**	**Severe**
• Local wound effects at the bite site • No systemic symptoms • No laboratory abnormalities	• Evidence of swelling, erythema, ecchymosis beyond the bite site • Minor systemic symptoms • No significant bleeding or significant laboratory abnormalities	• Swelling, erythema, ecchymosis of the entire body part • Systemic symptoms (significant hypotension, altered mental status, respiratory distress, tachycardia) • Significant bleeding, elevated prothrombin time, decreased fibrinogen level, thrombocytopenia ($<20,000\ \mu L^{-1}$)

Data from Gold BS, Dart RC, Barish RA. Bites of venomous snakes. N Engl J Med 2002;347(5):347–56.

Initial laboratory orders should focus on obtaining a complete blood cell count, a basic metabolic panel, serum transaminases, prothrombin time, fibrinogen level, and creatine kinase activity (see **Table 8**).

Infusing blood products for thrombocytopenia and hypofibrinogenemia is not necessary for pit viper envenomations unless life-threatening hemorrhage occurs. Circulating venom affects transfused blood products rendering them ineffective. Therefore, antivenom should be given before blood product administration unless a patient's condition warrants otherwise.

Antivenom administration should be initiated if a patient has moderate to severe symptoms, such as progressive swelling, uncontrolled pain, hematologic abnormalities, anaphylaxis, hypotension, and respiratory difficulties. Crotalidae polyvalent immune Fab antivenom (CroFab) is an ovine-derived immunoglobulin G (IgG) fragment made from 4 pit viper venoms: *Crotalus atrox, Crotalus adamanteus, Crotalus scutulatus,* and *Agkistrodon piscivorus*.[87] Antivenom cross-reactivity between pit viper species allows this antivenom to be used for all North American species. **Fig. 7** is a flow diagram of CroFab antivenom administration. Obtaining control of the swelling, pain, and hematologic effects is done by administering repeat doses of 4 to 6 vials. Control is defined as the end of progressive swelling and pain and improvement of hematologic effects. Maintenance therapy decreases the chance of recrudescence once control is achieved. Laboratory tests should be obtained after each dose of antivenom to monitor for worsening hematologic effects.

It is critical to explain to patients that antivenom does not reverse tissue damage and may not prevent further damage depending on the amount of venom in the tissue. Antivenom treatment helps correct hematologic effects and assist in the removal of circulating venom.

Other Treatment Considerations

Treatments, such as tissue excision, incision, and suction extraction; ice or heat application; electric shock; and so forth, have not proved useful and potentially may cause harm in envenomed patients.[65,88]

Constricting bands, tourniquets, and the Australian pressure immobilization technique are thought to reduce venom travel in the extremity to prevent worsening symptoms. The risk of tissue damage from the constricting band may cause more harm than

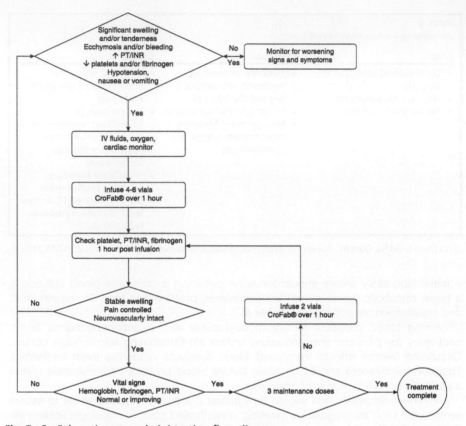

Fig. 7. CroFab antivenom administration flow diagram.

good. The pressure required to halt venom progression coupled with the difficulty to control the amount of pressure in the compartments make this technique dangerous. Because the tissue already has vascular compromise from swelling, it is not recommended in North American rattlesnake bites.[89–91]

Rattlesnake envenomations can cause severe tissue necrosis and impressive swelling. Swelling can lead to elevated compartment pressures and the risk of developing compartment syndrome. It is estimated that 2% to 8% of pit viper bites develop this limb-threatening problem.[92–94] Animal studies have shown that compartment pressures are decreased using antivenom.[95] In a recent review of the literature, Cumpston found no compelling evidence that fasciotomy or dermotomy may be tissue saving.[96] Fasciotomy is performed by making an incision into the skin and fascia to release pressure in the involved compartment. Decompressive dermotomy is an incision made into the skin to release compression made by skin. Until a properly designed study regarding the routine or prophylactic use of fasciotomy or dermotomy in crotaline envenomations occurs, this practice should be reserved only for extreme cases where antivenom therapy fails to decrease swelling and there is evidence of limb ischemia (**Box 3**).[97]

Both venom and antivenom may cause either anaphylaxis or anaphylactoid reactions. Standard measures using IV fluids, corticosteroids, antihistamines, epinephrine, and, if needed, vasopressors are recommended for treating these reactions.

> **Box 3**
> **Indications for fasciotomy or dermotomy despite antivenom treatment in crotaline envenomations**
>
> Pulselessness
>
> Persistently elevated measurements of intracompartamental pressure (>30 mm Hg) despite adequate antivenom treatment
>
> Pallor

Disposition, Follow-up, and Complications

Patients should be expected to improve over the next 2 to 4 weeks after the bite. Disability from pit viper bites may persist for weeks due to pain, swelling, and tissue damage. Function of the extremity may not totally recover depending on the type of wound. Severe wounds requiring amputation, fasciotomy, or dermotomy cause significant disability and reconstructive surgery may be necessary. Physical and occupational therapy may assist patients with performing activities of daily living and arranging for assistance equipment before discharge from the hospital. Pain control should be an integral part of discharge treatment.

Recurrent venom effects or recurrence is a phenomenon that may occur after completion of pit viper antivenom treatment. Circulating antivenom may be eliminated from the body before the venom diffusing into the circulation.[98] Thus, the signs and symptoms of pit viper envenoming can reappear, such as increased swelling, pain, and hematologic effects, such as prothrombin time elevation and falling platelet counts and fibrinogen levels. Patients are encouraged to have laboratory examinations at 2 to 4 days and at 7 days after antivenom treatment.[99] Patients at highest risk of late hematologic abnormalities are those with hypofibrinogenemia, elevated D-dimer levels, thrombocytopenia, or elevated prothrombin or partial thromboplastin times during the first 48 hours after envenomation.[100] Treatment of recurrence with antivenom depends on the clinician and the presentation of the patient. In general, patients with bleeding and severe hematologic abnormalities should be readmitted to the ICU for continued antivenom treatment and possible blood product transfusion. **Box 4** summarizes recommendations regarding recurrence.[101] Serum sickness is a possibility with antivenom administration (discussed later).

ANTIVENOM

Antivenom, also called antivenin, is made by injecting animals with venom obtained from the target animal. The injected animal's serum is later recovered and contains IgG antibodies directed to the venom. That serum is refined and processed to obtain antivenom suitable for human injection. **Table 10** summarizes the antivenoms

> **Box 4**
> **Consider additional antivenom administration in patients with recurrence and any of the following findings**
>
> Fibrinogen concentration <50 mg/dL, platelet count <25,000 μL^{-1}, international normalized ratio >3.0, or partial thromboplastin time >50 seconds
>
> Multicomponent coagulopathy with abnormal laboratory values of a lesser degree
>
> A clear worsening trend at follow-up in patients who had a severe early coagulopathy
>
> High-risk behavior or comorbid condition

Table 10
North American snake, scorpion, and black widow spider antivenom

Venom Source	Antivenom	Origin	Antibody Type	Preservatives and Additives
Agkistrodon piscivorus and *Crotalus atrox, Crotalus adamanteus,* and *Crotalus scutulatus* (pit vipers)	Crotalidae polyvalent immune Fab (CroFab, Protherics)	Ovine (sheep)	IgG Fab	Papain (from papaya), used as a cleavage agent[87]
Centruroides (scorpion)	Immune F(ab')$_2$ (Anascorp, Rare Disease Therapeutics)	Equine (horse)	IgG F(ab')$_2$	Thimerosal (mercury)[62]
Micrurus fulvius fulvius (Eastern coral snake) and *Micrurus fulvius tenere* (Texas coral snake)	North American coral snake antivenin (Wyeth, no longer manufactured)	Equine (horse)	Whole IgG	Thimerosal (mercury) and phenol[102]
Latrodectus mactans	Black widow spider antivenin (Merck and Co)	Equine (horse)	Whole IgG	Thimerosal (mercury)[50]

discussed in this article. Clinicians should determine if a patient has any hypersensitivity to the antivenom ingredients before its infusion. When giving antivenom, the risks and benefits of giving these drugs should be explained to patients, as outlined in **Box 5**.

Infusion of antivenom should be initiated slowly and the infusion rate gradually increased while monitoring for anaphylactoid or anaphylactic reactions. Anaphylactoid reactions may resemble anaphylaxis with skin flushing, dyspnea, bronchospasm, hypotension, tachycardia or bradycardia, tongue swelling, nausea, vomiting, and so forth. Cardiac monitoring and preparation with bedside IV medication infusions (epinephrine, antihistamines, and corticosteroids) may be helpful in these emergent situations. Consider having these medications at the bedside for faster administration should the need arise. For patients who are severely allergic to any component of antivenom, pretreatment with corticosteroids and antihistamines is necessary along with slow infusion of antivenom to monitor for adverse effects. The causes of antivenom reactions are thought to be mediated by complement activation against antivenom IgG, total protein concentration, antibody aggregation, additives and processing agents (eg, the cleaving agent papain used in F[ab']$_2$ processing), and previous exposure to the animal from which the antivenom is derived.[98]

Serum sickness is a type III (immune complex) hypersensitivity reaction that may occur with the administration of antivenom. Foreign proteins (antivenom IgG) can cause a delayed reaction due to immune complex formation between the antivenom and human IgG and collect in the joints and blood vessels.[103,104] Patients have fever, headaches, generalized rash, lymphadenopathy, and joint pain approximately 3 to 21 days after receiving antivenom.[105] Severe cases may present with nephritis, bronchospasm, and purpura.[65] Patients with this type of reaction are treated using a tapering course of corticosteroid and antihistamine medications.[104]

Skin testing was once advocated before the administration of some antivenom, especially horse-derived products. This routine practice has fallen out of favor because it did not predict which patients have a reaction to the antivenom.[106–108]

Special populations include pregnant patients and children. Most antivenoms have not been proved safe to give in pregnancy. The risk of fetal effects must be weighed when giving antivenom. The risk includes maternal symptoms that may cause hypoxia, increased circulating catecholamines, the length of illness, and the types of effects on the mother and fetus (eg, the hematologic effects of pit viper venom). The risk and benefits of administering antivenom to these individuals must be discussed with the

---

Box 5
Risks of antivenom administration

Risks

Anaphylaxis (type I hypersensitivity reactions)

Serum sickness (type III hypersensitivity reactions)

Anaphylactoid reactions

Hypersensitivity to components of the venom or venom processing

Possibility of transplacental passage (pregnant patients)

Unknown long-term effects, especially in children and pregnant patients

Precautions

Renal failure (unable to excrete venom-antivenom complexes)

patient and their families. Antivenom has not proved deleterious to a fetus, children, or pregnancy in the long term. There are few data to support withholding antivenom when it is required.[109–111]

SUMMARY

Care of envenomated patients can be challenging. Consultation with an experienced clinician or a poison control center (800-222-1222) can assist in the diagnosis and management of these bites and stings.

REFERENCES

1. Goddard J. Physician's guide to arthropods of medical importance. 3rd edition. Boca Raton (FL): CRC Press; 2000. p. 1–396.
2. Mebs D. Venomous and poisonous animals. Boca Raton (FL): CRC Press; 2002.
3. Steen CJ, Carbonaro PA, Schwartz RA. Arthropods in dermatology. J Am Acad Dermatol 2004;50(6):819–42.
4. Stafford CT. Hypersensitivity to fire ant venom. Ann Allergy Asthma Immunol 1996;77(2):87–95.
5. Sherman RA. What physicians should know about Africanized honeybees. West J Med 1995;163(6):541–6.
6. Taber S. Fire Ants. College Station (TX): Texas A&M University Press; 2000.
7. Kemp SF, de Shazo RD, Mofitt JE, et al. Expanding habitat of the imported fire ant (Solenopsis invicta): a public health concern. J Allergy Clin Immunol 2000; 105(4):683–91.
8. Klotz JH, Pinnas JL, Greenberg L, et al. What's eating you? Native and imported fire ants. Cutis 2009;83(1):17–20.
9. Conniff R. Stung: How tiny little insects get us to do exactly as they wish. Discover 2003;6:67.
10. Blaser K, Carballido J, Faith A, et al. Determinants and mechanisms of human immune responses to bee venom phospholipase A2. Int Arch Allergy Immunol 1998;117(1):1–10.
11. Lichtenstein LM, Valentine MD, Sobotka AK. Insect allergy: the state of the art. J Allergy Clin Immunol 1979;64(1):5–12.
12. Petroianu G, Liu J, Helfrich U, et al. Phospholipase A2-induced coagulation abnormalities after bee sting. Am J Emerg Med 2000;18(1):22–7.
13. Muller UR. Hymenoptera venom proteins and peptides for diagnosis and treatment of venom allergic patients. Inflamm Allergy Drug Targets 2011;10(5): 420–8.
14. Van der Linden PW, Struyvenberg A, Kraaijenhagen RJ, et al. Anaphylactic shock after insect-sting challenge in 138 persons with a previous insect-sting reaction. Arch Intern Med 1993;118(3):161–8.
15. Reisman RE. Natural history of insect sting allergy: relationship of severity of symptoms of initial anaphylaxis to re-sting reactions. J Allergy Clin Immunol 1992;90(3 Pt 1):335–9.
16. Erickson TB, Marquez A. Arthropod envenomation and parasitism. Wilderness medicine. 5th edition. Philadelphia: Mosby; 2007. p. 1051–85.
17. Meier J. Biology and distribution of hymenopterans of medical importance, their venom apparatus and venom composition. In: Meier J, White J, editors. Handbook of clinical toxicology of animal venoms and poisons. Boca Raton (FL): CRC Press; 1995. p. 331–48.

18. Schmidt JO. Allergy to venomous insects. In: Graham JM, editor. The hive and the honeybee. Hamilton (IL): Dadant & Sons; 1992. p. 1209–69.
19. Visscher PK, Vetter RS, Camazine S. Removing bee stings. Lancet 1996; 348(9023):301–2.
20. Available at: http://spiders.ucr.edu/images/colorloxmap.gif. Accessed April 2, 2012.
21. Chavez-Olortegui C, Zanetti VC, Ferreira AP, et al. ELISA for the detection of venom antigens in experimental and clinical envenoming by loxosceles intermedia spiders. Toxicon 1998;36(4):563–9.
22. Futrell JM. Loxoscelism. Am J Med Sci 1992;304(4):261–7.
23. Yarbrough B. Current treatment of brown recluse spiders. Curr Concepts Wound Care 1987;10(4):4–6.
24. Rees R, Campbell D, Rieger E, et al. The diagnosis and treatment of brown recluse spider bites. Ann Emerg Med 1987;16(9):945–9.
25. Gendron BP. Loxosceles reclusa envenomation. Am J Emerg Med 1990;8(1):51–4.
26. Vorse H, Seccareccio P, Woodruff K, et al. Disseminated intravascular coagulopathy following fatal brown spider bite (necrotic arachnidism). J Pediatr 1972;80(6):1035–7.
27. Bernstein B, Ehrlich F. Brown recluse spider bites. J Emerg Med 1986;4(6): 457–62.
28. Cacy J, Mold JW. The clinical characteristics of brown recluse spider bites treated by family physicians: an OKPRN Study. Oklahoma Physicians Research Network. J Fam Pract 1999;48(7):536–42.
29. Franca FO, Barbaro KC, Abdulkader RC. Rhabdomyolysis in presumed viscerocutaneous loxoscelism: report of two cases. Trans R Soc Trop Med Hyg 2002; 96(3):287–90.
30. Isbister GK, Fan HW. Spider bite. Lancet 2011;378(9808):2039–47.
31. King LE Jr, Rees RS. Dapsone treatment of a brown recluse bite. JAMA 1987; 250(5):648.
32. Hobbs GD, Anderson AR, Greene TJ, et al. Comparison of hyperbaric oxygen and dapsone therapy for loxosceles envenomation. Acad Emerg Med 1996; 3(8):758–61.
33. Phillips S, Kohn M, Baker D, et al. Therapy of brown spider envenomation: a controlled trial of hyperbaric oxygen, dapsone, and cyproheptadine. Ann Emerg Med 1995;25(3):363–8.
34. Rees RS, Altenbern DP, Lynch JB, et al. Brown recluse spider bites. A comparison of early surgical excision versus dapsone and delayed surgical excision. Ann Surg 1985;202(5):659–63.
35. Svendsen FJ. Treatment of clinically diagnosed brown recluse spider bites with hyperbaric oxygen: a clinical observation. J Ark Med Soc 1986;83(5):199–204.
36. Maynor ML, Moon RE, Klitzman B, et al. Brown recluse spider envenomation: a prospective trial of hyperbaric oxygen therapy. Acad Emerg Med 1997;4(3): 184–92.
37. Hobbs GD. Brown recluse spider envenomation: is hyperbaric oxygen the answer? Acad Emerg Med 1997;4(3):165–6.
38. Geppert M, Khvotchev M, Krasnoperov V, et al. Neurexin I alpha is a major alpha-latrotoxin receptor that cooperates in alpha-latrotoxin action. J Biol Chem 1998;273(3):1705–10.
39. van Renterghem C, Iborra C, Martin-Moutot N, et al. α-Latrotoxin forms calcium-permeable membrane pores via interactions with latrophilin or neurexin. Eur J Neurosci 2000;12(11):3953–62.

40. Clark RF. The safety and efficacy of antivenin Latrodectus mactans. J Toxicol Clin Toxicol 2001;39(2):125–7.
41. Clark RF, Wethern-Kestner S, Vance MV, et al. Clinical presentation and treatment of black widow spider envenomation: a review of 163 cases. Ann Emerg Med 1992;21(7):782–7.
42. Maretic Z. Latrodectism: variations in clinical manifestations provoked by latrodectus species of spiders. Toxicon 1983;21(4):457–66.
43. Sutherland SK, Trinca JC. Survey of 2144 cases of redback spider bites. Med J Aust 1978;2(14):620–3.
44. Hoover NG, Fortenberry JD. Use of antivenin to treat priapism after a black widow spider bite. Pediatrics 2004;114(1):e128–9.
45. Quan D, Ruha AM. Priapism associated with latrodectus mactans envenomation. Am J Emerg Med 2009;27(6):759.e1–2.
46. Russell FE, Marcus P, Streng JA. Black widow spider envenomation during pregnancy. Report of a case. Toxicon 1979;17(2):188–9.
47. Wolfe MD, Meyers O, Carvati EM, et al. Black widow spider envenomation in pregnancy. J Matern Fetal Neonatal Med 2011;24(1):122–6.
48. Sherman RP, Groll JM, Gonzalez DI, et al. Black widow spider (Latrodectus mactans) envenomation in a term pregnancy. Curr Surg 2000;57(4):346–8.
49. Handel CC, Izquierdo LA, Curet LB. Black widow spider (Latrodectus mactans) bite during pregnancy. West J Med 1994;160(3):261–2.
50. [Package insert]Antivenin (latrodectus mactans), black widow spider antivenin, equine origin. Whitehouse Station (NJ): Merck & Co; 2005.
51. Heard K, O'Malley GF, Dart RC. Antivenom therapy in the Americas. Drugs 1999;58(1):5–15.
52. Murphy CM, Hong JJ, Beuhler MC. Anaphylaxis with latrodectus antivenin resulting in cardiac arrest. J Med Toxicol 2011;7(4):317–21.
53. Offerman SR, Daubert GP, Clark RF. The treatment of black widow spider envenomation with Lactrodectus mactans: a case series. Permanente J 2011;15(3): 76–81.
54. Available at: http://www.upi.com/Odd_News/2009/07/20/Scorpions-on-a-plane/UPI-25831248119511/. Accessed January 15, 2012.
55. Available at: http://abcnews.go.com/US/scorpion-stings-man-flight-seattle-anchorage/story?id=13969984#.T00g3chXNY8. Accessed January 15, 2012.
56. Stachel SJ, Stockwell SA, van Vranken DL. The fluorescence of scorpions and cataractogenesis. Chem Biol 1999;6(8):531–9.
57. Bartholomew C. Acute scorpion pancreatitis in Trinidad. BMJ 1970;1(5967): 666–8.
58. LoVecchio F, McBride C. Scorpion envenomation in young children in central Arizona. Clin Toxicol 2003;41(7):937–40.
59. Chase P, Boyer-Hassen L, McNally J, et al. Serum levels and urine detection of Centruroides sculpturatus venom in significantly envenomated patients. Clin Toxicol 2009;47(1):24–8.
60. Curry SC, Vance MV, Ryan PJ, et al. Envenomation by the scorpion Centruroides sculpturatus. J Toxicol Clin Toxicol 1983–1984;21(4–5):417–49.
61. Bronstein AC, Spyker DA, Cantilena LR Jr, et al. 2010 annual report of the American Association of Poison Control Centers' National Poison Data System (NPDS): 28th annual report. Clin Toxicol 2011;49(10):910–41.
62. [Package insert]Anascorp® centruroides (scorpion) immune F(ab')2 (equine) injection. Franklin (TN): Rare Disease Therapeutics; 2011.

63. Boyer LV, Theodorou AA, Berg RA, et al. Antivenom for critically ill children with neurotoxicity from scorpion stings. N Engl J Med 2009;360(20):2090–8.
64. Riley BD, LoVecchio F, Pizon AF. Lack of scorpion antivenom leads to increased pediatric ICU admissions. Ann Emerg Med 2006;47(4):398–9.
65. Holstege CP, Miller MB, Wermuth M, et al. Crotalid snake envenomation. Crit Care Clin 1997;13(4):889–921.
66. Alape-Giron A, Stiles B, Schmidt J, et al. Characterization of multiple nicotinic acetylcholine receptor-binding proteins and phospholipases A2 from the venom of the coral snake Micrurus nigrocinctus. FEBS Lett 1996;380(1–2):29–32.
67. Rosso JP, Vargas-Rosso O, Gutierrez JM, et al. Characterization of alpha-neurotoxin and phospholipase A2 activities from Micrurus venoms. Determination of the amino acid sequence and receptor binding ability of the major alpha-neurotoxin from Micrurus nigrocinctus nigrocinctus. Eur J Biochem 1996; 238(1):231–9.
68. Ramsey GF, Klickstein GD. Coral snake bite: report of a case and suggested therapy. JAMA 1962;182(9):949–51.
69. Kitchens CS, Van Mierop LH. Envenomation by the Eastern coral snake (Micrurus fulvius fulvius): a study of 39 victims. JAMA 1987;258(12):1615–8.
70. Moseley T. Coral snake bite: recovery following symptoms of respiratory paralysis. Ann Surg 1966;163(6):943–8.
71. Morgan DL, Borys DJ, Stanford R, et al. Texas coral snake (Micrurus tener) bites. South Med J 2007;100(2):152–6.
72. Russell FE. Snake venom poisoning. 2nd edition. Great Neck (NY): Scholium International; 1983. p. 281.
73. Wingert WA, Wainschel J. Diagnosis and management of envenomation by poisonous snakes. South Med J 1975;68(8):1015–26.
74. Jansen PW, Perkin RM, VanStralen D. Mojave rattlesnake envenomation: prolonged neurotoxicity and rhabdomyolysis. Ann Emerg Med 1992;21(3): 322–5.
75. Walter FG, Chase PB, Fernandez MC, et al. Venomous snakes. In: Shannon MW, Borron SW, Burns M, editors. Haddad and winchester's clinical management of poisoning and drug overdose. 4th edition. Philadelphia: Saunders Elsevier; 2007. p. 399–422.
76. Carroll RR, Hall EL, Kitchens CS. Canebrake rattlesnake envenomation. Ann Emerg Med 1997;30(1):45–8.
77. Walker JP, Morrison RL. Current management of copperhead snakebite. J Am Coll Surg 2011;212(14):470–5.
78. Russell FE, Carlson RW, Wainschel J, et al. Snake venom poisoning in the United States experience with 550 cases. JAMA 1975;233(4):341–4.
79. Boyer LV, Seifert SA, Clark RF, et al. Recurrent and persistent coagulopathy following pit viper envenomation. Arch Intern Med 1999;159(7):706–10.
80. Guisto JA. Severe toxicity from crotalid envenomation after early resolution of symptoms. Ann Emerg Med 1995;26(3):387–9.
81. Swindel GM, Seaman KG, Arthur DC, et al. The six hour observation rule for grade I crotalid envenomation: is it sufficient? J Wilderness Med 1992;3(2):168–72.
82. Balestrieri F, Fisher S. Analgesics. In: Chernow B, editor. The pharmacologic approach to the critically ill patient. 3rd edition. Baltimore (MD): Williams & Wilkins; 1994. p. 640–50.
83. LoVecchio F, Klemens J, Welch S, et al. Antibiotics after rattlesnake envenomation. J Emerg Med 2002;23(4):327–8.

84. Clark RF, Selden BS, Furbee B. The incidence of wound infection following crotalid envenomation. J Emerg Med 1993;11(5):583–6.
85. Vomero VU, Marques MJ, Neto HS. Treatment with an anti-inflammatory drug is detrimental for muscle regeneration at Bothrops jararacussu envenoming: an experimental study. Toxicon 2009;54(3):361–3.
86. Nuchprayoon I, Pongpan C, Sripaiboonkij N. The role of prednisolone in reducing limb oedema in children bitten by green pit vipers: a randomized, controlled trial. Ann Trop Med Parasitol 2008;102(7):643–9.
87. [Package insert]CroFab® (crotalidae) polyvalent immune fab (ovine). Brentwood (TN): Protherics; 2011.
88. Norris RL, Bush SP. Bites by venomous reptiles in the Americas. In: Auerbach PS, editor. Wilderness medicine. 5th edition. Philadelphia: Mosby; 2007. p. 1051–85.
89. American College of Medical Toxicology, American Academy of Clinical Toxicology, American Association of Poison Control Centers, et al. Pressure immobilization after North American crotalinae snake envenomation. Clin Toxicol 2011;49(10):881–2.
90. Trevett AJ, Nwokolo N, Watters DA, et al. Tourniquet injury in a Papuan snakebite victim. Trop Geogr Med 1993;45(6):305–7.
91. Curry S, Kraner J, Kunkel D. Noninvasive vascular studies in management of rattlesnake envenomations to extremities. Ann Emerg Med 1985;14(11):1081–4.
92. Tanen D, Ruha A, Graeme K, et al. Epidemiology and hospital course of rattlesnake envenomations cared for at a tertiary referral center in Central Arizona. Acad Emerg Med 2001;8(2):177–82.
93. Smith TA II, Figge HL. Treatment of snakebite poisoning. Am J Hosp Pharm 1991;48(10):2190–6.
94. Tokish JT, Benjamin J, Walter F. Crotalid envenomation: the southern Arizona experience. J Orthop Trauma 2001;15(1):5–9.
95. Dart RC. Can steel heal a compartment syndrome caused by rattlesnake venom? Ann Emerg Med 2004;44(2):105–7.
96. Cumpston KL. Is there a role for fasciotomy in crotalinae envenomations in North America? Clin Toxicol 2011;49(5):351–65.
97. Hardy DL Sr, Zamudio KR. Compartment syndrome, fasciotomy, and neuropathy after a rattlesnake envenomation: aspects of monitoring and diagnosis. Wilderness Environ Med 2006;17(1):36–40.
98. Gutierrez JM, Leon G, Lomonte B, et al. Antivenoms for snakebite envenomings. Inflamm Allergy Drug Targets 2011;10(5):369–80.
99. Ruha AM, Curry SC, Albrecht C, et al. Late hematologic toxicity following treatment of rattlesnake envenomation with crotalidae polyvalent immune Fab antivenom. Toxicon 2011;57(1):53–9.
100. Seifert SA, I Kirschner R, Martin N. Recurrent, persistent, or late, new-onset hematologic abnormalities in crotaline snakebite. Clin Toxicol 2011;49(4):324–9.
101. Boyer LV, Seifert SA, Cain JS. Recurrence phenomena after immunoglobulin therapy for snake envenomations: part 2. guidelines for clinical management with crotaline Fab antivenom. Ann Emerg Med 2001;37(2):196–201.
102. [Package insert]Antivenin (micrurus fulvius), (equine origin). North American coral snake antivenin. Marietta (GA): Wyeth Laboratories; 2001.
103. Corrigan P, Russell FE, Wainschel J. Clinical reactions to antivenin. In: Rosenberg P, editor. Toxins: animal, plant and microbial. New York: Pergamon Press; 1978. p. 457–65.

104. LoVecchio F, Klemens J, Roundy EB, et al. Serum sickness following administration of antivenin (Crotalidae) polyvalent in 181 cases of presumed rattlesnake envenomation. Wilderness Environ Med 2003;14(4):200–21.

105. Warrell DA. WHO/SEARO guidelines for the clinical management of snake bites in Southeast Asian region. Southeast Asian J Trop Med Public Health 1999; 30(Suppl 1):1–85.

106. Jurkovich GJ, Luterman A, McCullar K, et al. Complications of crotalidae antivenin therapy. J Trauma 1988;28(7):1032–7.

107. Cupo P, Azevedo-Marques MM, de Menezes JB, et al. Immediate hypersensitivity reactions after intravenous use of antivenin sera: prognostic value of intradermal sensitivity tests. Rev Inst Med Trop Sao Paulo 1991;33(2):115–22.

108. Thiansookon A, Rojnuckarin P. Low incidence of early reactions to horse-derived F(ab')2 antivenom for snakebites in Thailand. Acta Trop 2008;105(2):203–5.

109. LaMonica GE, Seifert SA, Rayburn WF. Rattlesnake bites in pregnant women. J Reprod Med 2010;55(11–12):520–2.

110. Pizon AF, Riley BD, LoVecchio F, et al. Safety and efficacy of crotalidae polyvalent immune Fab in pediatric crotaline envenomations. Acad Emerg Med 2007; 14(4):373–6.

111. Offerman SR, Bush SP, Moynihan JA, et al. Crotaline Fab antivenom for the treatment of children with rattlesnake envenomation. Pediatrics 2002;110(5):968–71.

Methanol and Ethylene Glycol Intoxication

James A. Kruse, MD, FCCM[a,b,*]

KEYWORDS

- Methanol • Ethylene glycol • Intoxication • Ingestion

KEY POINTS

- More than 9000 cases of methanol and ethylene glycol ingestion were reported to the American Association of Poison Control Centers in 2010.
- Accidental or intentional ingestion of substances containing these agents can result in death, and some survivors are left with blindness, renal dysfunction, and chronic brain injury.
- Even in large ingestions, a favorable outcome is possible if the patient arrives at the hospital early enough and the poisoning is identified and appropriately treated in a timely manner.

The word alcohol is commonly used to specifically refer to ethyl alcohol or ethanol. However, in chemical terms, alcohol can refer to any hydroxyl derivative of a hydrocarbon. By extension, the suffix "-ol" is used in chemical nomenclature to designate any of various alcohols. Ethanol (CH_3-CH_2-OH) is derived from the 2-carbon hydrocarbon ethane (CH_3-CH_3) and is sometimes called grain alcohol because it can be produced by fermentation from various grains. It is the alcohol found in beer, wine, and distilled spirits such as whiskey. The simplest alcohol is methanol or methyl alcohol (**Table 1**),[1–9] derived from the 1-carbon hydrocarbon known as methane (CH_4). Methanol is also known as wood alcohol because it can be produced by the destructive distillation of wood.[2]

The worldwide demand for methanol is about 50 billion kg annually.[10] Methanol has many uses as a laboratory and industrial solvent and as a synthetic precursor. As a precursor, methanol is used in the production of certain plastics, synthetic textiles, and paints. Methanol also finds use as a fuel and antifreeze. It has been used, mainly in the past, as an antifreeze in automotive cooling systems.[6] Methanol is a constituent of certain other automotive fluids and household products (**Box 1**).[2,b] Two of particular note because of their availability at the residential level are many formulations of

[a] College of Physicians and Surgeons, Columbia University, 116 Broadway, New York, NY 10027, USA; [b] Critical Care Services, Bassett Medical Center, One Atwell Road, Cooperstown, NY 13326, USA
* Bassett Medical Center, One Atwell Road, Cooperstown, NY 13326.
E-mail address: james.kruse@bassett.org

Crit Care Clin 28 (2012) 661–711
http://dx.doi.org/10.1016/j.ccc.2012.07.002
0749-0704/12/$ – see front matter © 2012 Elsevier Inc. All rights reserved.

criticalcare.theclinics.com

Table 1
Properties of methanol and ethylene glycol

	Methanol	Ethylene Glycol
Molecular formula	CH_4O	$C_2H_6O_2$
Structural formula	CH_3-OH	$HO-CH_2-CH_2-OH$
Molecular mass (daltons)	32	62
Appearance	Clear, colorless	Clear, colorless
Physical state	Mobile liquid	Slightly viscous liquid
Aqueous solubility	Miscible	Miscible
Odor description	Slightly alcoholic	Practically odorless
Odor threshold (mg/m^3)	13.1	62.5
Taste description	Alcoholic	Sweet
Density (g/cm^3)	0.79	1.11
Vapor pressure at 20°C (torr)	96	0.06
Flammability	Highly	Slightly
Flash point (°C)	12	116
Boiling point (°C)	65	198
Freezing point (°C)	−98	−13
Freezing point, 50% solution (°C)[a]	−55	−35

[a] Aqueous solution, by weight.[1]
Data from Refs.[1–9] and other sources.

automotive windshield washer fluid, and a gelled formulation of methanol marketed in small cans for use as a food warmer under chaffing dishes (eg, Sterno brand, The Sterno Group, LLC Des Plaines, IL). Methanol is also found in many commercially available paint products, including various solvents and thinners.

Another major use of methanol is as a denaturant. Although ethanol has industrial uses other than in alcoholic beverages, potable ethanol-containing products, even if not intended for ingestion, are still subject to excise taxation and other governmental regulations. These taxes and restrictions are legally avoidable if the product contains a stipulated denaturant specifically to render the admixture unfit for human consumption. The resulting product is called denatured ethanol, or more commonly, denatured alcohol.[2] The US Code of Federal Regulations specifies many permissible denaturants and formulas, but a common one uses methanol, typically constituting 4% or 5% of the admixture.[14] Some alcoholics have been known to intentionally consume products containing denatured alcohol as a substitute for ethanol-containing beverages.[15,16] Certain countries have banned the use of methanol as a denaturant because of the health hazard posed by this practice.[17]

Methanol poisoning is most often caused by ingestions involving commercially available methanol-containing products, or from attempts to concoct alcoholic beverages from these products. Although methanol is found in small amounts in certain fruits and vegetables, and it is a metabolic product of the artificial sweetener aspartame, the quantities available from these sources do not pose a health hazard.[18,19] Similarly, small amounts of methanol are present as minor congeners in some legitimate fermented alcoholic beverages.[20,21]

The human toxicity of various alcohols depends on the specific chemical nature of the particular alcohol. The inebriating and sedative-hypnotic effects of ethanol are well known. Methanol can have similar effects, but it can also lead to substantial acute

---

Box 1
Products that may contain methanol

Denatured alcohol

Windshield washer fluids

Windshield deicers

Automotive antifreeze[a]

Carburetor cleaners

Gasohol (gasoline blends)

Race car fuels

Fuel cell fuels

Dry gas

Model airplane fuel

Portable torch fuel

Chafing-dish and camp-stove fuels

Various cleaning fluids

Embalming fluids

Octane booster in gasoline

Nonbeverage alcohol[b]

Surrogate alcohol[c]

Lacquer and paint thinners

Shellac thinners

Wood stains

Paints and varnishes

Shellacs

Dye-based wood stains

Furniture refinishers

Paint and varnish removers

Dewaxing preparations

Glass cleaners

Hobby and craft adhesives

Pipe sweeteners

Copy machine fluids

[a] Uncommon constituent of modern commercially available antifreeze products intended for automotive cooling systems, compared with ethylene glycol-based and propylene glycol-based formulations.
[b] Any alcohol not intended for human consumption.
[c] Illegally produced or homemade alcohol.
  Data from Refs.[2,5,7,11–13] and other sources.

toxicity or death if ingested in small amounts. Propyl alcohol, derived from the 3-carbon hydrocarbon propane, has 2 isomers: normal or *n*-propanol (CH_3-CH_2-CH_2-OH) and isopropanol (CH_3-CHOH-CH_3). The latter is commonly available in many rubbing alcohol formulations. Compared with methanol, isopropanol is less toxic and there are important differences in their toxicity.[11,12] Isopropanol ingestion is discussed elsewhere in this issue by Cartwright and colleagues.

Hydrocarbons containing 2 hydroxyl groups are called glycols. The glycol derived from ethane is called ethylene glycol (see **Table 1**). The estimated worldwide production of ethylene glycol exceeds 23 billion kg annually.[9] Ethylene glycol is used as the main ingredient in the most commonly available automotive antifreeze products.[1,2,6,9,22] Automotive antifreeze formulations may contain various additives such as anticorrosives, lubricants, antifoaming agents, and dyes. Sodium fluorescein, a compound that exhibits fluorescence on exposure to ultraviolet (UV) illumination, is commonly, but not universally, added to help identify automotive cooling system leaks.[2,23] Denatonium benzoate (Bitrex, Macfarlan Smith, Edinburgh, Scotland), a lidocaine derivative with an intensely disagreeable taste, is added to some antifreeze formulations and other products as an aversive agent to discourage accidental or intentional ingestion.[24] The same bittering agent is legally allowable in many countries, including the United States, as a denaturant (hence the generic name of the compound).[14] Some jurisdictions, including some states within the United States, require the addition of a bitterant in automotive antifreeze products, although a before-and-after study found no change in the frequency, severity, or rate of hospitalizations for antifreeze ingestions in children less than 5 years of age in areas where such statutes were enacted.[25]

Ethylene glycol is also found in various solvents and paint formulations, and other industrial and consumer products (**Box 2**).[2,5,7,11–13] The largest industrial use is as a synthetic precursor. For example, polyethylene terephthalate, the polymer used to make plastic carbonated beverage bottles and other containers, is produced from ethylene glycol, as is the familiar synthetic textile known as polyester (eg, Dacron brand).[2] Although these secondary products are made from ethylene glycol, they are distinct molecular entities that do not pose any direct toxic hazard. However, ethylene glycol itself, like methanol, can result in life-threatening poisoning if ingested.

The usefulness of ethylene glycol as an antifreeze derives from its low molecular mass, miscibility with water, and high boiling point (see **Table 1**). Whereas pure water freezes at 0°C, the addition of solute lowers the freezing point of the solution in proportion to the molal concentration of the solute (ie, moles of solute per kilogram of water). This colligative property requires dissolution of the solute, but is otherwise largely independent of the chemical nature of the solute. Thus, agents with limited aqueous solubility have a limited ability to affect the freezing point of water. Soluble agents that have a higher molecular mass also have limited capacity as antifreeze because for a given weight of added solute, the number of moles of solute decreases as the molecular mass of the solute increases. The lower molecular mass of methanol compared with ethylene glycol (see **Table 1**) makes methanol a more potent freezing point depressant on a weight basis.[1] However, methanol has a lower boiling point and a higher vapor pressure compared with ethylene glycol (see **Table 1**), making methanol less suitable for use in automobile cooling systems because the high running temperatures of internal combustion engines can lead to loss of the alcohol by vaporization.

Some automotive antifreeze formulations are made from propylene glycol and marketed as a less toxic alternative to ethylene glycol. Propylene glycol is considered generally safe by the US Food and Drug Administration,[26] and it is used as an additive in some food products, a base in some cosmetics and topical medicines, and a diluent

---

Box 2
Products that may contain ethylene glycol

Automotive antifreezes

Aircraft deicing fluids

Refrigerating fluids

Solar collector fluids

Automotive brake fluids

Car wash fluids

Hydraulic fluids

Heat transfer fluids

Coolants

Pesticides

Herbicides

Wood preservatives

Shoe polishes

Electrolytic capacitors

Theatrical fog generators

Paints, lacquers, paint products

Polishing compounds

Liquid detergents

Stamp-pad and ballpoint pen inks

Printer inks

Fire extinguisher (soybean oil-based) foam

Embalming fluids

Tobacco humectants

Adhesive humectants

Insect specimen killing-jar fluids

Cellophane softeners

Drywall joint compounds

Drying agents

Photographic developing fluids

Simulated smoke generators

Data from Refs.[2,5,7,11–13] and other sources.

---

in several parenteral pharmaceuticals. Propylene glycol is metabolized largely to lactic acid, which is metabolized to carbon dioxide and water. On the other hand, methanol and ethylene glycol are metabolized to toxic compounds that are responsible for their adverse effects. Although the metabolism and clinical manifestations of methanol and ethylene glycol differ from one another, both compounds can cause coma, severe metabolic acidosis, and death. Given the lethal potential of these 2 compounds, and given that antidotal therapy is available and potentially effective if administered in a timely fashion, clinical recognition of occult toxic ingestions with either compound can be of critical importance. There is substantial similarity but also some important differences in the clinical identification and treatment of poisoning with these 2 agents.

METABOLISM AND TOXICITY

Methanol and ethylene glycol are rapidly absorbed by the gastrointestinal (GI) tract, with peak plasma levels attained in 30 minutes to 1 hour and 1 to 4 hours, respectively. Methanol can penetrate skin to an extent, and it is mildly volatile.[27] As a result, there have been reported cases of poisoning by extensive dermal contact or inhalation, but these presentations are rare.[28–32] Unlike methanol, cutaneous contact and inhalation are not sources of acute systemic toxicity for ethylene glycol. Significant ethylene glycol absorption through intact skin does not occur with casual exposure. The vapor pressure of ethylene glycol is too low to lead to excessive inhalational exposure at room temperature (see **Table 1**). Inhalational exposure to ethylene glycol vapor is possible at increased temperatures or with aerosolized mists. However, airborne ethylene glycol concentrations high enough to theoretically result in significant inhalational absorption rapidly lead to intolerable throat and mucous membrane irritation, thereby preventing significant exposure.[33]

The minimal lethal doses of methanol and ethylene glycol are not well established. Available information suggests that there is considerable person-to-person variability. There are several known factors that can affect this variability, including the degree of dilution of the methanol or ethylene glycol contained in the specific formulation ingested, the presence of coingestants (notably ethanol), whether vomiting occurs, and renal function. A commonly cited minimum lethal dose for methanol is 15 mL, but there are case reports of patients surviving ingestions of hundreds of milliliters.[34] Similarly, the minimum lethal dose for ethylene glycol is commonly cited as 100 mL or 1 to 1.5 mL/kg, but also with considerable variability.[35] These reports are based either on animal experiments or from clinical reports that are mostly anecdotal, dependent on case histories, and probably often involve various degrees of unknown or unspecified dilutions rather than pure methanol or ethylene glycol. As described later, an important factor that can influence the response to a given volume of ingestion is the degree of concomitant ethanol ingestion, if any.

Taken internally, both compounds have volumes of distribution in the range of 0.5 to 0.8 L/kg body weight[35,36] and metabolism is chiefly hepatic. A minor fraction of both compounds is excreted in the urine. Because of its relatively high vapor pressure (see **Table 1**), some methanol is also eliminated by the lungs, affording the potential for recognizing ingestions by the breath odor of a poisoned patient, although the odor of methanol resembles ethanol. Untreated, the apparent elimination half-life of methanol ranges from 1 to 3 hours at low concentrations, and approximately 24 hours at high concentration. For ethylene glycol, the corresponding half-life ranges from 3 to 9 hours. These apparent half-lives are prolonged in the presence of ethanol.

Similar to ethanol, methanol and ethylene glycol have inebriating and sedating effects on the central nervous system (CNS), but the inherent toxicity of these compounds per se is low. However, both compounds are oxidized to intermediate metabolites that possess substantial cytotoxicity. Both compounds are initially metabolized chiefly by dehydrogenase enzymes in conjunction with the oxidized form of the cofactor nicotinamide adenine dinucleotide (NAD^+). The first reaction is catalyzed by alcohol dehydrogenase, which is capable of oxidizing certain hydroxyl-containing carbon atoms to aldehydes. A second enzyme, aldehyde dehydrogenase, then converts the aldehyde to a corresponding carboxylic acid. For methanol, this reaction sequence can be represented as[37]:

$$CH_3-OH \xrightarrow[\text{Alcohol dehydrogenase}]{NAD^+ \quad NADH + H^+} H-\overset{O}{\underset{}{C}}-H \xrightarrow[H_2O \quad \text{Aldehyde dehydrogenase}]{NAD^+ \quad NADH + H^+} H-\overset{O}{\underset{}{C}}-OH$$

Methanol   Formaldehyde   Formic acid

Conversion of methanol to formaldehyde occurs slowly, and constitutes the rate-limiting step of this reaction sequence. Both formaldehyde and formic acid are cytotoxic, but formaldehyde, with a half-life of 1 to 2 minutes, is present only transiently and does not accumulate. The formic acid molecule largely dissociates, releasing a hydrogen cation and a formate anion:

$$H-\overset{O}{\underset{}{C}}-OH \longrightarrow H^+ + H-\overset{O}{\underset{}{C}}-O^-$$

Formic acid   Formate

The released hydrogen ion lowers the pH of body fluids, and formate accumulates because it is only slowly metabolized to carbon dioxide or excreted by the kidney. Much of the resulting hydrogen ion production from this dissociation reaction is neutralized by bicarbonate ions present in body fluids, depleting bicarbonate and generating carbon dioxide, which is excreted by the lungs:

$$HCOOH + HCO_3^- \longrightarrow HCOO^- + H_2O + CO_2$$

Formic acid   Bicarbonate   Formate   exhaled

Because the buffering of hydrogen ions is incomplete, hydrogen ion accumulation also occurs, resulting in acidemia.

Formate exerts its cytotoxic effects, at least in part, by inhibiting cytochrome aa3 and cytochrome c oxidase and thereby interfering with intramitochondrial electron transport.[38–42] This interference does not cause cellular hypoxia, but it prevents oxygen use by mitochondria, slowing or stopping oxidative phosphorylation in the manner similar to that of cyanide or carbon monoxide.[42] Although tissue oxygenation may increase because of continued tissue oxygen delivery and decreased cellular uptake, the end effect is similar to that of hypoxia in that there is decreased aerobic production of adenosine triphosphate (ATP). Thus, formate inhibits and prevents ATP-requiring intracellular reactions from taking place, compromising cellular function and homeostasis. Critical degrees of interference with these cytochromes result in cellular injury and death. The CNS seems to be especially sensitive to the toxic effects of formate. Retinal and optic nerve neurons, perhaps because of peculiarities in their mitochondrial density, may be particularly susceptible to the adverse effects of formate.[38,43–49] The basal ganglia, particularly the putamen, and subcortical white matter also seem to have greater sensitivity to formate toxicity.[50–54]

The metabolism of ethylene glycol is more complex than methanol. As with methanol, alcohol dehydrogenase acts to oxidize a hydroxyl-containing carbon atom to a corresponding aldehyde[55]:

$$\begin{matrix} CH_2OH \\ | \\ CH_2OH \end{matrix} + NAD^+ \xrightarrow{\text{Alcohol dehydrogenase}} \begin{matrix} O_{\diagdown}\overset{}{C}\diagup^H \\ | \\ CH_2OH \end{matrix} + NADH + H^+$$

Ethylene glycol   Glycoaldehyde

This reaction constitutes 1 of 2 important rate-limiting steps of the overall metabolic pathway. Glycoaldehyde quickly undergoes further oxidation at either the aldehyde moiety by aldehyde dehydrogenase, or to a lesser extent, at the alcohol moiety by a cytochrome P450 enzyme (CYP2E1)[56,57]:

NADP$^+$ NADPH + H$^+$ → (CYP2E1, 2H$_2$O, O$_2$$^{\cdot-}$) → NAD$^+$ NADH + H$^+$ → (Aldehyde dehydrogenase, H$_2$O)

Glyoxal   Glycoaldehyde   Glycolic acid

resulting in production of glyoxal and glycolic acid. Glyoxal is then metabolized to glycolic acid or to glyoxylic acid[58,59]:

H$_2$O (Glutathione, Glyoxalase I and II) ←   NAD$^+$ NADH + H$^+$ → (α-Oxoaldehyde dehydrogenase, H$_2$O)

Glycolic acid   Glyoxal   Glyoxylic acid

Next, glycolic acid is converted to glyoxylic acid either by glycolate oxidase or lactate dehydrogenase (LDH), a conversion that constitutes the second important rate-limiting step of the overall sequence.[60] Glyoxylic acid is then converted to oxalic acid mainly by LDH but also to some degree by glycolate oxidase[61–64]:

NAD$^+$ NADH + H$^+$ (LDH and Glycolate oxidase, O$_2$, H$_2$O$_2$) →   NAD$^+$ NADH + H$^+$ (LDH and Glycolate oxidase, O$_2$, H$_2$O$_2$) →

Glycolic acid   Glyoxylic acid   Oxalic acid

Glycolic, glyoxylic, and oxalic acid all largely dissociate under physiologic conditions, releasing hydrogen ions from their carboxylic acid (R-COOH) moieties. Animal model and human autopsy examinations often reveal extensive crystal formation visible by light microscopy in various tissues including the renal tubules, brain, meninges, blood vessel walls, liver, spleen, pericardium, and cardiac conduction system.[65–74] These crystals have been identified as calcium oxalate, the poorly soluble calcium salt of oxalic acid, which forms in aqueous solutions of oxalic acid in the presence of calcium ions under certain chemicophysical conditions[61–63]:

+ Ca^{2+} → (H$_2$O) → Ca^{2+} + 2H$^+$

Oxalic acid   Calcium oxalate

Calcium oxalate cannot be further metabolized by humans and is effectively an end product of ethylene glycol metabolism.[63]

The pathologic finding of extensive oxalate crystal formation in the renal tubules was long accepted as the mechanism by which ethylene glycol poisoning resulted in the clinical manifestation of acute renal failure, either by causing renal tubular obstruction or by a direct cytotoxic effect of oxalate on the renal tubules. This putative mechanism was a logical presumption given that individuals with the autosomal-recessive inborn error of metabolism known as primary oxaluria or congenital oxalosis excrete large amounts of calcium oxalate and develop widespread crystal deposition, including nephrocalcinosis, which leads to renal failure, often in childhood.[63,75] Type I primary hyperoxaluria is caused by a gene mutation, resulting in genetic deficiency of hepatic peroxisomal alanine:glyoxylate aminotransferase, whereas type II is caused by deficiency of the cytosolic enzyme glyoxylate reductase.[76,77] Deficiency of either enzyme results in markedly increased oxalate excretion.

Besides micro-obstructive nephropathy by calcium oxalate, or oxalate-induced acute tubular necrosis, other postulated mechanisms of renal toxicity from ethylene glycol poisoning have included direct renal cytotoxicity from 1 or more of the intermediary metabolites, focal hemorrhagic cortical necrosis, other mechanisms of acute tubular necrosis, and interstitial nephritis.[75,78–82] Glycolate and glyoxylate are increased in primary oxalosis, and these or other intermediates may be factors in the pathogenesis of renal failure in that congenital disease.[75] In an isolated murine proximal tubular segment model and in cultured human tubular cells, incubation with ethylene glycol, glycolate, or oxalate had little overt effect on various measures of tubular injury. Conversely, glycoaldehyde and glyoxylate showed a high degree of toxicity, inducing profound ATP depletion, LDH release, and tubular cell death.[83] Glycoaldehyde also caused LDH and phospholipid degradation. Glyoxylate was shown to inhibit mitochondrial electron transport and oxidative phosphorylation, and inhibit the Krebs cycle.[84] Glyoxal also has cytotoxicity, forming reactive oxygen species, collapsing the mitochondrial membrane potential, inducing lipid peroxidation, and inhibiting cellular respiration.[58,59,85] The acid and aldehyde intermediates of ethylene glycol metabolism seem to have other toxic effects, such as interfering with glucose metabolism, blocking protein synthesis, and inhibiting nucleic acid synthesis and replication.[59,84,85]

CLINICAL HISTORY AND MANIFESTATIONS

Methanol and ethylene glycol ingestions occur under several different circumstances, either as isolated single cases or as epidemics. Individual cases occur sporadically and are either accidental (most cases) or intentional. Accidental cases may involve children or adults and arise from inadvertently drinking methanol-containing or ethylene glycol-containing products, often after the product has been transferred unwisely to a used beverage bottle or other container that suggests the liquid is potable.[67,86–88] Intentional cases have involved persons with suicidal intentions,[69,87,89] or rarely, cases in which the ingestion was unintentional on the part of the victim, but a matter of surreptitious or forced administration by another person with criminal intent.[65,90] Intentional ingestions also occur in desperate alcoholics who have no available ethanol-containing beverages and purposely ingest methanol-containing or glycol-containing products as a substitute, either not realizing that the substance is toxic, or with full awareness of the potential for harm.[70]

Many epidemics, some involving hundreds of people, have occurred involving either methanol[34,43,86,91–96] or ethylene glycol.[67,69,71,97] Most of these clusters resulted from preparing illicit beverages using methanol or ethylene glycol either in addition to or in place of ethanol, in some cases with the notion that the substitution would make for a more potent or fortified mixture. Cases of ethylene glycol intoxication have also occurred because of contaminated water systems.[97]

Determining that an accidental or intentional toxic ingestion has occurred is straightforward when the patient is willing and able to provide a firsthand historical account. Diagnosis can be more challenging when an accurate history cannot be obtained from the patient because of either an alteration in mental status or unwillingness on the part of the patient to divulge details of the history. In the case of intentional ingestion, this unwillingness may stem from the patient's notion that there could be adverse legal or social repercussions to their admission, or it may be inexplicable.[98,99]

The presentation in occult cases is often a patient with any of a large variety of symptoms, but most commonly there is some degree of alteration in mental status, with or without findings of metabolic acidosis on routine laboratory testing. Knowledge of the potential manifestations that can occur in methanol and ethylene glycol intoxication and a high index of suspicion are critically important in these occult cases because failure to recognize the problem and institute prompt treatment can lead to a poor outcome. On the other hand, a favorable outcome is possible even in large-volume ingestions if the patient arrives at the hospital without undue delay and appropriate therapy is initiated in a timely manner.

The clinical manifestations of both methanol and ethylene glycol poisoning depend on the amount ingested, the elapsed time since ingestion, and whether there was coingestion of ethanol or other toxic substances. The findings in early presentations can be similar to ethanol ingestion, namely epigastric distress or nausea caused by irritant effects on the gastric mucosa. These effects are soon followed by inebriation and CNS depression, which are caused by the parent compound and are proportional to the amount consumed. Further CNS depression, cytotoxicity to CNS tissue, and cardiopulmonary failure can evolve subsequently, stemming from the metabolic products of the parent compounds.

Manifestations of Methanol Poisoning

As with ethanol, methanol results in inebriation and can cause drowsiness. These are direct CNS effects of methanol per se, but methanol itself seems to cause no other important manifestations other than GI irritation. GI irritation frequently results in abdominal distress and vomiting. Hemorrhagic gastritis and diarrhea have also been described, but otherwise the parent compound, methanol, may be considered nontoxic.[93] If at this point, the patient's history does not explicitly reveal exposure to methanol, clinicians may mistakenly attribute the inebriation, sedation, and gastric symptoms solely to ethanol intake. Although the odor of methanol is fainter than that of ethanol, there is a resemblance that, if detected on the patient's breath, may promote this misconception. Subsequently, a latent period characteristically intervenes, during which the ingested methanol is slowly undergoing metabolism to formic acid. The inebriation may subside and in some cases there is a period in which the patient is relatively asymptomatic. This latent period can range from 6 to 30 hours, but is absent in some cases and longer in other cases.[36,43,93]

More serious effects follow this latent period, after a significant amount of methanol has been metabolized to formate. As formate accumulates, the most characteristic and often most prominent symptom is some type of visual disturbance marking the end of the latent period. These ocular manifestations can range from mildly impaired acuity, such as blurred vision or seeing spots, to total blindness with complete lack of light perception. A type of bright visual field blindness akin to snow-field blindness has been described. A wide variety of other ocular signs and symptoms may be seen (**Box 3**). In survivors, the ocular effects may be permanent or may resolve, partially or fully.

Hyperpnea (ie, Kussmaul respirations) may be seen secondary to the severe metabolic acidosis that eventually develops when enough methanol is metabolized.[34,93] Apart from the initial inebriation, CNS manifestation that can occur after the latent period may include headache, confusion, and stupor.[34,45,93,95,96,101–103,116] Seizures are a common manifestation if sufficient formate accumulation occurs.[47,93,104–106,117] In severe cases coma, cerebral edema, brain injury, and herniation may occur.[51] Severe reversible cardiac failure has also been reported in methanol intoxication,[101] and circulatory shock is not rare.[47,54,96,100,101,118] Respiratory arrest, sometimes dramatically sudden, has been described.[34,47,106]

The predilection of formate for injuring the basal ganglia and subcortical white matter has been shown by computed tomography and magnetic resonance imaging in numerous case reports of methanol poisoning.[52,53,104,106–109,119,120] The putamen is most often affected, with either hemorrhagic or nonhemorrhagic necrosis evident on imaging or at autopsy.[47,51,54,102,107–109,119,121]

Manifestations of Ethylene Glycol Poisoning

A useful model for understanding the evolution of ethylene glycol intoxication is to consider 3 sequential stages of effects. However, in practice, there is frequently overlap in these stages and the development, timing, and severity of each stage can vary. In some cases, a particular stage may not even occur. Nevertheless, the first stage, which often develops about 30 minutes to several hours after ingestion, begins with the symptoms and signs of inebriation and may be accompanied by headache, dizziness, euphoria, or strange behavior.[65,67,68,70,122–124] This inebriation may be indistinguishable on physical examination from that of ethanol intoxication. However, unless the patient has also recently ingested ethanol, there should be no odor of alcohol on the patient's breath.[70,82,125] GI and abdominal complaints may occur early on, because ethylene glycol, much as with ethanol and methanol, can produce gastric irritation, resulting in abdominal pain and in some cases vomiting. Subsequently, more serious CNS manifestations may develop and be superimposed on the initial inebriation. This first stage can persist beyond 12 hours, with the neurologic manifestations progressively worsening in severe cases. These serious CNS effects often include more severe depression in the level of consciousness, in some cases progressing to deep coma. Seizures, including status epilepticus, are common in severe cases,[68–70,72,82,90,126–135] along with a broad spectrum of other neurologic abnormalities (**Boxes 4** and **5**). Computed tomography and magnetic resonance imaging in ethylene glycol–poisoned patients have shown cerebral edema and hypodensities involving the medulla, pons, midbrain, thalamus, diencephalon, cerebellum, basal ganglia, temporal lobes, and periventricular and central white matter.[69,136–138] Sterile meningitis and encephalitis have also been observed on postmortem examination.[65,71,72]

Unlike methanol poisoning, ethylene glycol is not characteristically associated with ocular findings. Nevertheless, ocular abnormalities have been observed in some cases of ethylene glycol intoxication, and a wide variety of ocular signs and symptoms have been reported.[70–72,82,86,125,134,138,139] Some of these reports may have involved coingestion of methanol, although in most reports the history did not uncover concomitant methanol. Some reports are clear that the ingestant was antifreeze, but may not recognize that methanol has also been used for its antifreeze properties.[1,2,5,6,22,87,151,153] In other cases, cerebral edema, herniation, or widespread brain injury are likely responsible for the ocular findings, rather than any specific proclivity for ocular toxicity.[138]

The second stage, typically occurring 12 to 24 hours after ingestion, is characterized by cardiopulmonary manifestations. Hyperpnea is frequently evident early in this stage as a consequence of respiratory compensation for severe metabolic acidosis.[67,70,125,128,138] In some cases, endotracheal intubation is required for airway protection because of severe CNS depression. In other cases, pulmonary edema with attendant respiratory distress may occur and be the cause of frank respiratory failure.[140] Tachycardia or bradycardia, and either hypotension or hypertension can

Box 3
Clinical manifestations of methanol intoxication from case reports and case series

GI manifestations
- Abdominal distress
- Abdominal tenderness
- Nausea, vomiting
- Diarrhea
- Hyperamylasemia
- Pancreatitis
- Abnormal liver function tests

Ocular manifestations
- Impaired visual acuity
- Permanent visual acuity deficit
- Permanent blindness
- Blurred vision
- Total blindness
- Absent light perception
- Snow-field blindness
- Central scotomata
- Other visual field defects
- Photophobia
- Eye pain
- Burning eyes
- Seeing spots
- Optic disk hyperemia
- Retinal edema or papilledema
- Other funduscopic abnormalities
- Diminished pupillary light reflex
- Afferent pupillary defect
- Absent pupillary light reflex

Nonocular neurologic manifestations
- Inebriation
- Headache
- Dizziness
- Lightheadedness
- Fatigue
- Restlessness
- Confusion
- Lethargy
- Somnolence

- Stupor
- Agitation
- Impaired speech
- Pseudobulbar palsy
- Ataxia
- Seizures
- Coma

Other manifestations:

- Methanol or ethanol odor on breath
- Formalin odor on breath
- Kussmaul respirations
- Dyspnea
- Rhabdomyolysis
- Cardiac failure
- Hypotension
- Pulmonary edema
- Respiratory arrest
- Death

Data from Refs.[28,30,31,34,43,45,47,50,51,54,86,91,93,95,96,100–115]

occur, with some patients developing congestive heart failure.[70,82] Frank circulatory shock can ensue, in some cases unresponsive to intravascular volume expansion and requiring vasopressor administration.[69,72,100,130,135] These cardiopulmonary effects may be caused by deposition of oxalate crystals in the heart, lungs, and vasculature, or direct effects of other toxic intermediates at the cellular level in these organ systems. In fatal cases, death most often develops during this phase.

If the patient survives the neurologic and cardiopulmonary manifestations, severe acute renal failure often develops, marking the third stage of ethylene glycol poisoning, which typically develops 24 to 72 hours after ingestion.[67,69,82,90,99,122,123,130,139,141–143] The acute renal failure can be prolonged enough to necessitate hemodialysis, sometimes continuing long after the patient otherwise recovers.[99,130] The renal failure may be oliguric, anuric, or nonoliguric.[130] Conscious patients may complain of flank pain.[67,122] Microscopic or gross hematuria can occur.[67]

Delayed development of neurologic deficits involving various cranial nerves, particularly the facial and auditory nerves, has been observed in some patients (see **Box 5**). Although not included in classic descriptions of the temporal staging of ethylene glycol poisoning, some investigators have referred to this phenomenon as a fourth stage.[99,135]

LABORATORY FINDINGS

Measurements of plasma or serum methanol and ethylene glycol concentrations can provide confirmation of toxic exposure with these agents. However, quantitative assays for these substances are not available on-site at most hospital laboratories;

Box 4
Clinical manifestation of ethylene glycol intoxication from case reports and case series[a]

Stage I: predominately CNS manifestations (30 minutes–12 hours after ingestion)

Early manifestations

- Inebriation
- No odor of ethanol on patient's breath[b]
- Abdominal distress, nausea, vomiting

Later CNS manifestations[c]

- Headache
- Confusion
- Strange behavior
- Combative behavior
- Agitation
- Stupor
- Coma
- Seizures, status epilepticus
- Ataxia
- Hyporeflexia or areflexia
- Hyperreflexia
- Myoclonus
- Tetany
- Extensor plantar reflexes
- Decerebrate posturing
- Quadriplegia
- Cranial nerve deficits (see **Box 5**)
- Brain death

Stage II: cardiopulmonary manifestations (12–24 hours after ingestion)

- Hyperpnea
- Respiratory failure
- Tachycardia or bradycardia
- Hypertension
- Hypotension
- Pulmonary infiltrates or edema
- Congestive heart failure
- Circulatory shock
- Death

Stage III: renal manifestations (24–72 hours after ingestion)

- Acute renal failure
- Permanent renal failure (not typical)
- Flank pain

- Gross hematuria
- Death

Stage IV: delayed-onset neuropathy

- Cranial nerve deficits (see **Box 5**)
- Gait disturbance
- Dysmetria
- Ankle clonus
- Extensor plantar reflexes
- Ascending motor/sensory neuropathy

[a] There is frequently overlap in these depicted stages, and the development, timing, and severity of each stage can widely vary in practice.
[b] Odor of ethanol may be present if patient also consumed ethanol.
[c] Late CNS manifestations may overlap the initial inebriation.
   Data from Refs.[65,67–72,82,86,90,98,99,104,121–135,137–151]

and where they are available, there are important caveats to their interpretation. In cases in which there is credible history of methanol or ethylene glycol ingestion, with or without toxic clinical manifestations, simple laboratory testing available at most hospitals can provide important corroborative evidence for the exposure and also help evaluate whether toxic metabolites have begun to accumulate and which treatment modalities are indicated. For cases in which history is unavailable or incomplete, these screening laboratory tests are even more important, particularly if on-site measurements of methanol and ethylene glycol are not available.

Methanol and Ethylene Glycol Assays

Several assay methods have been developed for quantifying methanol and ethylene glycol concentrations in serum or plasma. There are colorimetric and enzymatic assays, but they have had major limitations with respect to specificity.[154–157] Colorimetric enzymatic assays have been commercially available recently in the United States for both methanol and ethylene glycol, but only for veterinary use (Catachem, Oxford, CT). Gas chromatography (GC) has been considered a criterion standard method for detection and quantification of methanol. Headspace GC is a common and potentially accurate technique in which a sample is introduced in the vapor phase into a chromatographic column. As the injectate moves through the column, the constituent compounds undergo separation according to their individual retention times. Headspace GC is commonly used for performing volatile alcohol screens, which often include methanol, ethanol, isopropanol, and acetone. Headspace GC is not usable for assaying ethylene glycol because of the high boiling point, high polarity, and low vapor pressure of this compound (see **Table 1**). This restriction can be circumvented by performing a preliminary chemical reaction to transform any ethylene glycol in the sample to a less polar and more volatile derivative (eg, various boronic esters). Actual detection and quantification of these analytes is best accomplished by coupling the exit port of the GC column to a flame ionization detector or mass spectrometer. Together, these techniques represent current state-of-the-art methods used to determine ethylene glycol and volatile alcohols concentrations. Although these methods can provide accurate results, the equipment is expensive, labor-intensive

---

Box 5
Cranial nerve deficits in ethylene glycol intoxication from case reports and case series

- Decreased visual acuity[a]
- Anisocoria[a]
- Pinpoint pupils
- Dilated pupils
- Nonreactive pupils
- Optic atrophy
- Papilledema[a]
- Absent corneal reflex[a]
- Ophthalmoplegia
- Absent oculocephalic reflex
- Absent oculovestibular reflex on caloric testing
- Diplopia
- Loss of accommodation
- Gaze paralysis
- Nystagmus[a]
- Facial diplegia[a]
- Facial droop[a]
- Facial sensory loss[a]
- Complete bilateral deafness[a]
- Dysarthria[a]
- Dysphagia[a]
- Vertigo or dizziness
- Absent gag reflex[a]

[a] Includes reported cases of delayed cranial neuropathy first occurring days to weeks after initial presentation.
   Data from Refs.[67,70–72,82,90,99,121,125,133–135,138,139,143,148,150,152]

---

to operate and maintain, and cannot be automated. As a result, these assays are available only at some, typically large, hospitals or medical centers, and at reference laboratories, but they are not available in the clinical chemistry laboratories of most hospitals in the United States.[155,158]

Even where these sophisticated GC methods are available, specific analytical precautions are necessary to avoid erroneous results. The type of column used and the internal reference standards selected are critical factors.[159–161] In addition, results must be interpreted cautiously. For example, false-positive results have been reported in patients with certain disease states and in patients with nontoxic levels of other glycols, such as 2,3-butanediol and propylene glycol.[162,163] False-positive ethylene glycol levels have been reported in patients with certain inborn errors of metabolism.[154,157,160] In 1 case, erroneous attribution of malicious poisoning led to criminal charges of homicide and imprisonment of a mother for allegedly poisoning her child, later overturned when ample evidence showed the assay findings to be false-positives.[164,165] Reports suggest that 2,3-butanediol, which may be produced in small amounts by chronic alcoholics or derived from methylethylketone ingested in surrogate alcoholic beverages, can be misinterpreted as ethylene glycol on gas chromatograms.[162,163,166] Propylene glycol is used as a vehicle in some parenteral drug formulations (eg, lorazepam, phenytoin, and nitroglycerin), and although usual doses of these drugs do not result in propylene glycol toxicity, plasma levels can be sufficient to trigger false-positive ethylene glycol levels when certain GC methods are used without suitable precautions.[159,161,167] In 1 report, false-positive ethylene glycol levels were explained by propylene glycol-containing medicines remaining in the dead space of a central venous catheter from which blood specimens were subsequently obtained for the ethylene glycol assay.[167]

Careful interpretation also requires consideration that the assay result may not represent the patient's peak plasma concentration. The circulating concentration could continue to increase because of ongoing GI absorption, or more commonly, the plasma level may have already peaked before obtaining the blood specimen. In the latter situation, even although the concentration of the parent compound may be relatively low, there potentially could be lethal concentrations of circulating toxic metabolites. Measurements of plasma formate, in the case of methanol ingestion, or glycolate in the case of ethylene glycol ingestion, would logically provide important information on the degree of intoxication, and this conclusion is supported by clinical observations.[116,168] Formate and glycolate assays are even less likely to be clinically available than methanol or ethylene glycol levels, especially on an urgent basis.[90,169]

Screening Laboratory Tests

The low molecular mass of methanol and ethylene glycol, coupled with their low intrinsic toxicity, at least for the untransformed molecules, allows for large molar concentrations of these substances to exist in the circulation in the immediate period after ingestion and GI absorption. In such cases, plasma osmolality, which represents the total molal concentration of all osmotically active solutes in plasma, increases in proportion to the concentration of methanol or ethylene glycol. Measurement of serum osmolality thus provides a clue to ingestion of these agents if the result is abnormally high and not explained by some other physiologic derangement. Azotemia, as well as hyperglycemia or hypernatremia, all tend to increase plasma osmolality as a result of increased urea, glucose, and sodium concentrations, respectively, in the absence of methanol or ethylene glycol. The serum osmole gap provides a simple screening method of checking for increased osmolality that is not explained by these other factors.[170] (See the toxidrome article elsewhere in this issue for further information on the serum osmole gap, including its calculation and important caveats and limitations regarding its interpretation.)

As methanol and ethylene glycol are metabolized, their plasma concentrations decrease and their contribution to plasma osmolality and the osmole gap also decline. Thus, even if the osmole gap was strikingly increased at some point, if the patient presents after much or all of the toxic alcohol or glycol has been metabolized, the serum osmole gap could have returned to a value within the normal range, yet there might be lethal concentrations of circulating toxic metabolites. In both their neutral and their anionic form, these toxic acid metabolites possess osmotic activity; however, in their anionic form they displace osmotically active bicarbonate anions and thus the acid anions have no net effect on osmolality. Nevertheless, the accumulating organic anions may be detectable by their associated effects on the serum anion gap and arterial pH.[171] Routine serum electrolyte panels include a measure of total carbon dioxide content (tCO_2) that, if low, should raise suspicion of metabolic acidosis. Low tCO_2 content and high anion gap together indicate a limited number of causes of metabolic acidosis, methanol, and ethylene glycol intoxication among them. Arterial blood gas analysis further helps to characterize the acid-base disturbance.[172] The interpretation, differential diagnosis, and limitations of a high anion gap metabolic acidosis are explained elsewhere in this issue, but both methanol and ethylene glycol intoxication are considerations in the appropriate clinical context.[173]

An increased serum osmole gap in conjunction with a normal serum anion gap and the absence of metabolic acidosis is expected early in the postingestion period, before there has been significant transformation of methanol to formate or ethylene glycol to glycolate. The serum osmole gap subsequently decreases toward normal as the metabolic acidosis develops and worsens, and as the anion gap increases, signifying accumulation of the toxic metabolites. In ethylene glycol intoxication, there is correlation between plasma glycolate (the predominant acid anion) and both arterial blood pH[60,126] and the serum anion gap.[90,131,174] Plasma formate levels in methanol intoxication correlate with blood pH[45,106,117,175–178] and serum anion gap.[91,116,118] Once developed, the acidosis of methanol and ethylene glycol poisoning is often severe and the serum anion gap is often increased to strikingly high levels (**Table 2**).

Table 2
Selected laboratory findings in methanol and ethylene glycol intoxication[a]

Finding	Methanol Intoxication	Ethylene Glycol Intoxication
Arterial pH		
>7.2	54,91,93,96,179	90,98,131,180
7.11–7.20	54,93,96,110,179,181	69,70,82,90,98,99,131,144,145,182
7.01–7.10	54,179	90,128,131,132,146
6.91–7.00	91,104,111,179	90,126–128,131–133,135,138,147,148,183
6.81–6.90	54,91,109,117,118,179	72,90,125,128,130,138,142,149,184
6.71–6.80	47,53,54,101,102,105,106,179	90,131,134,140
6.61–6.70	31,49,54,96,105,112,179	69
6.51–6.60	91,100	141
≤6.5	28,92,96	—
Serum anion gap (mEq/L)		
20–29	54,91,102	90,98,99,128,133,135,144,146,147,180,183
30–39	31,54,91,100,103,106,181	70,82,90,123,125,127–129,131,132,134,141,149,184,185
40–49	49,54,91,104	90,128,131,138,142,145
≥50	54,91,92	72
Blood lactate (mmol/L)		
1–1.9	—	98,125,131,147
2–2.9	91,104,106	180,185
3–3.9	91	129
4–4.9	—	82,131,132
≥5	91,106	72,98,128,131,184
Crystalluria	—	67–71,82,90,97,98,123,125–129,131,132,134,135,138,141,142,146–148,183,185–188

[a] From selected published reports and case series (see reference list). For reports with multiple values, most extreme reported values are listed. Early presentation cases treated by pharmacologic inhibition are generally not represented.

On the other hand, metabolic acidosis may be absent and the serum anion gap completely normal even in patients who have ingested large volumes of methanol or ethylene glycol. This situation occurs when the patient presents soon after the ingestion and there has not been sufficient time for transformation to the acid metabolites. History suggesting the possibility of methanol or ethylene glycol ingestion, or conducive physical findings in an appropriate clinical context, should therefore prompt further investigation even if there are no signs of metabolic acidosis or increased anion gap.

If the patient's history is incomplete, further efforts at obtaining history should be sought from any available sources. Evaluation of the serum osmole gap can provide important additional information. For hospitals that lack the capability to perform methanol and ethylene glycol assays on site, sending blood specimens to a reference laboratory for off-site analysis imposes an obligatory time delay, which can range to several days.[189] Given the potential for morbidity and mortality if the patient has ingested either methanol or ethylene glycol, withholding treatment while awaiting off-site assay results to confirm the diagnosis is potentially perilous. For cases in which the history of methanol or ethylene glycol exposure is obvious, prompt initiation of treatment is easily accomplished. However, when the history is incomplete but the possibility of exposure is a consideration, finding an otherwise unexplained high anion gap metabolic acidosis or an increased serum osmole gap can provide corroborating evidence for alcohol or glycol intoxication. Because delaying initiation of life-saving therapy could have lethal consequences, these alternative means of inferring the diagnosis can be useful, although they have limitations in sensitivity and specificity.[170,171,173]

Crystalluria

Methanol intoxication is not associated with crystalluria, but case reports and case series of patients with ethylene glycol poisoning have frequently documented observation of calcium oxalate crystals on urinalysis (see **Table 2**). In the appropriate setting, this finding is conducive to the diagnosis; however, false-positive and false-negative results can occur. For example, calcium oxalate crystalluria is observed in patients with certain intestinal disorders, and in patients with the rare disorder known as primary hyperoxaluria. Oxalate crystals have also been documented in unselected patients without known urologic disease.[190] Normal individuals may develop hyperoxaluria, with or without crystal formation, after ingesting foods that are high in oxalate and after large doses of ascorbic acid. On the other hand, the absence of oxalate crystalluria by urinalysis does not exclude ethylene glycol poisoning, as has been attested by case reports.[72,124,143,180,184] In some cases of ethylene glycol poisoning, urinalysis failed to reveal any crystals, but pathologic examination of the kidneys showed marked calcium oxalate crystal deposition within the renal tubules and interstitium and in some cases at extrarenal sites as well.[72,143] Absence of crystalluria may be caused by timing of obtaining the urine specimen, or particular physicochemical properties of the patient's urine that do not favor crystal formation.[129,191] Patients presenting soon after ethylene glycol ingestion and those who are given pharmacotherapy to prevent metabolic breakdown of the glycol may never develop oxaluria. Also, crystals may simply be overlooked or unreported on urinalysis, or they may be misidentified as crystals other than calcium oxalate.[129,132,182,188,192,193]

Calcium oxalate crystals take 2 forms, known as calcium oxalate monohydrate and calcium oxalate dihydrate. The former can appear in several different morphologies, as scattered individual crystals or clustered into aggregates (**Box 6**).[13,55,65,129,132,183,188,193,194] The dihydrate form is more familiar to many clinicians, appearing as regular, 8-sided polyhedrons. When the crystals are oriented at

Box 6
Comparison of monohydrate and dihydrate forms of calcium oxalate crystals

	Calcium Oxalate Monohydrate	Calcium Oxalate Dihydrate
Mineral name	Whewellite	Weddellite
Formula	$CaC_2O_4 \cdot H_2O$	$CaC_2O_4 \cdot 2H_2O$
Crystal system	Monoclinic	Tetragonal
Thermodynamic stability	Stable	Metastable

Crystal habit	*Pleomorphic (any of the following)*
	
	• Needlelike shapes
	• Elongated hexagons
	• Cigarlike shapes
	• Hempseed (orzolike) shapes
	• Biconcave ovoid shapes
	• Short prisms
	• Sheaf shapes
	• Dumbbell shapes
		Monomorphic
		
		• Dipyramidal (octahedral)
		  ○ Tentlike shapes
		  ○ Appear as a square circumscribing an X (envelopelike shape) or cross pattée pattern
		  ○ Interpenetrant twinning may occur

Crystal aggregation	Needle-shaped crystals may orient with 1 end directed to a central point forming a spheroidal aggregate	Crystals may be scattered or may appear in compactly interlocking aggregates
Crystal size[a] (μm)	9 ± 6	12 ± 8
Birefringence	Strong	Weak
Prevalence in ethylene glycol poisoning[b]	More common	Less common
Overall clinical prevalence[c]	Less common	More common
Other	Needle, prism, and elongated hexagonal forms may be misidentified as hippuric acid crystals	Greater tendency to form at higher calcium oxalate concentrations; may spontaneously transform to the monohydrate form

[a] Crystal size (mean ± standard deviation) data from freshly voided urine specimens of 27 unselected ambulatory outpatients with incidental oxalate crystalluria and no known urologic or toxicologic disorders.[190]
[b] Relative prevalence from animal models[195,196] and some clinical reports[132,186] of ethylene glycol poisoning.
[c] Relative clinical prevalence of isolated crystalluria without stone formation, outside the context of ethylene glycol poisoning.[190,197]
Data from Kruse JA. Ethanol, methanol, and ethylene glycol. In: Vincent JL, Abraham E, Moore FA, et al. editors. Textbook of Critical Care. Philadelphia: Elsevier; 2011. p. 1270–81; and Kruse JA. Ethylene glycol intoxication. J Intensive Care Med 1992;7(5):234–43.

particular angles under light microscopy, their two-dimensional projections can give the appearance of square envelopes (viewed flat, with the folded-paper edges showing).

Hippuric acid crystals have been reported in ethylene glycol–poisoned patients,[65,68,98,127–129,146,182] but most reports probably represent misidentification because the elongated hexagonal and needle-shaped forms of calcium oxalate monohydrate are easily mistaken for hippuric acid crystals.[13,55,89,98,129,132,188,192–194,196] Hippuric acid, a glycine-benzoate conjugate, is a normal constituent of the urine of many herbivorous mammals. The compound was first isolated from the urine of horses, hence the etymology of the name. Hippuric acid can also be present in human urine, in which case it is derived from the amino acid glycine in the presence of benzoic acid.[198] Benzoic acid is a metabolic product of toluene, and hippuric acid crystalluria has been reported after toluene intoxication.[11,199] Theoretically, hippuric acid may be formed in ethylene glycol poisoning in humans by a transamination reaction involving glyoxylic acid to form glycine, followed by conjugation of glycine to benzoic acid[13,56]:

| Glyoxylic acid | | Glycine | Benzoic acid | Hippuric acid |

Radiolabeled hippuric acid appears in the urine of rats injected with ^{14}C-labeled ethylene glycol and benzoic acid.[56] Pyridoxal (vitamin B_6) is required in the first reaction of this sequence, but because it serves as a cofactor it is not consumed by the reaction. On the other hand, the conjugation reaction requires a continuing source of benzoic acid or its anion, benzoate. As noted earlier, denatonium benzoate is an additive in some automotive antifreeze formulations, serving as an aversive agent; however, the concentration of the added benzoate is probably too low to serve as an appreciable source. Larger concentrations of benzoic acid or benzoate salts have been used as additives in some ethylene glycol-based antifreeze formulations for imparting anticorrosive properties.[6,128,192,200] Benzoate is also found in some vegetables and is added to some food and beverage products as a preservative.[201] It can also be synthesized by intestinal flora from dietary flavonoids, such as those found in black and green tea.[202] Theoretically, high urinary concentrations of hippuric acid could therefore occur, along with crystalluria, in some patients after ethylene glycol ingestion, but good documentary evidence is lacking. Godolphin and colleagues[129] found crystals in an ethylene glycol–poisoned patient that resemble hippuric acid, but using radiographic crystallography, a definitive method of crystal identification, they showed the crystals to be calcium oxalate monohydrate. Other investigators have identified calcium oxalate monohydrate crystalluria in ethylene glycol–poisoned patients using scanning electron microscopy, point radiographic fluorescence, and radiographic powder diffraction analysis.[188]

Blood Lactate Levels

Increased blood lactate levels have been described in both methanol and ethylene glycol poisoning, albeit inconsistently (see **Table 2**). Most of the enzyme-catalyzed dehydrogenation reactions involved in the metabolism of methanol and ethylene glycol require the enzyme cofactor NAD$^+$, producing the reduced version of the cofactor, NADH. Normally, excess NADH is reoxidized back to NAD$^+$ by the intramitochondrial electron transport system. This regeneration of NAD$^+$ may be impeded if additional ATP is not needed by the cell, or if the involved toxic molecules interfere with the operation of the electron transport system or its associated upstream pathway reactions (eg, the Krebs cycle). Under these circumstances, transformation of pyruvate to lactate can serve as a means of replenishing NAD^+.[203] At rest, lactate concentrations in body fluid are normally in steady-state equilibrium with the glycolytic intermediate pyruvate, produced by the metabolism of glucose. The conversion of pyruvate to lactate is catalyzed by the enzyme LDH and requires NADH:

$$
\underset{\text{Pyruvate}}{\overset{\displaystyle CH_3}{\underset{\displaystyle \overset{O}{\underset{O^-}{\overset{|}{C}}}}{\overset{|}{\underset{}{C}}=O}}} + NADH + H^+ \overset{LDH}{\rightleftharpoons} \underset{\text{Lactate}}{\overset{\displaystyle CH_3}{\underset{\displaystyle \overset{O}{\underset{O^-}{\overset{|}{C}}}}{H-\overset{|}{\underset{}{C}}-OH}}} + NAD^+
$$

Thus, excess accumulation of NADH from metabolism of large amounts of methanol or ethylene glycol might be expected to raise the ratio of NADH to NAD^+, tending to drive this reaction in the direction of lactate and increasing blood lactate concentration, to replenish NAD^+.

However, the inconsistent levels of blood lactate in case reports of these ingestions, including in cases in which large amounts of toxic metabolites have been generated, argues against this mechanism as an appreciable source of lactate generation. The metabolism of ethanol also uses NAD^+ and similarly alters the redox state of the cell secondary to increased NADH accumulation, but systematic clinical observations have shown that lactate levels do not increase appreciably unless there is another reason for lactic acidosis, such as seizures or circulatory shock.[204] Seizures are a common manifestation in both methanol–poisoned[47,93,104–106,117] and ethylene glycol–poisoned[68–70,72,82,90,126–135] patients with acidosis, and lactic acidosis is expected during ictus and in the postictal period, stemming from the imbalance between tissue oxygen availability and demand.[205] Circulatory shock, which also represents an imbalance between tissue oxygen supply and demand and is a common cause of lactic acidosis,[206] is a frequent concomitant in critical cases of methanol[47,54,96,100,101,118] and ethylene glycol[69,72,126,130,135] poisoning. Furthermore, experimental models of ethylene glycol poisoning using rats, dogs, and monkeys, as well as some human case reports (see **Table 2**), have not shown substantial lactate increases.[60,131,193] Given the potential severity of cardiopulmonary effects that can occur in these poisonings, a common mechanism of associated hyperlactatemia is anaerobic metabolism from circulatory failure, hypoperfusion, hypoxia, or related explanations.[184]

Another possible contributing factor to hyperlactatemia is decreased aerobic ATP production caused by inhibition of cellular respiration, thereby promoting anaerobic ATP production via glycolysis.[40–42,58,59,83,84]

Blood lactate levels may be artifactually increased in ethylene glycol poisoning, sometimes to extreme levels.[141,149] A common automated method of assaying lactate uses a coupled enzymatic reaction sequence, the first step of which involves conversion of L-lactate to pyruvate catalyzed by L-lactic oxidase[203]:

$$
\underset{\text{L-Lactate}}{\overset{\displaystyle CH_3}{\underset{\displaystyle \overset{O}{\underset{O^-}{\overset{|}{C}}}}{H-\overset{|}{\underset{}{C}}-OH}}} + O_2 \overset{\textit{L-Lactate oxidase}}{\longrightarrow} \underset{\text{Pyruvate}}{\overset{\displaystyle CH_3}{\underset{\displaystyle \overset{O}{\underset{O^-}{\overset{|}{C}}}}{\overset{|}{\underset{}{C}}=O}}} + H_2O_2
$$

The second step involves colorimetric or amperometric assay of the peroxide product. In the electrochemical version, the following reactions take place at silver and platinum electrodes within the reaction chamber:

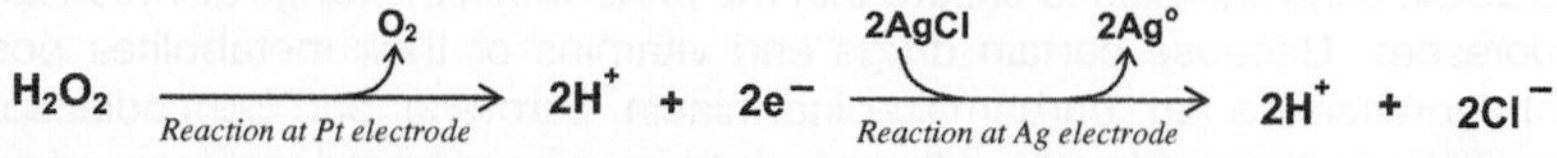

$$H_2O_2 \xrightarrow[\textit{Reaction at Pt electrode}]{O_2} 2H^+ + 2e^- \xrightarrow[\textit{Reaction at Ag electrode}]{2AgCl \quad 2Ag^\circ} 2H^+ + 2Cl^-$$

These reactions generate an electrical current that flows through an external circuit connecting the 2 electrodes, and that current is stoichiometrically proportional to the amount of lactate transformed to pyruvate. Glycolate, which is the chief metabolite of ethylene glycol that accumulates in plasma, is structurally similar to lactate, differing only by a methyl group on the α carbon:

Glycolate   Lactate

As a result, depending on the species from which the enzyme is derived, certain L-lactate oxidase variants may also react with glycolate, oxidizing it to glyoxylate:

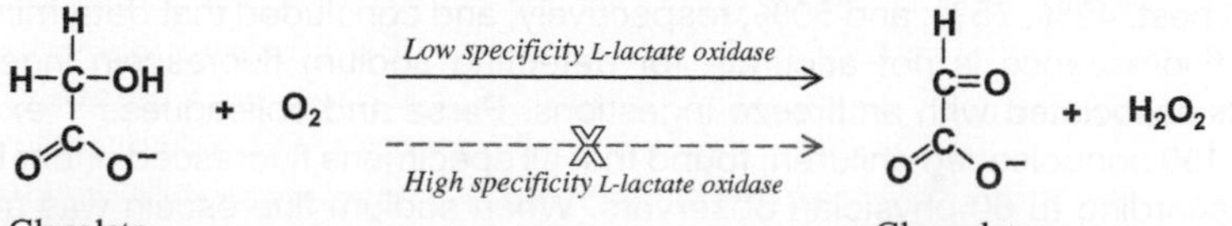

Glycolate   Glyoxylate

The hydrogen peroxide product reacts at the platinum electrode, generating an electrical current, in this case proportional to the combined amount of lactate and glycolate in the sample, yielding a falsely increased lactate determination.[207] As an example, in 1 reported case of a patient surviving ethylene glycol intoxication, the blood lactate level was found to be 60 mmol/L using this assay method.[141]

If recognized, this specificity limitation of certain enzymatic methods for measuring blood lactate may serve as an advantage for some institutions that lack the ability to measure ethylene glycol or glycolate. If the institution has at its disposal more than 1 available method for assaying lactate, and 1 method is known to be sensitive to glycolate whereas the other method is not, glycolate-containing specimens that are analyzed on both instruments yield a discrepancy, the degree of which approximates the plasma glycolate concentration. (Suitable glycolate calibration standards are necessary for quantitative application.) This phenomenon has been termed the lactate gap.[208–211]

Urine Fluorescence

In 1990, Winter and colleagues[212] reported their findings from a simulation test designed to test whether the sodium fluorescein additive included in many automotive antifreeze formulations could be detected in human urine by observing whether the urine fluoresces on exposure to UV illumination. Urine specimens were obtained from 6 healthy volunteers after they ingested 600 μg of sodium fluorescein. Urine collected within 2 hours of ingestion was found to contain an average of 32 ng/mL of fluorescein by fluorimetric assay. Blinded evaluators rated the urine as visually fluorescent under a Wood lamp in 100% of the samples from volunteers ingesting fluorescein, but gave a nonfluorescent rating to all of the control urine samples. The investigators were careful to point out the many potential pitfalls of the test, including lower identification rates for urine obtained more than 2 to 4 hours after ingestion, the high native fluorescence of some plastic urine specimen containers, and the necessity of adding alkali to acidic urine samples to ensure that the pH is within the range at which fluorescein fluoresces. Because certain drugs and vitamins or their metabolites possess inherent fluorescence (eg, carbamazepine, niacin, carotene, and benzodiazepines), false-positive results could occur if these substances have been ingested and appear in the urine. False-negative results could occur if the urine specimen is obtained more than a few hours after ingestion, or if the ingested antifreeze happened to be a formulation that does not contain sodium fluorescein. The test was subsequently advocated or used as a means of surrogate identification of ingested antifreeze in the urine, of antifreeze splashes on skin or clothing, or of antifreeze in gastric aspirate.[213,214]

Subsequently, Casavant and colleagues[215] studied 16 healthy children and 30 children hospitalized for reasons other than a toxic ingestion, and found that most of the urine specimens fluoresced. These investigators concluded that fluorescent urine is not an indicator of antifreeze ingestion by children, and recommended that urine testing for fluorescence be abandoned. Wallace and colleagues[214,216] performed a blinded, randomized, controlled comparison of the accuracy of Wood lamp examination for urinary fluorescence, similar to the original study of Winters and colleagues. Wallace and colleagues reported mean examiner sensitivity, specificity, and accuracy to be, at best, 42%, 75%, and 50%, respectively, and concluded that determination of urinary fluorescence is not accurate for detecting sodium fluorescein ingestion in amounts associated with antifreeze ingestions. Parsa and colleagues,[217] examining urine of 150 nonpoisoned children, found that all specimens fluoresced under UV radiation, according to 60 physician observers. When sodium fluorescein was added to urine samples to generate a wide range of urine fluorescein concentrations (10–1256 ng/mL), there were no observable differences in fluorescence compared with unadulterated urine samples until reaching a concentration of 312 ng/mL. The investigators also found poor interrater agreement regarding fluorescence. Taken together, the available information suggests that determination of urine fluorescence is not a reliable screening tool for suspected antifreeze ingestion.

Other Laboratory Abnormalities

Methanol and ethylene glycol can result in several other laboratory manifestations besides the metabolic acidosis, increased anion gap, and increased osmole gap. Hypocalcemia is described in many case reports of ethylene glycol poisoning,[72,82,123,124,132,136,138] and may be caused by calcium oxalate crystal deposition occurring throughout the body. Increased plasma activity of amylase caused by pancreatitis or salivary gland inflammation has been reported.[113,179] Azotemia develops during the classic third stage of ethylene glycol poisoning. Renal failure is not a characteristic feature of methanol poisoning, but is nevertheless observed occasionally. These occurrences of renal injury correlate with the degree of metabolic acidosis and may be secondary to rhabdomyolysis, acute tubular necrosis caused by perfusion failure, or other factors.[218] Abnormal erythrocyte indices, specifically increased mean corpuscular volumes, have been described in methanol intoxication.[95] Thrombocytopenia has been described in ethylene glycol poisoning.[140]

TREATMENT

Severity of illness in methanol and ethylene glycol poisoning varies over a wide spectrum depending on the ingested dose, time from ingestion to presentation, concomitant ethanol ingestion, and other factors. In late presentations after a substantial ingested volume, the patient may be in extremis, with rapidly evolving multiple organ system failure. Supportive treatment includes those measures that are widely applicable to seriously poisoned patients or critically ill patients in general. However, a key principle of therapy in methanol or ethylene glycol poisoning hinges on the use of specific pharmacologic antidotes to delay further production of toxic metabolic intermediates and allow or hasten bodily elimination of both the parent compound and already produced toxic by-products. There are 2 primary forms of specific antidotal pharmacotherapy available, namely ethanol and fomepizole. These pharmacologic treatments work by similar mechanisms and may be equally effective if properly administered. They should be considered mutually exclusive forms of treatment (ie, they are not used together in the same patient). Indications for initiating therapy with ethanol or fomepizole are given in **Box 7**.

Supportive Measures and Gut Decontamination

Initial therapy always begins with ensuring adequacy of the patient's airway, ventilation, and perfusion. Endotracheal intubation may be necessary for late presentations in which the patient is already in coma or having active seizures. For patients with an altered sensorium, blood glucose should be assessed with a point-of-care assay instrument. If the blood glucose measurement results are not available within a minute or so, an intravenous (IV) bolus of dextrose should be administered empirically. Induction of vomiting is contraindicated, even in conscious patients, because of the potential for sensorial depression developing. Gastric lavage might be a consideration in a large-volume ingestion if the patient presented less than 1 hour after ingestion and had an endotracheal tube in place, although this scenario contradicts the expected time course of significant CNS depression in these poisonings. There are limited data concerning the usefulness of activated charcoal for methanol and ethylene glycol, but it is probably not useful.[35,36] Charcoal may be given if there is an applicable coingestant.

Seizures are treated with parenteral anticonvulsant therapy (eg, lorazepam followed by either phenytoin or fosphenytoin loading). Screening blood tests should include

---

Box 7
Criteria for ethanol or fomepizole administration for the treatment of methanol or ethylene glycol poisoning

- Serum methanol or ethylene glycol level >20 mg/dL

or

- Documented history of recent ingestion of toxic amounts of methanol or ethylene glycol in conjunction with a serum osmole gap >10 mosmol/L

or

- History or strong clinical suspicion of methanol or ethylene glycol poisoning in conjunction with at least 2 of the following criteria:

  ○ Arterial blood pH <7.3

  ○ Plasma bicarbonate or serum CO_2 content <20 mmol/L

  ○ Serum osmole gap >10 mosmol/L

  ○ Calcium oxalate crystalluria (ethylene glycol poisoning)

Data from Refs.[35,36,219]

serum electrolytes (including calcium), anion gap, osmolality (by the freezing point depression method), urea nitrogen, glucose, arterial blood gas analysis, and urinalysis. Serum amylase, lipase, transaminase, and creatine kinase activity levels should be assessed. If the diagnosis of methanol or ethylene glycol poisoning is uncertain, a differential diagnosis should be formulated and consideration given for other diagnostic studies. Emergency computed tomography should be performed if there is an altered sensorium, seizures, or a focal neurologic deficit.

Thiamine

Thiamine is routinely given to hospitalized patients with chronic ethanol use, particularly those with altered mental status. The rationale for this is to prevent or treat Wernicke-Korsakoff syndrome, for which there is an increased incidence in patients with chronic alcoholism. Although that syndrome is uncommon, parenteral thiamine administration is inexpensive and safe, and the potential adverse consequences of foregoing treatment can be severe. Given the increased (albeit still low) incidence of both intentional and unintentional methanol and ethylene glycol poisoning in patients with alcoholism, an argument can be made for routinely administering thiamine to patients with known or suspected poisoning with either of these 2 agents.

If present, thiamine deficiency could play a more specific albeit minor role in ethylene glycol poisoning. As depicted earlier, glyoxylic acid, one of the toxic intermediates of ethylene glycol metabolism, is converted to oxalic acid, but glyoxylic acid can also be enzymatically transformed to α-hydroxy-β-ketoadipic acid as:

$$
\underset{\text{Glyoxylic acid}}{\begin{array}{c}\text{CHO}\\|\\\text{COOH}\end{array}} + \underset{\text{α-Ketoglutaric acid}}{\begin{array}{c}\text{COOH}\\|\\(\text{CH}_2)_2\\|\\\text{C=O}\\|\\\text{COOH}\end{array}} \xrightarrow[\text{Thiamine, Mg}]{\text{2-Hydroxy-3-oxo-adipate synthase}} \underset{\text{α-Hydroxy-β-ketoadipic acid}}{\begin{array}{c}\text{COOH}\\|\\\text{CH-OH}\\|\\\text{C=O}\\|\\(\text{CH}_2)_2\text{-COOH}\end{array}} + CO_2
$$

This reaction requires both thiamine (vitamin B_1) and magnesium as obligatory cofactors. The resulting product, a derivative of the 6-carbon dicarboxylic acid adipic acid, can be considered nontoxic. This minor pathway is not capable of handling the large amounts of glyoxylic acid expected in clinical poisoning cases, but hypothetically could be of some therapeutic value in thiamine-deficient patients, who would be expected to lack any advantage available by this minor pathway. Thus, thiamine should be given (eg, 100 mg IV) to patients with a history of alcohol abuse or suspicion of thiamine deficiency. Similarly, magnesium should be administered if there is hypomagnesemia.

Sodium Bicarbonate

IV administration of sodium bicarbonate has been a conventional element of the supportive treatment of diverse causes of metabolic acidosis in critically ill patients for many decades. However, the use of sodium bicarbonate for treating common forms of acute metabolic acidosis, such as the lactic acidosis associated with circulatory shock,[220] mild to moderate diabetic ketoacidosis,[221] and most cases of cardiac arrest,[222] has been increasingly questioned in recent years. Although bicarbonate is nevertheless often still used in treating lactic and ketoacidosis, contemporary use tends to be limited to severe cases, usually without the intention of fully correcting the acidemia. In the acidosis associated with methanol and ethylene glycol poisoning, controlled trial data are lacking but uncontrolled observations, animal studies, and pathophysiologic considerations suggest that alkali administration may be of value.

First, the acidosis of methanol and ethylene glycol poisoning can be profound, and large amounts of sodium bicarbonate may be required (see **Table 2**). There are numerous reports in which the arterial blood pH is in the 6.3 to 6.9 range. Such striking degrees of acidemia argue for empiric administration of alkali, but there are also theoretic reasons that argue for correction of acidosis. Given that the toxic metabolites are largely carboxylic acids, and that many of the most severe adverse effects are those affecting the CNS, any measure that would decrease accessibility of the toxic molecules to the CNS would seem rationale. In the case of methanol, the toxic acid is formic acid. The dissociation equation for formic acid is reversible, and thus the acid exists either in equilibrium or some nonsteady state with its conjugate anion, formate, as:

$$H-\overset{\overset{O}{\|}}{C}-OH \;\rightleftharpoons\; H^+ + H-\overset{\overset{O}{\|}}{C}-O^-$$

Formic acid   Formate

Because the pK_a of formic acid is 3.7,[2] most of the molecules assume the ionic form within the physiologic or pathophysiologic pH range. However, the lower the pH (and thus the higher the hydrogen ion concentration), the greater the fraction of the protonated (acid) form. The nonionic acid form is capable of crossing biologic membranes, including the blood-brain barrier. Thus, a more acidic environment favors CNS penetration with likely greater adverse consequences for the patient. Administering sodium bicarbonate tends to drive this chemical equation to the right, favoring anion formation and limiting tissue penetration, including into the CNS, and limiting formate-induced inhibition of cytochrome c oxidase and other cytotoxicity.[38–42] The same principle should logically apply to the acid intermediates of ethylene glycol metabolism.

In addition, animal studies suggest a benefit from alkali administration. In a rat model of ethylene glycol poisoning, Borden and Bidwell[66] reported a 71% survival rate in rats given ethylene glycol and treated with sodium bicarbonate (0.2 g/kg every 6 hours for 6 doses) versus 14% survival in untreated controls. Renal cortical oxalate crystallization was also decreased from a 94% incidence in control animals to 55% in bicarbonate-treated animals. Case series of methanol intoxication have reported that the incidence and severity of permanent ocular abnormalities and death correlate with the incidence and severity of metabolic acidosis.[34,43,86,92,93,105] Although the severity of acidosis may represent an epiphenomenon signifying greater toxin generation rather than a mechanism per se for morbidity and mortality, and although the clinical data are uncontrolled, there are reports of rapid improvement in visual acuity immediately after sodium bicarbonate administration, and reports correlating symptomatic improvement and survival with the degree of correction of acidosis using sodium bicarbonate.[34,43,130] The American Academy of Clinical Toxicology guidelines[35,36] recommend administering sodium bicarbonate to methanol-poisoned and ethylene glycol–poisoned patients with arterial pH levels less than 7.30 to normalize arterial pH (ie, to increase pH to between 7.35 and 7.45).

Ethanol

For many years, ethanol has been the conventional pharmacologic antidote for both methanol and ethylene glycol poisoning. It has been successfully used by both the oral and IV routes. The basis for ethanol therapy is the following endogenous reaction sequence, which represents the main pathway for ethanol metabolism in the body:

$$CH_3-CH_2-OH \xrightarrow[\text{Alcohol dehydrogenase}]{NAD^+ \quad NADH + H^+} CH_3-\overset{O}{\overset{\|}{C}}-H \xrightarrow[\substack{H_2O \\ \text{Aldehyde} \\ \text{dehydrogenase}}]{NAD^+ \quad NADH + H^+} CH_3-\overset{O}{\overset{\|}{C}}-OH$$

Ethanol   Acetaldehyde   Acetic acid

The same 2 enzymes, alcohol dehydrogenase and aldehyde dehydrogenase, along with nicotinamide cofactors, are involved in the breakdown of ethanol as with methanol (compare with the first reaction presented in this review). For both alcohols, the first step converts the alcohol to an aldehyde and the second step converts the aldehyde to a carboxylic acid. The resulting aldehydes differ in that acetaldehyde is less toxic than formaldehyde. The acids differ in that formic acid has considerable human toxicity, whereas acetic acid can be considered nontoxic. Acetic acid is conjugated to coenzyme A (CoA) to form acetyl-CoA, a normal intermediate metabolite present in all aerobic cells. As a physiologic intermediary metabolite of aerobic glucose, fatty acid, and amino acid metabolism, acetyl-CoA serves as the main point of entry into the Krebs cycle.

Both ethanol and methanol are substrates for these 2 dehydrogenase enzymes, and the 2 alcohols compete for the active sites on these enzymes. However, the affinity and catalytic efficiency of alcohol dehydrogenase for ethanol are generally orders of magnitude higher than for methanol or ethylene glycol.[223] Thus, the enzyme has a higher specificity for ethanol over either methanol or ethylene glycol. In the presence of ethanol and either or both of the other 2 substrates, the enzyme, in effect, preferentially catalyzes the breakdown of ethanol, functionally inhibiting the activity of the enzyme as far as methanol or ethylene glycol oxidation is concerned.

The efficacy of ethanol as a competitive inhibitor of alcohol dehydrogenase has been shown in animal models. For example, rats poisoned with 10 mL/kg ethylene glycol and then treated with ethanol (0.4 g/kg every 6 hours for 6 doses) had a 73% survival rate compared with 14% survival in untreated control animals.[66] Survival further increased to 89% if treatment consisted of sodium bicarbonate and ethanol. Similar, albeit less impressive, results were reported in canine models of ethylene glycol poisoning.[73] Renal cortical oxalate crystallization was also decreased from a 94% incidence in control animals to 25% in ethanol-treated animals, whereas renal oxalate crystallization was not detected in animals treated with both ethanol and sodium bicarbonate. Case reports and uncontrolled case series of patients with ethylene glycol ingestion also support the clinical efficacy of ethanol treatment, in some cases preventing significant acidemia and any apparent renal impairment despite repeatedly documented high serum ethylene glycol levels.[124]

Administering ethanol to a methanol-poisoned patient is therapeutic in that the ethanol greatly impedes the breakdown of methanol to formic acid, allowing time for the methanol to be slowly excreted by the lungs and kidneys or to be slowly converted to carbon dioxide by metabolic pathways that would otherwise be overwhelmed by large amounts of formate. Ethanol treatment is of no value if administered after the ingested methanol dose has already been fully metabolized to formic acid. If ethanol is given after a portion of the ingested methanol has been metabolized, the ethanol is potentially effective only for that portion of the toxic alcohol that has not undergone metabolic conversion. Ethanol is also effective at inhibiting the metabolism of ethylene glycol by the same mechanisms (ie, by inhibition of alcohol dehydrogenase).

The standard recommendation is to target a serum or blood alcohol concentration in the range of 100 to 150 mg/dL (22–33 mmol/L), which is sufficient to fully inhibit alcohol dehydrogenase. Ethanol is miscible with water and diffuses into all body fluid compartments, with a volume of distribution of about 0.68 L/kg in men and 0.63 L/kg in women.[224,225] The conventional loading dose recommended to rapidly achieve a blood ethanol level within the range described earlier is 0.6 g of ethanol per kilogram body weight,[35,36,110] equivalent to 0.76 mL of absolute (ie, 100%, anhydrous) ethanol per kilogram body weight. Loading can be accomplished by IV administration using a 10% (volume/volume) solution of ethanol in sterile water for injection, and also containing 5 g/dL dextrose. Using that formulation, a 70-kg man requires 532 mL of 10% ethanol as a loading dose, administered over 1 hour. This dose assumes that the patient's blood ethanol level is zero to begin with. The baseline ethanol level should be assessed because some patients already have ethanol on board from having consumed ethanol along with or around the time the ethylene glycol or methanol was ingested. No loading dose is necessary if the baseline blood ethanol level is within or in excess of the target level. For patients with detectable but lower baseline blood ethanol concentration, a proportionately smaller loading dose is administered.

Oral loading doses, consisting of commercial whiskey or prepared from suitable pharmaceutical-grade ethanol, have also been used therapeutically.[226] This route is not advised in patients with an altered sensorium because of the high risk of aspiration if vomiting should occur. The oral route is also not advised in patients unaccustomed to consuming hard liquor because of the likelihood of vomiting, even if the preparation is diluted. The ethanol content of whiskey and similar distilled spirits are commonly given in proof units, derived from the antiquated practice of testing for potency and dilution of the alcoholic beverage by dousing gunpowder with the beverage and then attempting ignition using a flame. Combustion was taken as proof of sufficient alcohol content. In the United States, each proof unit is equivalent to 0.5 percentage units (ie, volume/volume percent). Thus, 100 proof liquor is equivalent to 50% ethanol by volume. The density of ethanol is 0.79 g/mL at 20° C; therefore, 100 proof whiskey contains 40 g of ethanol per 100 mL. This figure translates to an oral loading dose of 1.5 mL of 100 proof whiskey per kilogram body weight. Oral dosing is best given with additional diluent (eg, to a final concentration of ≤20%) to minimize abdominal discomfort and vomiting, side effects that can be avoided by using IV ethanol.

Clinical experience and data from studies in healthy volunteers suggest that these loading doses, which were based on limited patient data, commonly undershoot the targeted serum ethanol concentration, especially when administered by the oral route.[227] As a result, some sources advise routinely using 0.7 g/kg instead of 0.6 g/kg, and note that even this higher loading dose may fail to achieve a serum ethanol level of 100 mg/dL.[13,35,227] Loading doses of up to 0.8 g/kg have also been recommended.[36]

Ongoing ethanol dosing is necessary to maintain the blood ethanol concentration within the targeted range. The average maintenance ethanol dose required to sustain blood ethanol concentration within the targeted range is approximately 66 mg/kg/h in individuals not habituated to ethanol, and 154 mg/kg/h in chronic users.[110] These values should be considered starting points for maintenance dosing, with the dose then determined by titration to blood or serum ethanol assays performed every 1 or 2 hours. Once a near steady state has been reached and the necessary maintenance dose determined, the ethanol assay frequency may be decreased to every 2 to 3 hours. Assay frequencies of every 1 to 2 hours should be resumed if an ethanol level is obtained that is out of the targeted range, if the maintenance dosing is interrupted, or if dialysis is undertaken.

Five percent and 10% (volume/volume) parenteral ethanol solutions in 5% (weight/volume) dextrose in water have been used for IV maintenance dosing. If commercial pharmaceutical solutions are unavailable, they may be prepared using

95% (volume/volume) ethanol or anhydrous or absolute (100%) ethanol and 5% dextrose in water. Denatured ethanol must not be used. Using the 10% solution, a continuous IV infusion given at 0.83 mL/kg/h is selected for nondrinkers and 1.96 mL/kg/h for chronic ethanol users. For 5% ethanol solutions, the infusion rates would be 1.66 and 3.92 mL/kg/h, respectively. Intermediate infusion rates may be selected initially for patients with chronic alcohol intake that is between these extremes. To maintain targeted blood ethanol levels, maintenance doses higher than those cited here may be necessary, particularly in chronic alcoholics who are accustomed to large daily volumes of alcoholic beverages.[110,226]

For oral maintenance dosing in alcohol-naive patients using 100 proof commercially available spirits, 0.17 mL/kg is administered as hourly doses, initially. If the liquor is not 100 proof, the volumetric dose must be adjusted accordingly. Although the loading dose is theoretically unaffected by chronic ethanol exposure, heavy ethanol users may require double to triple this oral maintenance recommendation. Whether administered intravenously or orally, the maintenance dose needs to be further increased if hemodialysis is initiated during ethanol administration.[54,110,145,226] This increase is necessary to compensate for the ethanol removed by dialysis. In some cases, the dose may need to be doubled or tripled during hemodialysis, but the required increase is affected by various factors and is difficult to predict. A typical maintenance ethanol dose during hemodialysis is 169 mg/kg/h, in terms of absolute ethanol. This dose is equivalent to 2.13 mL/kg/h if using a 10% parenteral ethanol solution. For patients who regularly consume ethanol on a chronic basis, a representative ethanol dose on hemodialysis is 257 mg/kg/h, equivalent to 3.26 mL/kg/h using a 10% ethanol solution.

Whether hemodialysis is used or not, the key to effective maintenance dosing of ethanol is obtaining frequent blood ethanol assays and using that information to titrate the ethanol infusion rate. Typically, ethanol levels are obtained every 1 hour initially and during dialysis, and every 2 hours when the patient is off dialysis once a stable ethanol level has been achieved. The ethanol infusion is titrated as needed to maintain the blood ethanol concentration between 100 and 150 mg/dL. Higher levels are not needed and can cause unnecessary sedation, inebriation, and impairment of protective reflexes. Lower levels are avoided because they may be insufficient to fully inhibit enzymatic conversion of the ingested methanol or ethylene glycol.

The 10% (10 mL/dL) ethanol in 5% (5 g/dL) dextrose and water formulation is hyperosmolar, having an osmolarity of approximately 1995 mosmol/L,[228] similar to that of many total parenteral nutrition solutions. A central venous catheter is therefore necessary for sustained IV administration at this concentration. Lower dilutions have the disadvantage of requiring twice the volume, which is considerable given the doses of ethanol that are typically required. For example, using a 5% (volume/volume) ethanol solution and IV administration, a 70-kg man requires a loading dose of more than 1 L. If this patient had a history of regular heavy ethanol consumption, then using a 5% (volume/volume) parenteral ethanol solution, he might require a continuous IV infusion rate of 300 mL or more per hour just to maintain the appropriate blood ethanol concentration. Careful attention to fluid balance is necessary, particularly for patients with impaired cardiac or renal function. In later presentations of ethylene glycol poisoning, evolving renal dysfunction with oliguria could develop despite ethanol administration, further increasing the potential for fluid overload.

Although parenteral ethanol solutions have regulatory approval for clinical use by the US Food and Drug Administration, there is no approved labeling for use in treating methanol or ethylene glycol poisoning. Nevertheless, ethanol has a long history of clinical use for this purpose. Animal models, clinical case reports, and case series attest to the effectiveness of ethanol treatment, given either orally or parenterally, but controlled human trials are lacking. There are known drawbacks to ethanol therapy (**Table 3**). Ethanol has well-known sedating effects, including at the doses and targeted blood levels advocated for treating toxic alcohol and glycol ingestions. These effects can interfere with neurologic assessments and increase the risk of falls and pulmonary aspiration. Ethanol-induced inebriation with its attendant emotional lability can also affect patient cooperation and compliance with treatment or otherwise complicate management. Hypoglycemia has been documented during controlled ethanol administration to healthy individuals, and particular concerns have been raised regarding children and malnourished individuals.[227] However, recent studies have not found hypoglycemia to be an issue in the therapeutic context, perhaps because ethanol in dextrose infusions is used and glucose monitoring is commonly used.[229,230] Oral administration potentially poses additional side effects, including abdominal pain, nausea, gastritis, GI bleeding, vomiting, and aspiration pneumonitis.

Dosing calculations for ethanol are complex and unfamiliar to some clinicians because of infrequent occasion for use. The variety of ethanol solutions available (eg, 5%, 10%, and 95% solutions), descriptive nomenclature applied to ethanol (eg, absolute ethanol, anhydrous ethanol, denatured ethanol), and differing concentration units (eg, volume/volume units, mass/volume units, proof units) for ethanol may all be unfamiliar and confusing to some clinicians. These factors increase the risk for errors in prescribing, dispensing, and administering ethanol solutions. There is much patient-to-patient variability in ethanol pharmacokinetics, depending on the patient's size, gender, age, hepatic function, and, most importantly, chronic ethanol exposure history. This variability and clinician unfamiliarity with ethanol dose titration can sometimes make it difficult to achieve and maintain ethanol levels within the targeted range.

Criteria for initiating inhibitor therapy are given in **Box 7**. Ethanol treatment should continue until methanol or ethylene glycol levels are undetectable; or alternatively, until

Table 3
Summary comparison of ethanol versus fomepizole for the treatment of methanol and ethylene glycol poisoning

	Ethanol	Fomepizole
Inebriation effect	Yes	No
Sedation effect	Yes	No
Hypoglycemia potential	Yes	No
Acquisition cost of drug	Low	High
Laboratory monitoring required	Yes	No
Duration of action	Short	Long
Potency for ADH inhibition	High	Low
Pharmacokinetics	Unpredictable	Predictable
Ease of administration	More difficult	Less difficult
Gastritis, nausea, vomiting	Yes (if by mouth)	No
Volume overload potential	Yes (if IV)	No
Dialyzable	Yes	Yes
Dose adjustment during dialysis	Yes	Yes
Dose adjustment in alcoholism	Yes	No
Availability	Wide	May be limited
Clinical experience	Long-term	Less, but increasing

Abbreviation: ADH, alcohol dehydrogenase.

levels are less than 20 mg/dL and the patient's arterial pH is normal. Additional continuation criteria are applicable if hemodialysis is used (see later discussion).

Fomepizole

Some of the drawbacks of ethanol therapy for methanol and ethylene glycol are obviated or mitigated by use of the alternative inhibitor of alcohol dehydrogenase, fomepizole. Fomepizole is the international nonproprietary name for 4-methylpyrazole:

$$CH_3 \quad \underset{NH}{\overset{N}{\diagup}}$$

Fomepizole

The drug has been studied in animal models of ethylene glycol poisoning, and in numerous case reports and case series.[60,74,231–235] Based on data from an uncontrolled clinical trial involving 19 patients, fomepizole (Antizol, Jazz Pharmaceuticals, Inc., Palo Alto, CA) was approved by the US Food and Drug Administration in 1997 for the treatment of ethylene glycol poisoning. In 2000, based on data from a trial involving 11 methanol-poisoned patients, the approved labeling was modified to allow its use for the treatment of methanol poisoning as well.[117,126,219] Like ethanol, fomepizole is a competitive inhibitor of alcohol dehydrogenase, but has several advantages over ethanol (see **Table 3**). The drug has a complicated dosing regimen. The first dose constitutes a loading dose, whereas the second to fourth doses represent smaller maintenance doses. Because the drug induces its own metabolism, subsequent doses are increased to that of the original loading dose to offset this metabolic induction. Like ethanol, the drug is dialyzable and must therefore be given more frequently during hemodialysis. In addition, the transition onto and off hemodialysis potentially alters the dose and dosing schedule (see **Box 8**). Despite these complexities, fomepizole is simpler to administer than ethanol because therapeutic drug levels are not required and because the dosing regimen is predetermined rather than empirically titrated. Furthermore, calculation and preparation of the fomepizole doses are simplified compared with ethanol. These advantages, coupled with the improved side effect profile of fomepizole, make it preferable to ethanol, where available. On the other hand, the drug acquisition cost for a course of fomepizole is substantial. In some cases, the cost may be offset by decreased use of other services.[236]

Lepik and coworkers[237] reviewed 189 cases treated with either ethanol or fomepizole and found at least 1 medication error associated with 78% of the ethanol-treated patients compared with 45% of the fomepizole-treated patients ($P = .0001$). The most common error-related harms were delayed antidote initiation and excessive antidote dose. The same group found fewer drug-related adverse events associated with fomepizole use compared with ethanol.[230]

Criteria for initiating fomepizole therapy are identical to ethanol therapy (see **Box 7**). Details of fomepizole administration are given in **Box 8**. As with ethanol therapy, fomepizole treatment is continued until methanol or ethylene glycol levels are undetectable; or alternatively, until levels are less than 20 mg/dL and the patient's arterial pH is normal. Additional continuation criteria are applicable if hemodialysis is used (see next section).

Hemodialysis

Inhibitor therapy does not completely stop generation of toxic by-products of methanol and ethylene glycol, but it does substantially slow their production. To an extent,

---

Box 8
Fomepizole administration for treatment of methanol or ethylene glycol poisoning[a]

- Initiating dosing if patient is not on hemodialysis:
  - Give a loading dose of 15 mg/kg IV over 30 minutes
  - Give 10 mg/kg IV over 30 minutes every 12 hours for 4 doses, then
  - Give 15 mg/kg IV over 30 minutes every 12 hours until (1) the plasma toxin level is undetectable, or (2) the plasma toxin level is <20 mg/dL, the arterial blood pH is within normal limits, and the patient is asymptomatic.
- On initiation of hemodialysis:
  - If <6 hours have elapsed since the last dose, skip the next scheduled dose.
  - If >6 hours have elapsed since the last dose, give the next scheduled dose (15 mg/kg) immediately.
- During ongoing hemodialysis:
  - Give 15 mg/kg IV over 30 minutes every 4 hours.
- At time of stopping hemodialysis:
  - If <1 hour has elapsed since the last dose, do not give a dose at the end of hemodialysis.
  - If 1 to 3 hours have elapsed since the last dose, give a half-dose (7.5 mg/kg) at the end of hemodialysis.
  - If >3 hours have elapsed since the last dose, give the next scheduled dose (15 mg/kg).
- Postdialysis dosing:
  - Beginning 12 hours after the last dose, give 15 mg/kg IV over 30 minutes every 12 hours until plasma toxin level is <20 mg/dL.

[a] Toxin level refers to methanol or ethylene glycol plasma concentration.
Data from Refs.[35,36,219]

---

the human body is capable of safely metabolizing these toxins, such as formate, glycolate, and glyoxylate; the problem is that large amounts of the parent compound easily overwhelm the downstream portions of these metabolic pathways, resulting in accumulation of toxic intermediates faster than they can be physiologically eliminated. In the presence of normal renal function, methanol and ethylene glycol are also excreted in the urine to a limited extent. Some methanol is also excreted by the lungs. During this ongoing physiologic elimination, the presence of therapeutic concentrations of either ethanol or fomepizole prevents excessive formation and accumulation of the toxic intermediates. However, neither ethanol nor fomepizole hastens the elimination of methanol or ethylene glycol from the body. Rather, these antidotes serve to delay or slow conversion of the parent compounds to their toxic metabolic products. Toxic intermediates already elaborated from the ingested compound before initiation of inhibitor therapy continue to exert their adverse effects despite inhibition of alcohol dehydrogenase. Methanol, ethylene glycol, and their toxic metabolites are all small molecules and are readily dialyzable. For these reasons, treatment of methanol-poisoned and ethylene glycol–poisoned patients has conventionally included hemodialysis to remove both the ingested parent compound as well as any toxic metabolites.[123] The conventional view has been that delay in further generation of toxic intermediates, as afforded by inhibitor therapy, provides time for dialytic removal of the ingestant before further transformation to toxic molecules.

Hemodialysis constitutes a potentially vital therapeutic intervention in patients for whom there has been sufficient delay between the time of ingestion and the time at which either ethanol or fomepizole treatment is initiated, during which time significant concentrations of formate or glycolate have accumulated. In some cases, the history may be unreliable or not available for gauging this time delay, but the clinical picture and the presence of either metabolic acidosis or an increased anion gap provide important information for determining whether metabolic conversion has occurred and to what degree. These features constitute indications for initiating hemodialysis (**Box 9**). Conventional indications advised hemodialysis for all patients with serum methanol or ethylene glycol levels exceeding 50 mg/dL. However, more recent evidence and guideline recommendations from the American Academy of Clinical Toxicology suggest that dialysis is not necessarily required for levels above this threshold if ethanol or fomepizole is being administered and the patient is asymptomatic, has a normal arterial pH, and has no other indication for dialysis.[35,36,233,236,238–242]

Hemodialysis remains an important therapeutic adjunct to inhibitor therapy for patients with signs of toxicity and laboratory findings of significant acidosis. Hemodialysis may also be considered in asymptomatic patients without acidosis who are receiving inhibitor therapy if the methanol or ethylene glycol level is high enough that prolonged ethanol or fomepizole is required (eg, several days). In those cases, the potential benefits, risks, and inconvenience of prolonged inhibitor treatment should be weighed against the use of hemodialysis.

Hemodialysis not only removes methanol, ethylene glycol, and their toxic metabolites from the blood stream but it also removes ethanol and fomepizole. Therefore, initiation of dialysis requires higher maintenance dosing of either form of inhibitor therapy.[35,36,110,145,219] In the case of fomepizole, this goal is accomplished as part of the labeled dosing recommendations (see **Box 8**). In the case of ethanol, the maintenance dose, either the hourly oral doses or the IV infusion rate, needs to be increased as previously described and then titrated according to hourly serum ethanol levels. An alternative method for ethanol administration during hemodialysis is to discontinue oral dosing or IV infusion and instead add ethanol to the dialysate at a concentration of 100 mg/dL.[54,181,243]

Conventional recommendations have been to continue hemodialysis until either (1) the methanol or ethylene glycol level is undetectable, (2) the methanol level is less than 25 mg/dL and there is no significant acidosis, or (3) the ethylene glycol level

---

Box 9
Indications for hemodialysis in methanol and ethylene glycol poisoning[a]

- Worsening clinical status
- Significant metabolic acidosis (arterial blood pH <7.30)
- Renal failure
- Visual disturbance
- Electrolyte abnormalities
- Serum methanol or ethylene glycol level >50 mg/dL[b]

[a] Any of the listed criteria are considered indications if unresponsive to standard measures and supportive treatment.[35,36]
[b] This is a conventional indication, but recent evidence and guidelines suggest that hemodialysis may not be necessary in some cases if this is the only criterion that is satisfied, the patient is asymptomatic, and the arterial pH is normal (see text).

is less than 20 mg/dL, renal function is normal, and there is no significant acidosis. An additional consideration is continuing until there are no signs of systemic toxicity, but this criterion requires recognition that some ocular, neurologic, and renal manifestations may persist or be permanent. Compared with measurements of plasma methanol or ethylene glycol, measurement of plasma formate (in the case of methanol ingestion) or glycolate (in the case of ethylene glycol ingestion), logically provides important information regarding the value of initiating or discontinuing hemodialysis.[116,174] However, these assays are not commonly available on an urgent basis.

For patients with high methanol or ethylene glycol levels, a prolonged dialysis session is often necessary to reach these goals. The required duration of hemodialysis (in hours) may be estimated by[244–246]:

$$\text{Required hemodialysis time} = \frac{-TBW \times \ln(5/C_0)}{0.06 \times k}$$

where C_0 is the initial plasma concentration of methanol or ethylene glycol in (mmol/L); k is 80% of the manufacturer-specified dialyzer urea clearance (mL/min) at the initial observed blood flow rate; and TBW represents total body water (L), determined using[247]:

$$TBW(\text{men}) = 2.447 - 0.09516 \times A + 0.1074 \times H + 0.3362 \times W$$
$$TBW(\text{women}) = -2.097 + 0.1069 \times H + 0.2466 \times W$$

where A represents age (years), H is height (cm), and W is weight (kg). Methanol and ethylene glycol concentrations may be converted from conventional units (mg/dL) to Système International units (mmol/L) using the molecular mass of the compound (see **Table 1**) and the following conversion formula:

$$\text{Concentration in mmol/L} = \frac{\text{concentration in mg/dL}}{\text{molecular mass}/10}$$

Initial formate or glycolate plasma levels, if available, may alternatively be used in lieu of the parent compound concentration in the formula for required dialysis time.

Rebound increase in the plasma methanol or ethylene glycol level has been described within the 12-hour to 36-hour period after termination of dialysis in some cases, ascribed to redistribution from tissue compartments to the plasma compartment.[35,36,112,124] Because this rebound phenomenon is unpredictable and the increase in concentration may be significant, ethanol or fomepizole should be continued after dialysis with ongoing monitoring of serum osmolality, electrolytes, anion gap, and osmole gap reassessment at intervals (eg, every 2–4 hours) for a period of 12 to 36 hours after discontinuing dialysis. The patient should continue to receive inhibitor therapy (fomepizole or ethanol) until the methanol or ethylene glycol level is undetectable, or alternatively, until the level is less than 20 mg/dL, the arterial pH and serum anion gap are normal, and the patient is asymptomatic. If methanol or ethylene glycol levels are unavailable, the serum osmole gap should also remain normal before discontinuation of inhibitor therapy. Redevelopment of an osmole gap points to a rebound increase that should prompt continued inhibitor therapy. In addition, reassessment of the plasma methanol or ethylene glycol level (if available) or repeat hemodialysis may be considered.

As noted earlier, higher methanol or ethylene glycol levels may not require dialysis if there is no acidosis and inhibitor therapy is being given appropriately. Administration of sodium bicarbonate may have completely corrected academia, yet significant concentrations of circulating formate or glycolate may still be present. This situation may be detectable as an increased anion gap, even although there is no sign of acidosis by arterial blood gas analysis. Assessment for metabolic acidosis should therefore routinely include evaluation of the serum anion gap.

Folic and Folinic Acid

Although rats and dogs develop severe acidosis and die when given large doses of ethylene glycol,[66,73,74] early studies found that otherwise healthy rats given methanol did not develop acidosis, organ failure, or death.[176,248,249] Methanol is metabolized to toxic formic acid in both humans and rodents; however, rats have the ability to more rapidly break down formic acid via a tetrahydrofolate (THF)-dependent pathway:

$$\text{HCOOH} + \text{THF} \xrightarrow[\textit{Formate-THF ligase}]{\overset{\text{ATP} \qquad \text{ADP} + \text{Pi}}{}} N^{10}\text{-formyl-THF}$$

where ADP and P_i represent adenosine diphosphate and phosphate, respectively. THF is a reduced form of the vitamin folic acid and it is an obligatory cofactor required by the enzyme catalyzing this reaction. THF is regenerated by the following reaction[37]:

$$N^{10}\text{-formyl-THF} \xrightarrow[\substack{\text{H}_2\text{O} \quad \textit{dehydrogenase}}]{\overset{\text{NADP}^+ \quad \text{NADPH} + \text{H}^+}{\textit{Formyl-THF}}} \text{CO}_2 + \text{THF}$$

The enzymes catalyzing these reactions are present in humans, but either because of insufficient enzyme activity or constrained availability of THF, the rate of formate detoxification by this route is slow and limited in humans. On the other hand, folate-depleted rats develop metabolic acidosis, accumulate formate, and develop pathologic retinal changes.[44,176,250] Similarly, higher concentrations of formate have been reported in folate-deprived macaques given methanol compared with control animals given methanol.[178] Methanol poisoning has been modeled successfully in nonfolate-deprived macaques, which oxidize formate to CO_2 at less than half the rate of rats, because of species differences in this folate-dependent pathway.[248,250,251] Folate pretreatment in healthy macaques results in a higher rate of oxidation of formate to CO_2.[178] Administration of folinic acid, an activated form of the vitamin, after giving toxic doses of methanol to these nonhuman primates, has been shown to mitigate formate accumulation, prevent metabolic acidosis, and reverse established toxicity.[251] There are no controlled clinical trials investigating the efficacy of folic or folinic acid in human methanol poisoning. However, given the compelling animal findings, along with the recognized safety of parenterally administered water-soluble vitamins, folinic acid (or, if unavailable, folic acid) is recommended for patients with methanol poisoning.[36]

It has been proposed that limited amounts of glyoxylic acid produced in ethylene glycol poisoning might undergo decarboxylation in vivo to form CO_2 and formic acid, hypothetically catalyzed by an uncharacterized dehydrogenase enzyme such as:

$$\underset{\text{Glyoxylic acid}}{\overset{\text{CHO}}{\underset{\text{COOH}}{|}}} \xrightarrow[\text{H}_2\text{O}]{\overset{\text{NAD}^+ \quad \text{NADH} + \text{H}^+}{?}} \underset{\text{Formic acid}}{\overset{\text{H}}{\underset{\text{COOH}}{|}}} + \underset{\text{Carbon dioxide}}{\text{O=C=O}}$$

Studies in rat liver slices incubated with ^{14}C-labeled ethylene glycol have shown that $^{14}CO_2$ is generated.[56] On the other hand, Clay and Murphy[60] administered ^{14}C-labeled ethylene glycol to pigtail macaques and found that blood and urine formate concentrations, as well as exhaled $^{14}CO_2$ production (the expected breakdown product of formate), did not differ from control values. These findings are evidence against appreciable in vivo decarboxylation of glyoxylic acid to produce formate in primates. Although folinic (or folic) acid is recommended as adjunctive therapy in human methanol poisoning, there is no empiric evidence that folate compounds are useful for treating ethylene glycol intoxication and they are not recommended for routine use unless there is suspicion of concomitant methanol ingestion or folic acid deficiency.[35,36]

Typical recommendations in methanol poisoning are to administer IV folinic acid at a dose of 1 mg/kg, up to 50 mg, at 4-hour intervals.[36] Folic acid should be used if folinic acid is unavailable. Folinic acid is the international nonproprietary name approved by the World Health Organization for the compound 5-formyl-THF. Before elucidating its structure, it was first described as a required growth factor for the bacterium *Leuconostoc citrovorum* and therefore it was historically called citrovorum factor.[252] In the United States, its official generic pharmaceutical name is leucovorin, and it has been used primarily in oncology (eg, as rescue therapy after administration of toxic doses of the antineoplastic agent methotrexate, which is a folic acid antagonist).

Pyridoxine

Vitamin B$_6$ (pyridoxine) has been cited for its hypothetical therapeutic value in ethylene glycol intoxication. The rationale is that limited amounts of glyoxylic acid can be metabolized to the amino acid glycine through a transamination reaction catalyzed by alanine:glyoxylate aminotransferase, the enzyme that is deficient in type I primary hyperoxaluria[63,253]:

$$\underset{\text{Glyoxylic acid}}{\overset{\displaystyle CHO}{\underset{\displaystyle COOH}{|}}} \quad + \quad \underset{\text{Alanine}}{\overset{\displaystyle CH_3}{\underset{\displaystyle COOH}{\overset{|}{\underset{|}{CH-NH_2}}}}} \quad \xrightarrow[\text{B6}]{\text{Aminotransferase}} \quad \underset{\text{Pyruvic acid}}{\overset{\displaystyle CH_3}{\underset{\displaystyle COOH}{\overset{|}{\underset{|}{C=O}}}}} \quad + \quad \underset{\text{Glycine}}{\overset{\displaystyle NH_2}{\underset{\displaystyle COOH}{\overset{|}{\underset{|}{CH_2}}}}}$$

This aminotransferase requires vitamin B$_6$ (pyridoxine) as a cofactor. This step may be considered a detoxification reaction because the resulting pyruvic acid and glycine are normal metabolic intermediates.[63] Pyruvate can be metabolized by way of the Krebs cycle, and glycine can be metabolized to serine, carbon dioxide, or under some circumstances (see earlier discussion), hippuric acid. Although the capabilities of this pathway for handling glyoxylic acid are limited and are likely overwhelmed if there is significant ethylene glycol exposure and metabolism, pyridoxine deficiency is expected to hamper this reaction. Outside the context of ethylene glycol intoxication, increased urinary concentrations of oxalate have been observed in pyridoxine deficiency, whereas large doses of pyridoxine have been shown to decrease urinary oxalate excretion.[75,254] Pyridoxine is also a necessary cofactor in an alternative pathway for regenerating THF from N^{10}-formyl-THF in the metabolism of formate.[37] Based on these observations, some investigators have recommended pyridoxine administration (eg, single or multiple 50-mg doses IV) to cover for the possibility of the vitamin deficiency in ethylene glycol and methanol poisoning.[12] Routine use of vitamin B$_6$ in methanol or ethylene glycol ingestions otherwise lacks an evidence base, but is indicated in patients at risk for pyridoxine deficiency and hence in patients known or suspected of having a history of chronic alcoholism or malnutrition.

Calcium

There are reports of hypocalcemia in ethylene glycol poisoning.[72,82,123,124,136,138] Extensive deposition of calcium oxalate crystals in renal and other tissues may be the mechanism that leads to this electrolyte disturbance. Sodium bicarbonate administration also may promote or worsen hypocalcemia. Calcium supplementation is not recommended in hypocalcemic patients with ethylene glycol intoxication unless there are manifestations of hypocalcemia. The concern is that calcium administration could increase calcium oxalate formation, with resulting crystal deposition in the brain, heart, kidneys, and other vital organs and tissues, leading to untoward effects. In the face of hypocalcemia, manifestations warranting calcium administration (eg, IV calcium gluconate) may include Chvostek or Trousseau sign, tetany, intractable seizures, or significant electrocardiographic QT interval prolongation.

PROGNOSIS

Permanent visual impairment, including complete blindness, has occurred in some patients surviving methanol poisoning, and many deaths have also occurred (**Table 4**). In the 1951 Atlanta, Georgia, outbreak of methanol poisoning that followed widespread distribution of bootleg whiskey containing methanol, there were 41 deaths among 323 patients, and among the evaluated survivors there were 9 patients with permanent blindness (acuity ≤20/200 in 1 or, more usually, both eyes).[43] Among a more recent but smaller methanol poisoning outbreak in Papua New Guinea involving 24 patients, there were no ocular abnormalities in 9 patients and only transient abnormalities in 7 patients, but 8 suffered permanent ocular deficits (complete blindness in 2 and severe deficits in 4 patients).[86] In another series of 12 cases of methanol ingestion, there was 1 death and 1 patient with permanent blindness.[54] A fairly consistent finding of these and other reports is that coma, respiratory arrest, and severity of metabolic acidosis (eg, pH <7.0) correlated with poor prognosis for survival and, in survivors, permanent visual impairment.[34,43,86,92,93,103,105] Both early hospital presentation after the ingestion and a finding of respiratory compensation for metabolic acidosis have been associated with survival in methanol poisoning.[92] Detection of ethanol in the blood at the time of admission has also been associated with better outcome, as is expected from its antidotal properties.[105] Paasma and colleagues[114] followed up survivors of a 2001 outbreak of methanol poisoning and concluded that visual and neurologic sequelae present at the time of hospital discharge were still present 6 years later, suggesting that these cases represented irreversible damage. Permanent nonocular neurologic findings, including polyneuropathy, encephalopathy, ataxia, sensory loss, and extrapyramidal manifestations resembling parkinsonism have been described in some survivors of methanol intoxication.[52,53,82,103,109,114] In some cases, appearance of significant neurologic derangements occurred after a delay of some days beyond the acute presentation.[82,114]

Table 4
Outcomes in methanol and ethylene glycol intoxication[a]

Sequelae	Methanol Intoxication	Ethylene Glycol Intoxication
Ocular	31,34,43,45,54,86,91–93,96,101–103,105,107,108, 112,114,115,179	139
Neurologic	53,91–93,103,109,114	133,143,144
Renal	—	126,132,133,139,143,144
Death	31,34,43,47,49–51,53,54,69,87,91–93,96,100, 104–106,108,109,112,114,117–120,179,255	65,68–70,72,90,126,127,129–131,134,143,185,187

[a] Selected published cases and series (see reference list) reporting death or apparently permanent sequelae.

Many deaths have also occurred from ethylene glycol poisoning (see **Table 4**). Porter and colleagues[90] reviewed a series of 39 patients treated for ethylene glycol poisoning and found that 8 died, all with acute renal failure; whereas of the 31 survivors, 15 had acute renal failure. In a series of 36 ethylene glycol cases in Sweden, 24 patients developed acute renal failure and 6 patients died.[69] Although most patients surviving ethylene glycol ingestion, even if they develop acute anuric renal failure and require prolonged hemodialysis, eventually recover renal function, there are case reports of apparently permanent renal impairment.[82,122,126,133,139,141–144] There are reports of cerebral infarction and other neurologic impairments after recovery from ethylene glycol ingestion, often but not invariably resolving over time (see **Table 4**).[133,138,139,143] A wide variety of cranial nerve deficits have been described (see **Box 5**), also with variability in outcome in survivors. In some reports, severe cranial nerve or other neurologic deficits developed up to a week or more after the toxic ingestion in patients who had not had neurologic impairments before that point.[82,99,133,135,139,143,150] The most common delayed cranial nerve deficit is facial diplegia.

REFERENCES

1. Conrad FH, Hill EF, Ballman EA. Freezing points of the system ethylene glycol-methanol-water. Ind Eng Chem 1940;32(4):542–3.
2. Budavari S, O'Neil MJ, Smith A, et al, editors. The Merck Index. 11th edition. Rahway (NJ): Merck; 1989. p. 594–9, 651, 662–3, 939.
3. Dow Chemical Co. Dow ethylene glycols: physical properties. Midland (MI): Dow Chemical; 2012.
4. Gibbard HF, Creek JL. Vapor pressure of methanol from 288.15 to 337.65K. J Chem Eng Data 1974;19(4):308–10.
5. Lucius JE, Olhoeft GR, Hill PL, et al. Properties and hazards of 108 selected substances. Open-File Report 90–408. 1990 edition. Washington, DC: US Department of the Interior, Geological Survey; 1990.
6. Munro LA. Antifreeze; radiator compounds; brake fluids. In: Chemistry in Engineering. Englewood Cliffs (NJ): Prentice-Hall; 1964. p. 243–52.
7. National Institute for Occupational Safety and Health. The emergency response safety and health database. Atlanta (GA): US Centers for Disease Control and Prevention; 2008. Available at. http://www.cdc.gov/niosh/ershdb/. Accessed June 12, 2012.
8. Ruth JH. Odor thresholds and irritation levels of several chemical substances: a review. Am Ind Hyg Assoc J 1986;47(3):A142–51.
9. Yue H, Zhao Y, Ma X, et al. Ethylene glycol: properties, synthesis, and applications. Chem Soc Rev 2012;41(11):4218–44.
10. Methanol Institute. The clear alternative for transportation. Methanol fuel and FFV technology. Arlington (VA): Methanol Institute; 2011.
11. Kruse JA. Methanol, ethylene glycol, and related intoxications. In: Carlson RW, Geheb MA, editors. Principles and practice of medical intensive care. Philadelphia: WB Saunders; 1993. p. 1714–23.
12. Kruse JA. Alcohol and glycol intoxications. In: Kruse JA, Fink MP, Carlson RW, editors. Saunders manual of critical care. Philadelphia: WB Saunders; 2003. p. 233–9.
13. Kruse JA. Ethanol, methanol, and ethylene glycol. In: Vincent JL, Abraham E, Moore FA, et al, editors. Textbook of critical care. Philadelphia: Elsevier; 2011. p. 1270–81.

14. Alcohol, tobacco and firearms. Formula for denatured alcohol and rum. 27 CFR §21, 1983.

15. Egbert AM, Liese BA, Powell BJ, et al. When alcoholics drink aftershave: a study of nonbeverage alcohol consumers. Alcohol Alcohol 1986;21(3): 285–94.

16. Lachenmeier DW, Rehm J, Gmel G. Surrogate alcohol: what do we know and where do we go? Alcohol Clin Exp Res 2007;31(10):1613–24.

17. European Commission. Commission Regulation (EC) No. 3199/93 of 22 November 1993 on the mutual recognition of procedures for the complete denaturing of alcohol for the purposes of exemption from excise duty. Off J Eur Community L288:12–15.

18. Leon AS, Hunninghake DB, Bell C, et al. Safety of long-term large doses of aspartame. Arch Intern Med 1989;149(10):2318–24.

19. Stegink LD, Brummel MC, McMartin K, et al. Blood methanol concentrations in normal adult subjects administered abuse doses of aspartame. J Toxicol Environ Health 1981;7(2):281–90.

20. Greizerstein HB. Congener contents of alcoholic beverages. J Stud Alcohol 1981;42(11):1030–7.

21. Malandain H, Cano Y. Serum methanol in the absence of methanol ingestion. Ann Emerg Med 1996;28(1):102–3.

22. Green DH, Lamprey H, Sommer EE. Properties vs. performance of present-day anti-freeze solutions. J Chem Educ 1941;18(1):488–92.

23. Davis L. Pinpointing vehicle leaks faster with ultraviolet light. Mater Eval 1989; 47(11):1248–50.

24. Payne HA. Bitrex–a bitter solution to safety. Chem Ind 1988;21:721–3.

25. White NC, Litovitz T, Benson BE, et al. The impact of bittering agents on pediatric ingestions of antifreeze. Clin Pediatr 2009;48(9):913–21.

26. US Food and Drug Administration. Substances generally recognized as safe. 21 CFR §582.1666, 2011.

27. Dutkiewicz B, Konczalik J, Karwacki W. Skin absorption and per os administration of methanol in men. Int Arch Occup Environ Health 1980;47(1): 81–8.

28. Kahn A, Blum D. Methyl alcohol poisoning in an 8-month-old boy: an unusual route of intoxication. Pediatrics 1979;94(5):841–3.

29. Frenia ML, Schauben JL. Methanol inhalation toxicity. Ann Emerg Med 1993; 22(12):1919–23.

30. Bebarta VS, Heard K, Dart RC. Inhalational abuse of methanol products: elevated methanol and formate levels without vision loss. Am J Emerg Med 2006;24(6):725–8.

31. Kleiman R, Nickle R, Schwartz M. Inhalational methanol toxicity. J Med Toxicol 2009;5(3):158–64.

32. Aufderheide TP, White SM, Brady WJ, et al. Inhalational and percutaneous methanol toxicity in two firefighters. Ann Emerg Med 1993;22(12):1916–8.

33. Wills JH, Coulston F, Harris ES, et al. Inhalation of aerosolized ethylene glycol by man. Clin Toxicol 1974;7(5):463–76.

34. Bennett IL Jr, Cary FH, Mitchell GL Jr, et al. Acute methyl alcohol poisoning: a review based on experiences in an outbreak of 323 cases. Medicine 1953; 32(4):431–63.

35. Barceloux DG, Krenzelok EP, Olson K, et al. American Academy of Clinical Toxicology practice guidelines on the treatment of ethylene glycol poisoning. Ad Hoc Committee. J Toxicol Clin Toxicol 1999;37(5):537–60.

36. Barceloux DG, Bond GR, Krenzelok EP, et al. American Academy of Clinical Toxicology practice guidelines on the treatment of methanol poisoning. J Toxicol Clin Toxicol 2002;40(4):415–46.
37. Kruse JA. Methanol poisoning. Intensive Care Med 1992;18(7):391–7.
38. Jacobsen D, McMartin KE. Methanol and ethylene glycol poisonings. Mechanism of toxicity, clinical course, diagnosis and treatment. Med Toxicol 1986;1(5): 309–34.
39. Jacobsen D, Webb R, Collins TD, et al. Methanol and formate kinetics in late diagnosed methanol intoxication. Med Toxicol Adverse Drug Exp 1988;3(5): 418–23.
40. Keyhani J, Keyhani E. EPR study of the effect of formate on cytochrome C oxidase. Biochem Biophys Res Commun 1980;92(1):327–33.
41. Nicholls P. The effect of formate on cytochrome aa3 and on electron transport in the intact respiratory chain. Biochim Biophys Acta 1976;430(1):13–29.
42. Liesivuori J, Savolainen H. Methanol and formic acid toxicity: biochemical mechanisms. Pharmacol Toxicol 1991;69(3):157–63.
43. Benton CD Jr, Calhoun FP Jr. The ocular effects of methyl alcohol poisoning: report of a catastrophe involving 320 persons. Am J Ophthalmol 1953;36(12):1677–85.
44. Eells JT, Salzman MM, Lewandowski MF, et al. Formate-induced alterations in retinal function in methanol-intoxicated rats. Toxicol Appl Pharmacol 1996; 140(1):58–69.
45. Hantson P, de Tourtchaninoff M, Simoens G, et al. Evoked potentials investigation of visual dysfunction after methanol poisoning. Crit Care Med 1999;27(12): 2707–15.
46. Seme MT, Summerfelt P, Neitz J, et al. Differential recovery of retinal function after mitochondrial inhibition by methanol intoxication. Invest Ophthalmol Vis Sci 2001;42(3):834–41.
47. Sharpe JA, Hostovsky M, Bilbao JM, et al. Methanol optic neuropathy: a histopathological study. Neurology 1982;32(10):1093–100.
48. Tephly TR. The toxicity of methanol. Life Sci 1991;48(11):1031–41.
49. Treichel JL, Murray TG, Lewandowski MF, et al. Retinal toxicity in methanol poisoning. Retina 2004;24(2):309–12.
50. Andresen H, Schmoldt H, Matschke J, et al. Fatal methanol intoxication with different survival times—morphological findings and postmortem methanol distribution. Forensic Sci Int 2008;179(2–3):206–10.
51. Karayel F, Turan AA, Sav A, et al. Methanol intoxication. Pathological changes of central nervous system (17 cases). Am J Forensic Med Pathol 2010;31(1):34–6.
52. Ley CO, Gali FG. Parkinsonian syndrome after methanol intoxication. Eur Neurol 1983;22(6):405–9.
53. McLean DR, Jacobs H, Mielke BW. Methanol poisoning: a clinical and pathological study. Ann Neurol 1980;8(2).161–7.
54. Pappas SC, Silverman M. Treatment of methanol poisoning with ethanol and hemodialysis. CMAJ 1982;126(12):1391–4.
55. Kruse JA. Ethylene glycol intoxication. J Intensive Care Med 1992;7(5):234–43.
56. Gessner PK, Parke DV, Williams RT. Studies in detoxification: 86. The metabolism of ^{14}C-labelled ethylene glycol. Biochem J 1961;79(Pt 3):482–9.
57. O'Brien PJ, Siraki AG, Shangari N. Aldehyde sources, metabolism, molecular toxicity mechanisms, and possible effects on human health. Crit Rev Toxicol 2005;35(7):609–62.
58. Shangari N, O'Brien PJ. The cytotoxic mechanism of glyoxal involves oxidative stress. Biochem Pharmacol 2004;68(7):1433–42.

59. Kun E. A study on the metabolism of glyoxal in vitro. J Biol Chem 1952;194(2): 603–11.
60. Clay KL, Murphy RC. On the metabolic acidosis of ethylene glycol intoxication. Toxicol Appl Pharmacol 1977;39(1):39–49.
61. Murray MS, Holmes RP, Lowther WT. Active site and loop 4 movements within human glycolate oxidase: implications for substrate specificity and drug design. Biochemistry 2008;47(8):2439–49.
62. Murray MS, Holmes RP, Lowther WT. Human glycolate oxidase 1: a structural and biochemical examination of a possible target for hyperoxaluria treatment. Urol Res 2007;35(5):264–5.
63. Danpure CJ. Primary hyperoxaluria type I: AGT mistargeting highlights the fundamental differences between peroxisomal and mitochondrial protein import pathways. Biochim Biophys Acta 2006;1763(12):1776–84.
64. Pennati A, Gadda G. Involvement of ionizable groups in catalysis of human liver glycolate oxidase. J Biol Chem 2009;284(45):31214–22.
65. Armstrong EJ, Engelhart DA, Jenkins AJ, et al. Homicidal ethylene glycol intoxication. A report of a case. Am J Forensic Med Pathol 2006;27(2): 151–5.
66. Borden TA, Bidwell CD. Treatment of acute ethylene glycol poisoning in rats. Invest Urol 1968;6(3):205–10.
67. Goldsher M, Better OS. Antifreeze poisoning during the October 1973 war in the Middle-East: case reports. Mil Med 1979;144(5):314–5.
68. Hagemann PO, Chiffelle TR. Ethylene glycol poisoning. A clinical and pathologic study of three cases. J Lab Clin Med 1948;33(5):573–84.
69. Karlson-Stiber C, Persson H. Ethylene glycol poisoning: experiences from an epidemic in Sweden. Clin Toxicol 1992;30(4):565–74.
70. Miskovitz PF. Metabolic acidosis in a somnolent alcoholic. Drug Ther 1980; 10(12):33–9.
71. Pons CA, Custer RP. Acute ethylene glycol poisoning; a clinico-pathologic report of 18 fatal cases. Am J Med Sci 1946;211(5):544–52.
72. Scully RE, Galdabini JJ, McNeely BU. Case records of the Massachusetts General Hospital. N Engl J Med 1979;201(12):650–7.
73. Szabuniewicz M, Bailey EM, Wiersig DO. A new approach to the treatment of ethylene glycol poisoning in dogs. Southwest Vet 1975;28(1):7–11.
74. Van Stee EW, Harris AM, Horton ML, et al. The treatment of ethylene glycol toxicosis with pyrazole. J Pharmacol Exp Ther 1975;192(2):251–9.
75. Boquist L, Lindqvist B, Östberg Y, et al. Primary oxalosis. Am J Med 1973;54(5): 673–81.
76. Danpure CJ. Molecular and clinical heterogeneity in primary hyperoxaluria type I. Am J Kidney Dis 1991;17(4):366–9.
77. Williams HE, Smith LH Jr. L-Glyceric aciduria—a new genetic variant of primary hyperoxaluria. N Engl J Med 1968;278(5):233–9.
78. Bove KE. Ethylene glycol toxicity. Am J Clin Pathol 1966;45(1):46–50.
79. Aquino HC, Leonard CD. Ethylene glycol poisoning: report of three cases. J Ky Med Assoc 1972;70(6):463–5.
80. Walker JT, Keller MS, Katz SM. Computed tomography and sonographic findings in acute ethylene glycol poisoning. J Ultrasound Med 1983;2(9):429–31.
81. Munro KM, Adams JH. Acute ethylene glycol poisoning: report of a fatal case. Med Sci Law 1967;7(4):181–4.
82. Parry MF, Wallach R. Ethylene glycol poisoning. Am J Med 1974;57(1): 143–50.

83. Poldelski V, Johnson A, Wright S, et al. Ethylene glycol-mediated tubular injury: identification of critical metabolites and injury pathways. Am J Kidney Dis 2001; 38(2):339–48.

84. Bachmann E, Goldberg L. Reappraisal of the toxicology of ethylene glycol. III. Mitochondrial effects. Food Cosmet Toxicol 1971;9(1):39–55.

85. Klamerth OL. Influence of glyoxal on cell function. Biochim Biophys Acta 1968; 155(1):271–9.

86. Dethlefs R, Naraqi S. Ocular manifestations and complications of acute methyl alcohol intoxication. Med J Aust 1978;2(10):483–5.

87. Liu JJ, Daya MR, Mann NC. Methanol-related deaths in Ontario. Clin Toxicol 1999;37(1):69–73.

88. Mårtensson E, Olofsson U, Heath A. Clinical and metabolic features of ethanol-methanol poisoning in chronic alcoholics. Lancet 1988;1(8581):327–8.

89. Roberts J. Ethylene glycol intoxication and multiple trauma. Emerg Med 2000; 32(1):8–10.

90. Porter WH, Rutter PW, Bush BA, et al. Ethylene glycol toxicity: the role of serum glycolic acid in hemodialysis. Clin Toxicol 2001;39(6):607–15.

91. Hovda KE, Hunderi OH, Rudberg N, et al. Anion and osmolal gaps in the diagnosis of methanol poisoning: clinical study in 28 patients. Intensive Care Med 2004;30(9):1842–6.

92. Hovda KE, Hunderi OH, Tafjord A-B, et al. Methanol outbreak in Norway 2002–2004: epidemiology, clinical features and prognostic signs. J Intern Med 2005;258(2):181–90.

93. Naraqi S, Dethlefs RF, Slobodniuk RA, et al. An outbreak of acute methyl alcohol intoxication. Aust N Z J Med 1979;9(1):65–8.

94. Pincus F. Die Massenerkrankungen im städtischen Asyl für Obdachlose in Berlin 24, bis 31 December 1911. Med Klin 1912;1:41 [in German].

95. Swartz RD, Millman RP, Billi JE, et al. Epidemic methanol poisoning: clinical biochemical analysis of a recent episode. Medicine 1981;60(5):373–82.

96. Teo SK, Lo KL, Tey BH. Mass methanol poisoning: a clinico-biochemical analysis of 10 cases. Singapore Med J 1996;37(5):485–7.

97. Schultz S, Kinde M, Johnson D, et al. Ethylene glycol intoxication due to contamination of water systems. MMWR Morb Mortal Wkly Rep 1987; 36(36):611–4.

98. Eder AF, McGrath CM, Dowdy YG, et al. Ethylene glycol poisoning: toxicokinetic and analytical factors affecting laboratory diagnosis. Clin Chem 1998;44(1): 168–77.

99. Glossop AJ, Bryden DC. Case report: an unusual presentation of ethylene glycol poisoning. J Intensive Care Soc 2009;10(2):118–21.

100. Kinoshita H, Ijiri I, Ameno S, et al. Combined toxicity of methanol and formic acid: two cases of methanol poisoning. Int J Legal Med 1998;111(6):334–5.

101. Cavalli A, Volpi A, Maggioni AP, et al. Severe reversible cardiac failure associated with methanol intoxication. Postgrad Med J 1987;63(744):867–8.

102. Fontenot AP, Pelak VS. Development of neurologic symptoms in a 26-year-old woman following recovery from methanol intoxication. Chest 2002;122(4): 1436–9.

103. Lu JJ, Kalimullah EA, Bryant SM. Unilateral blindness following acute methanol poisoning. J Med Toxicol 2010;6(4):459–60.

104. Girault C, Tamion F, Moritz F, et al. Fomepizole (4-methylpyrazole) in fatal methanol poisoning with early CT scan cerebral lesions. Clin Toxicol 1999;37(6): 777–80.

105. Hassanian-Moghaddam H, Pajoumand A, Dadgar SM, et al. Prognostic factors in methanol poisoning. Hum Exp Toxicol 2007;26(7):583–6.
106. Shahangian S, Ash KO. Formic and lactic acidosis in a fatal case of methanol intoxication. Clin Chem 1986;32(2):395–7.
107. Chattopadhyay S, Chandra P. Putaminal necrosis. N Engl J Med 2007;356(22):e23.
108. Önder F, İlker S, Kansu T, et al. Acute blindness and putaminal necrosis in methanol intoxication. Int Ophthalmol 1999;22(2):81–4.
109. Sefidbakht S, Rasekhi AR, Kamali K, et al. Methanol poisoning: acute MR and CT findings in nine patients. Neuroradiology 2007;49(5):427–35.
110. McCoy HG, Cipolle RJ, Ehlers SM, et al. Severe methanol poisoning: application of a pharmacokinetic model for ethanol therapy and hemodialysis. Am J Med 1979;67(5):804–7.
111. Harviel JD, Meth BM, Bray JG, et al. Management of methanol poisoning in an environment with limited facilities. Intensive Care World 1994;11(1):39–42.
112. Hantson P, Haufroid V, Wallemacq P. Formate kinetics in methanol poisoning. Hum Exp Toxicol 2005;24(2):55–9.
113. Eckfeldt JH, Kerhaw M. Hyperamylasemia following methyl alcohol intoxication. Source and significance. Arch Intern Med 1986;146(1):193–4.
114. Paasma R, Hovda KE, Jacobsen D. Methanol poisoning and long term sequelae–a six year follow-up after a large methanol outbreak. BMC Clin Pharmacol 2009;9(5):1–5.
115. Sanaei-Zadeh H, Zamani N, Shadnia S. Outcomes of visual disturbances after methanol poisoning. Clin Toxicol 2011;49(2):102–7.
116. Osterloh JD, Pond SM, Grady S, et al. Serum formate concentrations in methanol intoxication as a criterion for hemodialysis. Ann Intern Med 1986;104(2):200–3.
117. Brent J, McMartin K, Phillips S, et al. Fomepizole for the treatment of methanol poisoning. N Engl J Med 2001;344(6):424–9.
118. McMartin KE, Ambre JJ, Tephly TR. Methanol poisoning in human subjects. Role of formic acid accumulation in the metabolic acidosis. Am J Med 1980;68(3):414–8.
119. Suit PF, Estes ML. Methanol intoxication: clinical features and differential diagnosis. Cleve Clin J Med 1990;57(5):464–70.
120. Babu KM, Rosenbaum CD, Boyer EW. Head CT in patient with metabolic acidosis. J Med Toxicol 2008;4(4):275.
121. Anderson B, Adams QM. Facial-auditory nerve oxalosis. Am J Med 1990;88(1):87–8.
122. Davis DP, Bramwell KJ, Hamilton RS, et al. Ethylene glycol poisoning: case report of a record-high level and a review. J Emerg Med 1997;15(5):653–7.
123. Hagstam K-E, Ingvar DH, Paatela M, et al. Ethylene-glycol poisoning treated by hemodialysis. Acta Med Scand 1965;178(5):599–606.
124. Stokes JB, Aueron F. Prevention of organ damage in massive ethylene glycol ingestion. JAMA 1980;243(20):2065–6.
125. Kassirer JP, Kopelman RL. A comatose alcoholic. Hosp Pract 1985;20(1):26–32.
126. Brent J, McMartin K, Phillips S, et al. Fomepizole for the treatment of ethylene glycol poisoning. Methylpyrazole for Toxic Alcohols Study Group. N Engl J Med 1999;340(11):832–8.
127. Cadnapaphornchai P, Taher S, Bhathena D, et al. Ethylene glycol poisoning: diagnosis based on high osmolal and anion gaps and crystalluria. Ann Emerg Med 1981;10(2):94–7.

128. Gabow P, Clay K, Sullivan JB, et al. Organic acids in ethylene glycol intoxication. Ann Intern Med 1986;105(1):16–20.
129. Godolphin W, Meagher EP, Sanders HD, et al. Unusual calcium oxalate crystals in ethylene glycol poisoning. Clin Toxicol 1980;16(4):479–86.
130. Hylander B, Kjellstrand CM. Prognostic factors and treatment of severe ethylene glycol intoxication. Intensive Care Med 1996;22(6):546–52.
131. Jacobsen D, Ovrebo S, Ostborg J, et al. Glycolate causes the acidosis in ethylene glycol poisoning and is effectively removed by hemodialysis. Acta Med Scand 1984;216(4):409–16.
132. Jacobsen D, Hewlett TP, Webb R, et al. Ethylene glycol intoxication: evaluation of kinetics and crystalluria. Am J Med 1988;84(1):145–52.
133. Lewis LD, Smith BW, Mamourian AC. Delayed sequelae after acute overdoses or poisonings: cranial neuropathy related to ethylene glycol ingestion. Clin Pharmacol Ther 1997;61(6):692–9.
134. Momont SL, Dahlberg PJH. Ethylene glycol poisoning. Wis Med J 1989;88(9): 16–20.
135. Takayesu JK, Bazari H, Linshaw M. Case 7-2006: a 47-year-old man with altered mental status and acute renal failure. N Engl J Med 2006;354(10):1065–72.
136. Caparros-Lefebvre D, Policard J, Sengler C, et al. Bipallidal haemorrhage after ethylene glycol intoxication. Neuroradiology 2005;47(2):105–7.
137. Dribben W, Furbee B, Kirk M. Brainstem infarction and quadriplegia associated with ethylene glycol ingestion. J Toxicol Clin Toxicol 1999;37(5):657.
138. Morgan BW, Ford MD, Follmer R. Ethylene glycol ingestion resulting in brainstem and midbrain dysfunction. Clin Toxicol 2000;38(4):445–51.
139. Berger JR, Ayyar R. Neurological complications of ethylene glycol intoxication. Arch Neurol 1981;38(11):724–5.
140. Piagnerelli M, Carlier E, Lejeune P. Adult respiratory distress syndrome and medullary toxicity: two unusual complications of ethylene glycol intoxication. Intensive Care Med 1999;25(10):1200.
141. Castanares-Zapatero D, Fillée C, Philippe M, et al. Survival with extreme lactic acidosis following ethylene glycol poisoning? Can J Anaesth 2008;55(5): 318–9.
142. Olivero JJ. A comatose man with marked acidosis and crystaluria. Hosp Pract 1993;28(7):86–8.
143. Palmer BF, Eigenbrodt EH, Henrich WL. Cranial nerve deficit: a clue to the diagnosis of ethylene glycol poisoning. Am J Med 1989;87(1):91–2.
144. Baldwin F, Sran H. Delayed ethylene glycol poisoning presenting with abdominal pain and multiple cranial and peripheral neuropathies: a case report. J Med Case Rep 2010;4:220–4.
145. Peterson CD, Collins AJ, Himes JM, et al. Ethylene glycol poisoning. Pharmacokinetics during therapy with ethanol and hemodialysis. N Engl J Med 1981; 304(1):21–3.
146. Wendland E, Yamase H, Adams N, et al. Hippuric acid not calcium oxalate crystals in the urine of a patient with ethylene glycol ingestion. Am J Kidney Dis 2011;57(4):A104.
147. Catchings TT, Beamer WC, Lundy L, et al. Adult respiratory distress syndrome secondary to ethylene glycol ingestion. Ann Emerg Med 1985;14(6):594–6.
148. Wacker WE, Haynes H, Druyan R, et al. Treatment of ethylene glycol poisoning with ethyl alcohol. JAMA 1965;194(11):1231–3.
149. Fijen JW, Kemperman H, Tessa Ververs FF, et al. False hyperlactatemia in ethylene glycol poisoning. Intensive Care Med 2006;32(4):626–7.

150. Broadley SA, Ferguson IT, Walton B, et al. Severe sensorimotor polyradiculo-neuropathy after ingestion of ethylene glycol. J Neurol Neurosurg Psychiatry 1997;63(2):261.
151. Ahmed MM. Ocular effects of antifreeze poisoning. Br J Ophthalmol 1971; 55(12):854–5.
152. Reddy NJ, Sudini M, Lewis LD. Delayed neurological sequelae from ethylene glycol, diethylene glycol and methanol poisonings. Clin Toxicol 2010;48(10): 967–73.
153. Yant WP, Schrenk HH, Sayers RR. Methanol antifreeze and methanol poisoning. Ind Eng Chem 1931;23(5):551–5.
154. Pien K, van Vlem B, van Coster R, et al. An inherited metabolic disorder present-ing as ethylene glycol intoxication in a young adult. Am J Forensic Med Pathol 2002;23(1):96–100.
155. Porter WH. Ethylene glycol poisoning: quintessential clinical toxicology; analyt-ical conundrum. Clin Chim Acta 2012;413(3–4):365–77.
156. Standefer J, Blackwell W. Enzymatic method for measuring ethylene glycol with a centrifugal analyzer. Clin Chem 1991;37(10):1734–6.
157. Wax P, Branton T, Cobaugh D, et al. False positive ethylene glycol determination by enzyme assay in patients with chronic acetaminophen hepatotoxicity. J Toxicol Clin Toxicol 1999;37(5):604.
158. Kearney J, Rees S, Chiang W. Availability of serum methanol and ethylene glycol levels: a national survey. J Toxicol Clin Toxicol 1997;35(5):509.
159. Robinson CA Jr, Scott JW, Ketchum C. Propylene glycol interference with ethylene glycol procedures. Clin Chem 1983;29(4):727.
160. Bjellerup P, Kallner A, Kollind M. GLC determination of serum-ethylene glycol, interferences in ketotic patients. Clin Toxicol 1994;32(1):85–7.
161. Apple FS, Googins M, Resen D. Propylene glycol interference in gas-chromatographic assay of ethylene glycol. Clin Chem 1993;39(1):167.
162. Casazza JP, Song BJ, Veech RL. Short chain diol in human disease states. Trends Biochem Sci 1990;15(1):26–30.
163. Rutstein DD, Veech RL, Nickerson RJ, et al. 2,3-butanediol: an unusual metab-olite in the serum of severely alcoholic men during acute intoxication. Lancet 1983;2(8349):534–7.
164. Shoemaker JD, Lynch RE, Hoffmann JW, et al. Misidentification of propionic acid as ethylene eglycol in a patient with methylmalonic academia. J Pediatr 1992; 120(3):417–21.
165. Hoffman M. Scientific sleuths solve a murder mystery. Science 1991;254(5034): 931.
166. Jones AW, Nilsson L, Gladh SÅ, et al. 2,3-Butanediol in plasma from an alcoholic mistakenly identified as ethylene glycol by gas-chromatography analysis. Clin Chem 1991;37(8):1453–5.
167. Hilliard NJ, Robinson CA, Hardy R, et al. Repeated positive ethylene glycol levels by gas chromatography. Arch Pathol Lab Med 2004;128(6): e79–80.
168. Hewlett TP, McMartin KE, Lauro AJ, et al. Ethylene glycol poisoning: the value of glycolic acid determinations for diagnosis and treatment. Clin Toxicol 1986; 24(5):389–402.
169. Fraser AD. Importance of glycolic acid analysis in ethylene glycol poisoning. Clin Chem 1998;44(8):1769.
170. Kruse JA, Cadnapaphornchai P. The serum osmole gap. J Crit Care 1994;9(3): 185–97.

171. Kruse JA. Clinical utility and limitations of the anion gap. Int J Intensive Care 1997;4(2):51–66.
172. Kruse JA. Acid-base interpretations. In: Prough DS, Traystman RJ, editors. Critical care: state of the art, vol. 14. Anaheim (CA): Society of Critical Care Medicine, and Baltimore (MD): Williams & Wilkins; 1993. p. 275–97.
173. Kruse JA. Use of the anion gap in intensive and care and emergency medicine. In: Vincent JL, editor. Yearbook of intensive care and emergency medicine. New York: Springer-Verlag; 1994. p. 685–96.
174. Moreau CL, Kerns W II, Tomaszewski CA, et al. Glycolate kinetics and hemodialysis clearance in ethylene glycol poisoning. META Study Group. J Toxicol Clin Toxicol 1998;36(7):659–66.
175. Kerns W II, Tomaszewski C, McMartin K, et al. Formate kinetics in methanol poisoning. Clin Toxicol 2002;40(2):137–43.
176. Makar AB, Tephly TR. Methanol poisoning in the folate-deficient rat. Nature 1976;261(5562):715–6.
177. Martin-Amat G, Tephly TR, McMartin KE, et al. Methyl alcohol poisoning. II. Development of a model for ocular toxicity in methyl alcohol poisoning using the rhesus monkey. Arch Ophthalmol 1977;95(10):1847–50.
178. McMartin KE, Martin-Amat G, Makar AB, et al. Methanol poisoning. V. Role of formate metabolism in the monkey. J Pharmacol Exp Ther 1977;201(3):564–72.
179. Hantson P, Mahieu P. Pancreatic injury following acute methanol poisoning. Clin Toxicol 2000;38(3):297–303.
180. Haupt MC, Zull DN, Adams SL. Massive ethylene glycol poisoning without evidence of crystalluria: a case for early intervention. J Emerg Med 1988;6(4):295–300.
181. Chow MT, Di Silvestro VA, Yung CY, et al. Treatment of acute methanol intoxication with hemodialysis using an ethanol-enriched, bicarbonate-based dialysate. Am J Kidney Dis 1997;30(4):568–70.
182. Buell JF, Sterling R, Mandava S, et al. Ethylene glycol intoxication presenting as a metabolic acidosis associated with a motor vehicle crash: case report. J Trauma 1998;45(4):811–3.
183. Morfin J, Chin A. Urinary calcium oxalate crystals in ethylene glycol intoxication. N Engl J Med 2005;353(24):e21.
184. Singh M, Murtaza M, D'souza N, et al. Abdominal pain and lactic acidosis with ethylene glycol poisoning. Am J Emerg Med 2001;19(6):529–30.
185. Verrilli MR, Deyling CL, Pippenger CE, et al. Fatal ethylene glycol intoxication. Report of a case and review of the literature. Cleve Clin J Med 1987;54(4):289–95.
186. Jacobsen D, Åkesson I, Shefter E. Urinary calcium oxalate monohydrate crystals in ethylene glycol poisoning. Scand J Clin Lab Invest 1982;42(3):231–4.
187. Reddy NJ, Suriawinata AA, Sedlacek M. The importance of recognizing whewellite. Nephrol Dial Transplant 2006;21(9):2667.
188. Terlinsky AS, Grochowski J, Geoly KL, et al. Identification of atypical calcium oxalate crystalluria following ethylene glycol ingestion. Am J Clin Pathol 1981;76(2):223–6.
189. Juenke JM, Hardy L, McMillin GA, et al. Rapid and specific quantification of ethylene glycol levels. Adaptation of a commercial enzymatic assay to automated chemistry analyzers. Am J Clin Pathol 2011;136(2):318–24.
190. Elliot JS, Rabinowitz IN. Calcium oxalate crystalluria: crystal size in urine. J Urol 1980;123(3):324–7.

191. Carvalho M, Vieira MA. Changes in calcium oxalate crystal morphology as a function of supersaturation. Int Braz J Urol 2004;30(3):205–9.
192. Gabow P, Clay K, Sullivan JB, et al. Organic acids in ethylene glycol intoxication. Ann Intern Med 1986;105(5):800.
193. Jacobsen D. Organic acids in ethylene glycol intoxication. Ann Intern Med 1986; 105(5):799–800.
194. Willis MS, Wians FH, Kroft S, et al. The case of the needle-shaped urine crystals. Lab Med 2002;33(8):637–40.
195. Khan SR, Hackett RL. Crystal-matrix relationships in experimentally induced urinary calcium oxalate monohydrate crystals, an ultrastructural study. Calcif Tissue Int 1987;41(3):157–63.
196. Thrall MA, Dial SM, Winder DR. Identification of calcium oxalate monohydrate crystals by X-ray diffraction in urine of ethylene glycol-intoxicated dogs. Vet Pathol 1985;22(6):625–8.
197. Wesson JA, Worcester EM, Wiessner JH, et al. Control of calcium oxalate crystal structure and cell adherence by urinary macromolecules. Kidney Int 1998;53(4): 952–7.
198. Pero RW. Health consequences of catabolic synthesis of hippuric acid in humans. Curr Clin Pharmacol 2010;5(1):67–73.
199. Carlisle EJ, Donnelly SM, Vasuvattakul S, et al. Glue-sniffing and distal renal tubular acidosis: sticking to the facts. J Am Soc Nephrol 1991;1(8): 1019–27.
200. Weon JI, Woo HS. Corrosion mechanism of aluminum alloy by ethylene glycol-based solution. Mat Corr 2011;62(9999):1–10.
201. Bælum J. Human solvent exposure factors influencing the pharmacokinetics and acute toxicity. Pharmacol Toxicol 1991;68(Suppl 1):1–36.
202. Mulder TP, Rietveld AG, van Amelsvoort JM. Consumption of both black tea and green tea results in an increase in the excretion of hippuric acid into urine. Am J Clin Nutr 2005;81(Suppl):256S–60S.
203. Kruse JA. Lactic acidosis. In: Carlson RW, Geheb MA, editors. Principles and practice of medical intensive care. Philadelphia: WB Saunders; 1993. p. 1231–45.
204. MacDonald L, Kruse JA, Levy D, et al. Lactic acidosis and acute ethanol intoxication. Am J Emerg Med 1994;12(1):32–5.
205. Orringer CE, Eustace JC, Wunsch CD, et al. Natural history of lactic acidosis after grand-mal seizures. A model for the study of an anion gap acidosis not associated with hyperkalemia. N Engl J Med 1977;297(15):796–9.
206. Kruse JA. Lactic acidosis: understanding pathogenesis and causes. J Crit Illn 1999;14:456–66.
207. Morgan TJ, Clark C, Clague A. Artifactual elevation of measured plasma L-lactate concentration in the presence of glycolate. Crit Care Med 1999;27(10): 2177–9.
208. Woo MY, Greenway DC, Nadler SP, et al. Artifactual elevation of lactate in ethylene glycol poisoning. J Emerg Med 2003;25(3):289–93.
209. Porter WH, Crellin M, Rutter PW, et al. Interference by glycolic acid in the Beckman Synchron method for lactate: a useful clue for unsuspected ethylene glycol intoxication. Clin Chem 2000;46(6):874–5.
210. Brindley PG, Butler MS, Cembrowski G, et al. Falsely elevated point-of-care lactate measurement after ingestion of ethylene glycol. CMAJ 2007;176(8): 1097–9.
211. Pernet P. False elevation of blood lactate reveals ethylene glycol poisoning. Am J Emerg Med 2009;27(1):132.e1–2.

212. Winter ML, Ellis MD, Snodgrass WR. Urine fluorescence using a Wood's lamp to detect the antifreeze additive sodium fluorescein: a qualitative adjunctive test in suspected ethylene glycol ingestions. Ann Emerg Med 1990;19(6):663–7.
213. Curtin L, Kraner J, Wine H, et al. Complete recovery after massive ethylene glycol ingestion. Arch Intern Med 1992;152(6):1311–3.
214. Wallace K, Suchard J, Curry S, et al. Accuracy and reliability of urine fluorescence by Wood's lamp examination for antifreeze ingestion. Clin Toxicol 1999; 37(5):669.
215. Casavant MJ, Shah MN, Battels R. Does fluorescent urine indicate antifreeze ingestion by children? Pediatrics 2001;109(1):113–4.
216. Wallace KL, Suchard JR, Curry SC, et al. Diagnostic use of physicians' detection of urine fluorescence in a simulated ingestion of sodium fluorescein-containing antifreeze. Ann Emerg Med 2001;38(1):49–54.
217. Parsa T, Cunningham SJ, Wall SP, et al. The usefulness of urine fluorescence for suspected antifreeze ingestion in children. Am J Emerg Med 2005;23(6): 787–92.
218. Verhelst D, Moulin P, Haufroid V, et al. Acute renal injury following methanol poisoning: analysis of a case series. Int J Toxicol 2004;23(4):267–73.
219. Jazz Pharmaceuticals. Antizole–fomepizole injection, solution [package insert]. Palo Alto (CA): Jazz Pharmaceuticals; 2006.
220. Cooper DJ, Walley KR, Wiggs BR, et al. Bicarbonate does not improve hemodynamics in critically ill patients who have lactic acidosis. Ann Intern Med 1990; 112(7):492–8.
221. American Diabetes Association. Hyperglycemic crises in diabetes. Diabetes Care 2004;27(Suppl 1):S94–102.
222. Neumar RW, Otto CW, Link MS, et al. Part 8: Adult advanced cardiovascular life support: 2010 American Heart Association guidelines for cardiopulmonary resuscitation and emergency cardiovascular care. Circulation 2010;122(Suppl 3):S729–67.
223. Wagner FW, Burger AR, Ballee BL. Kinetic properties of human liver alcohol dehydrogenase: oxidation of alcohols by class I isoenzymes. Biochemistry 1983;22(8):1857–63.
224. Baraona E, Abittan CS, Dohmen K, et al. Gender differences in pharmacokinetics of alcohol. Alcohol Clin Exp Res 2001;25(4):502–7.
225. Cowan JM Jr, Weathermon A, McCutcheon JR, et al. Determination of volume of distribution for ethanol in male and female subjects. J Anal Toxicol 1996;20(5): 287–90.
226. Peterson CD. Oral ethanol doses in patients with methanol poisoning. Am J Hosp Pharm 1981;38(7):1024–7.
227. Cobaugh DJ, Gibbs M, Shapiro DE, et al. A comparison of the bioavailabilities of oral and intravenous ethanol in healthy male volunteers. Acad Emerg Med 1999; 6(10):984–8.
228. Kendall McGaw Laboratories. Alcohol and dextrose injections USP hypertonic [package insert]. Irvine (CA): Kendall McGaw Laboratories; 1986.
229. Roy M, Bailey B, Chalut D, et al. What are the adverse effects of ethanol used as an antidote in the treatment of suspected methanol poisoning in children. J Toxicol Clin Toxicol 2003;41(2):155–61.
230. Lepik KJ, Levy AR, Sobolev BG, et al. Adverse drug events associated with the antidotes for methanol and ethylene glycol poisoning: a comparison of ethanol and fomepizole. Ann Emerg Med 2009;53(4):439–50.
231. Baud FJ, Galliot M, Astier A, et al. Treatment of ethylene glycol poisoning with intravenous 4-methylpyrazole. N Engl J Med 1988;319(2):97–100.

232. Blomstrand R, Ellin Å, Löf A, et al. Biological effects and metabolic interactions after chronic and acute administration of 4-methylpyrazole and ethanol to rats. Arch Biochem Biophys 1980;199(2):591–605.

233. Borron SW, Mégarbane B, Baud FJ. Fomepizole in treatment of uncomplicated ethylene glycol poisoning. Lancet 1999;354(4):831.

234. De Brabander N, Wojciechowski M, De Decker K, et al. Fomepizole as a therapeutic strategy in paediatric methanol poisoning. A case report and review of the literature. Eur J Pediatr 2005;164(3):158–61.

235. Jobard E, Harry P, Turcant A, et al. 4-Methylpyrazole and hemodialysis in ethylene glycol poisoning. J Toxicol Clin Toxicol 1996;34(4):373–7.

236. Boyer EW, Mejia M, Woolf A, et al. Severe ethylene glycol ingestion treated without hemodialysis. Pediatrics 2001;107(1):172–3.

237. Lepik KJ, Sobolev BG, Levy AR, et al. Medication errors associated with the use of ethanol and fomepizole as antidotes for methanol and ethylene glycol poisoning. Clin Toxicol 2011;49(5):391–401.

238. Buchanan JA, Alhelail M, Cetaruk EW, et al. Massive ethylene glycol ingestion treated with fomepizole alone—a viable therapeutic option. J Med Toxicol 2010;6(2):131–4.

239. Buller GK, Moskowitz CB. When is it appropriate to treat ethylene glycol intoxication with fomepizole alone without hemodialysis? Semin Dial 2011;24(4): 441–2.

240. Hovda KE, Jacobsen D. Expert opinion: fomepizole may ameliorate the need for hemodialysis in methanol poisoning. Hum Exp Toxicol 2008;27(7):539–46.

241. Levine M, Curry SC, Ruha AM, et al. Ethylene glycol elimination kinetics and outcomes in patients managed without hemodialysis. Ann Emerg Med 2012; 59(6):527–31.

242. Velez LI, Shepherd G, Lee LC, et al. Ethylene glycol ingestion treated only with fomepizole. J Med Toxicol 2007;3(3):125–8.

243. Nzerue CM, Harvey P, Volcy J, et al. Survival after massive ethylene glycol poisoning: role of an ethanol enriched, bicarbonate-based dialysate. Int J Artif Organs 1999;22(11):744–6.

244. Hirsch D, Jindal K, Wong P, et al. A simple method to estimate the required dialysis time for cases of alcohol poisoning. Kidney Int 2001;60(5):2021–4.

245. Mégarbane B, Borron SW, Baud FJ. Current recommendations for treatment of severe toxic alcohol poisonings. Intensive Care Med 2005;31(2):189–95.

246. Youssef GM, Hirsch DJ. Validation of a method to predict required dialysis time for cases of methanol and ethylene glycol poisoning. Am J Kidney Dis 2005; 46(3):509–11.

247. Watson P, Watson I, Batt R, et al. Total body water volumes for adult males and females estimated from anthropometric measurements. Am J Clin Nutr 1980; 33(1):27–39.

248. McMartin KE, Makar AB, Martin A, et al. Methanol poisoning. I. The role of formic acid in the development of metabolic acidosis in the monkey and the reversal by 4-methylpyrazole. Biochem Med 1975;13(4):319–33.

249. Anonymous Use of folate analogue in treatment of methyl alcohol toxic reactions is studied. JAMA 1979;242(18):1961–2.

250. Black KA, Eells JT, Noker PE, et al. Role of hepatic tetrahydrofolate in the species difference in methanol toxicity. Proc Natl Acad Sci U S A 1985; 82(11):3854–8.

251. Noker PE, Eells JT, Tephly TR. Methanol toxicity: treatment with folic acid and 5-formyl tetrahydrofolic acid. Alcohol Clin Exp Res 1980;4(4):378–83.

252. Sauberlich HE, Baumann CA. A factor required for the growth of *Leuconostoc citrovorum*. J Biol Chem 1948;176(1):165–73.
253. Salido E, Pey AL, Rodriguez R, et al. Primary hyperoxalurias: disorders of glyoxylate detoxification. Biochim Biophys Acta 2012;1822(9):1453–64.
254. Gibbs DA, Watts RW. The action of pyridoxine in primary hyperoxaluria. Clin Sci 1970;38(2):277–86.
255. Ferrari LA, Arado MG, Nardo CA, et al. Post-mortem analysis of formic acid disposition in acute methanol intoxication. Forensic Sci Int 2003;133(1–2):152–8.

Index

Note: Page numbers of article titles are in **boldface** type.

Crit Care Clin 28 (2012) 713–723
http://dx.doi.org/10.1016/S0749-0704(12)00071-1
0749-0704/12/$ – see front matter © 2012 Elsevier Inc. All rights reserved.

criticalcare.theclinics.com

United States Postal Service

Statement of Ownership, Management, and Circulation
(All Periodicals Publications Except Requestor Publications)

1. Publication Title
Critical Care Clinics

2. Publication Number
0 0 0 - 7 0 8

3. Filing Date
9/14/12

4. Issue Frequency
Jan, Apr, Jul, Oct

5. Number of Issues Published Annually
4

6. Annual Subscription Price
$193.00

7. Complete Mailing Address of Known Office of Publication (Not printer) (Street, city, county, state, and ZIP+4®)

Elsevier Inc.
360 Park Avenue South
New York, NY 10010-1710

Contact Person
Stephen R. Bushing

Telephone (Include area code)
215-239-3688

8. Complete Mailing Address of Headquarters or General Business Office of Publisher (Not printer)

Elsevier Inc., 360 Park Avenue South, New York, NY 10010-1710

9. Full Names and Complete Mailing Addresses of Publisher, Editor, and Managing Editor (Do not leave blank)

Publisher (Name and complete mailing address)

Kim Murphy, Elsevier, Inc., 1600 John F. Kennedy Blvd. Suite 1800, Philadelphia, PA 19103-2899

Editor (Name and complete mailing address)

Patrick Manley, Elsevier, Inc., 1600 John F. Kennedy Blvd. Suite 1800, Philadelphia, PA 19103-2899

Managing Editor (Name and complete mailing address)

Barbara Cohen-Kligerman, Elsevier, Inc., 1600 John F. Kennedy Blvd. Suite 1800, Philadelphia, PA 19103-2899

10. Owner (Do not leave blank. If the publication is owned by a corporation, give the name and address of the corporation immediately followed by the names and addresses of all stockholders owning or holding 1 percent or more of the total amount of stock. If not owned by a corporation, give the names and addresses of the individual owners. If owned by a partnership or other unincorporated firm, give its name and address as well as those of each individual owner. If the publication is published by a nonprofit organization, give its name and address.)

Full Name	Complete Mailing Address
Wholly owned subsidiary of	1600 John F. Kennedy Blvd., Ste. 1800
Reed/Elsevier, US holdings	Philadelphia, PA 19103-2899

11. Known Bondholders, Mortgagees, and Other Security Holders Owning or Holding 1 Percent or More of Total Amount of Bonds, Mortgages, or Other Securities. If none, check box ☐ None

Full Name	Complete Mailing Address
N/A	

12. Tax Status (For completion by nonprofit organizations authorized to mail at nonprofit rates) (Check one)
The purpose, function, and nonprofit status of this organization and the exempt status for federal income tax purposes:
☐ Has Not Changed During Preceding 12 Months
☐ Has Changed During Preceding 12 Months (Publisher must submit explanation of change with this statement)

PS Form 3526, September 2007 (Page 1 of 3 (Instructions Page 3)) PSN: 5530-01-000-9931 **PRIVACY NOTICE:** See our Privacy policy in www.usps.com

---

13. Publication Title
Critical Care Clinics

14. Issue Date for Circulation Data Below
July 2012

15. Extent and Nature of Circulation

			Average No. Copies Each Issue During Preceding 12 Months	No. Copies of Single Issue Published Nearest to Filing Date
a. Total Number of Copies (Net press run)			1168	1021
b. Paid Circulation (By Mail and Outside the Mail)	(1)	Mailed Outside-County Paid Subscriptions Stated on PS Form 3541 (Include paid distribution above nominal rate, advertiser's proof copies, and exchange copies)	650	632
	(2)	Mailed In-County Paid Subscriptions Stated on PS Form 3541 (Include paid distribution above nominal rate, advertiser's proof copies, and exchange copies)		
	(3)	Paid Distribution Outside the Mails Including Sales Through Dealers and Carriers, Street Vendors, Counter Sales, and Other Paid Distribution Outside USPS®	214	225
	(4)	Paid Distribution by Other Classes Mailed Through the USPS (e.g. First-Class Mail®)		
c. Total Paid Distribution (Sum of 15b (1), (2), (3), and (4))		▶	864	857
d. Free or Nominal Rate Distribution (By Mail and Outside the Mail)	(1)	Free or Nominal Rate Outside-County Copies Included on PS Form 3541	77	71
	(2)	Free or Nominal Rate In-County Copies Included on PS Form 3541		
	(3)	Free or Nominal Rate Copies Mailed at Other Classes Through the USPS (e.g. First-Class Mail)		
	(4)	Free or Nominal Rate Distribution Outside the Mail (Carriers or other means)		
e. Total Free or Nominal Rate Distribution (Sum of 15d (1), (2), (3) and (4))		▶	77	71
f. Total Distribution (Sum of 15c and 15e)		▶	941	928
g. Copies not Distributed (See instructions to publishers #4 (page #3))		▶	227	93
h. Total (Sum of 15f and g)		▶	1168	1021
i. Percent Paid (15c divided by 15f times 100)			91.82%	92.35%

16. Publication of Statement of Ownership
☐ If the publication is a general publication, publication of this statement is required. Will be printed in the October 2012 issue of this publication. ☐ Publication not required

17. Signature and Title of Editor, Publisher, Business Manager, or Owner

[signature] September 14, 2012

Stephen R. Bushing – Inventory Distribution Coordinator   **Date**

I certify that all information furnished on this form is true and complete. I understand that anyone who furnishes false or misleading information on this form or who omits material or information requested on the form may be subject to criminal sanctions (including fines and imprisonment) and/or civil sanctions (including civil penalties).

PS Form 3526, September 2007 (Page 2 of 3)

Moving?

Make sure your subscription moves with you!

To notify us of your new address, find your **Clinics Account Number** (located on your mailing label above your name), and contact customer service at:

Email: journalscustomerservice-usa@elsevier.com

800-654-2452 (subscribers in the U.S. & Canada)
314-447-8871 (subscribers outside of the U.S. & Canada)

Fax number: 314-447-8029

Elsevier Health Sciences Division
Subscription Customer Service
3251 Riverport Lane
Maryland Heights, MO 63043

*To ensure uninterrupted delivery of your subscription, please notify us at least 4 weeks in advance of move.

Printed and bound by CPI Group (UK) Ltd, Croydon, CR0 4YY

03/10/2024

01040452-0010